Disorders of Movement

Disorders of Movement

Edited by

A. Barbeau

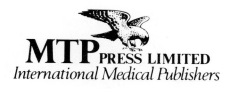
MTP PRESS LIMITED
International Medical Publishers

LR J DODDE

Published by
MTP Press Limited
Falcon House
Lancaster, England

Copyright © 1981 MTP Press Limited

First published 1981

ISBN 0-85200-212-2

Printed in Great Britain by
Mather Bros (Printers) Ltd, Preston

Contents

CONTENTS

List of Contributors

A. BARBEAU
Department of Neurobiology, Clinical Research Institute of Montreal, Montreal, Quebec, Canada H2W 1R7

C. BERTRAND
Department of Neurosurgery, Hôpital Notre-Dame (Université de Montréal), Montreal, Quebec, Canada

D. B. CALNE
Experimental Therapeutics Branch, National Institute of Neurological and Communicative Disorders of Health, National Institutes of Health, Bethesda, MD20205, USA

C. G. GOETZ
Department of Neurological Sciences, Rush–Presbyterian–St Luke's Medical Center, Chicago, IL 60612, USA

E. CHUNG HWANG
Department of Neurology, Mount Sinai School of Medicine, New York, NY 10029, USA

H. L. KLAWANS
Department of Neurological Sciences, Rush–Presbyterian–St Luke's Medical Center, Chicago, IL 60612, USA

C. D. MARSDEN
University Department of Neurology, Institute of Psychiatry and King's College Hospital Medical School, London SE5 8AF

T. J. MURRAY
Dalhousie University, Halifax, Nova Scotia, Canada

G. W. PAULSON
Department of Neurology, Riverside Hospital and Ohio State University, Columbus, Ohio, USA

A. K. SHAPIRO
Tourette and Tic Laboratory and Clinic, Mount Sinai School of Medicine, New York, NY 10029, USA

E. SHAPIRO
Tourette and Tic Laboratory and Clinic, Mount Sinai School of Medicine, New York, NY 10029, USA

R. D. SWEET
One Old Mamaroneck Road, White Plains, NY 10605, USA

M. H. VAN WOERT
Department of Neurology and Pharmacology, Mount Sinai School of Medicine, New York, NY 10029, USA

W. J. WEINER
Department of Neurological Sciences, Rush–Presbyterian–St Luke's Medical Center, Chicago, IL 60612, USA

A. WILLIAMS
Experimental Therapeutics Branch, National Institutes of Neurological and Communicative Disorders and Stroke, National Institutes of Health, Bethesda, MD 20205, USA

Consultant Editor's Note

CURRENT STATUS OF MODERN THERAPY

The *Current Status of Modern Therapy* is a major series with the purpose of providing a definitive view of modern therapeutic practice in those areas of clinical medicine in which important changes are occurring. The series consists of monographs specially commissioned under the individual editorship of internationally recognized experts in their fields. Their selection of a panel of contributors from many countries ensures an international perspective on developments in therapy.

The series aims to review the growth areas of clinical pharmacology and therapeutics in a systematic way. It is a continuing series in which the same subject areas will be covered by revised editions as advances make this desirable.

Our understanding of the pathophysiology of many of the disorders of movement has been advanced by the dramatic discoveries of the past two decades in the field of chemical neurotransmitters and their specific receptors. These advances have given rise to parallel development in the therapy of these ills. For this reason, the present volume is a natural topic for the *Current Status of Modern Therapy* series.

Dr Barbeau's own contributions to the basic science in this field have been enormous but throughout he has maintained his concern and interest for the practical value of the discoveries. This is shown very clearly by his selection of topics and authors for this volume, and I feel confident that André Barbeau's wish that this book 'will be of help to physicians involved in the management of patients . . .' will be fulfilled.

J. MARKS
Girton College
Cambridge

Series Editor

ix

Preface

Disorders of movement constitute one of the most important groups of entities in the fields of neurology and psychiatry. Taken together, and even excluding hemiplegias from cerebrovascular accidents and paraplegias from spinal cord trauma, they involve at least two individuals in every 1000 members of the population. It is in their study that some of the outstanding contributions to neurology have been achieved during the last quarter century.

In the present volume we will adopt Denny-Brown's definition of movement as fundamentally a change in posture. Posture itself is the result of the constant adjustments of a series of attitudinal reflexes in order to maintain the upright position or to recover equilibrium after passive or active displacements. In this context involuntary movements should be viewed as attitudinal instabilities. They will, however, frequently be called dyskinesias.

Our purpose is to review the state of the art in the treatment of these various disorders where dyskinesias are present (Parkinson's disease, Wilson's disease, tardive dyskinesia) and, less specifically, to consider the general approach to identifiable symptoms such as: rest, intention or postural tremor, chorea, athetosis, myoclonias, tics or dystonias.

As in all such endeavours, it is impossible to be thorough and at the same time to simplify the presentation of the present approach to each disorder. This problem was partially circumvented by choosing as contributors the outstanding researchers on the subject, neurologists or psychiatrists who, collectively, have created the field and whose judgement is buttressed by long experience. We hope that this balanced presentation will be of help to physicians involved in the management of patients with disorders of movement.

Our thanks are due to Suzanne Gariepy and Diane Magnan for their editorial help with the manuscripts and to the staff of MTP Press Limited for their encouragement and patience.

1980   ANDRÉ BARBEAU

1

History of movement disorders and their treatment*

A. Barbeau

INTRODUCTION

In man's eternal quest for knowledge, nothing is insignificant. From the atoms to the stars, his search goes on for an understanding of nature, and, perhaps, of God.

In this adventure, the physician holds a privileged position. From the bedside, he is a witness to human misery and to human hope. He must tend to the former and fortify the other. But to do this properly, he must have knowledge and understanding, faith and wisdom.

The physician's philosophy of life cannot, and must not, be materialistic if he is to remain true to his oath. Ambroise Paré used to say, '*Je le pansai, Dieu le guérit*' and despite the formidable advances of modern science, this is still realistic.

But, a philosophy of life is not built in one day. It comes from the daily contact with human frailty, from the treasures of human relationships and from the teachings of history.

To the student of medicine, the complexity of disease is such that a purely descriptive and psuedo-scientific approach often becomes the easiest way to knowledge. One can treat paralysis agitans without knowing about James Parkinson, and one could conceivably do research on the functions of the globus pallidus without having heard of Cecile and Oskar Vogt, but one will never understand the true nature of diseases without reading the original descriptions and the most important contributions.

In the light of history, the miseries of man become more human, more

---

* Large portions of this chapter are reproduced with permission, from a paper published in 1958 in *The Journal of Nervous and Mental Disease* (Ref. 1). More complete references are to be found in that paper.

understandable and the failures of physicians and patients alike do not appear so useless. When the overall picture is considered, signs of progress and improvement are more evident—a ray of hope is more justified.

We propose in this paper to review a few pages of the story of involuntary movements. This, in one way, is the story of man's credulity and ignorance, but it is also the story of one of the most difficult problems confronting neurologists and physiologists. For the most part, it is not the story of great men, but that of astute observers, simple and honest practitioners, devoted to the care of sufferers. Very few of the heroes we will mention knew the reward of fame during their lives and many contributors, whose names we do not even remember, lie forgotten behind the tombstones of the more famous.

THE MIDDLE AGES

The story of involuntary movement does not, as one would expect, go back to the Greeks. Hippocrates makes no mention of this kind of disorder. Occasionally the word 'Scelotyrben' appears in the literature and probably derives from the Greek σχελοσ—leg and θυρβη—weakness or perturbation, but there is doubt as to its true meaning. Some of the miracles reported in the Bible undoubtedly represent the cure of types of involuntary movements, whether physiological or hysterical in nature. The great Galen himself only mentions a form of incomplete paralysis of the lower limbs and gives no explanation of abnormal movements.

Strangely enough, our story is born in one of the most ancient expressions of man's religion and joy—dancing. Man dances to celebrate his victories, to excercise his limbs, to demonstrate his love. He uses dances to tell stories and to worship his gods. To the pace of music he can be melodious or lose himself in complete intoxication. Man has expressed his most beautiful sentiments in the form of music and dances but he has also used the stimulation of mass imitation to gather courage for his battles. The Indians of America, like the natives of Africa and Polynesia, always dance before a hunt or a raid. Gradually kindled by the shamans or medicine men, the intoxication becomes such that the meeker are driven to frenzy. Autointoxication is induced intentionally or incidentally by dancing and certainly the best known examples are the wild excesses of the bacchanals or the sexual dances of the Polynesians. Some dances are known to imitate the gambol of the wolf and bear or other wild beasts. The Ostyak tribes of northern Asia dance sudden leaps and violent turns, which exhaust the muscular power of the whole body. The bushmen also dance in long irregular jumps.

But the strangest dances of all are certainly the ones that the world witnessed in the darkest hours of the Middle Ages. The phenomenom of the

Dark Ages is a strange one indeed and a sad one at that. One shudders at the memory of the Inquisition and the fight against heresy, and one is almost unable to believe the miseries of the great epidemics that destroyed large portions of the living world. Only in a period of total ignorance and blind credulity can such events occur, but the centuries before the Renaissance were ripe for the strangest of maladies.

The first sign of the impending epidemic occurred in the year 1027 in Kolbig, but the worst disaster the world had ever known struck in 1348. The extent of the Plague, known as the black death, cannot be understood nowadays, even with the accounts of Hecker and Petrarch. The story in all its horror and ominous memories is told in one of the world's most widely read books, Boccaccio's *Decameron*.

The logical explanation of such a calamity could only be found in the belief that man was suffering in expiation of his sins and the Church used the uncontrollable fear of the nations to establish more firmly its control. People were nervous and confused and it is not surprising that at Aix-la-Chapelle, in the year 1374, a strange new disease was born.

In that year, the fear that gripped most of humanity was so great that the occasion of the famous festival of St John the Baptist soon created wild orgies:

> People formed circles hand in hand, and appearing to have lost all control over their senses, continued dancing regardless of the bystanders, for hours together, in wild delirium, until at length they fell to the ground in a state of exhaustion. They then complained of extreme oppression, and groaned as if in the agonies of death, until they were swathed in cloths bound tightly round their waists, upon which they again recovered and remained free from complaint until the next attack[2].

Most of the sufferers had vivid hallucinations, generally of the Saviour or the Virgin Mary and encouraged by the priests who tried to stop them, they formed processions, dancing and jumping and singing, 'St John so, so, brisk and cheerful St John'.

This new and strange epidemic spread rapidly to many countries where it was known under different names. In Germany it was called St John's or St Vitus' Dance; in France, 'Dance de St Guy.' The Latin name of *Chorea Sancti Viti* is the best known. The disease, obviously mainly hysterical in nature, did not completely disappear for it was still described in the sixteenth century and episodic occurrences were still known in parts of the world till the last century, being variously known as tarantism, astaragaza, 'leaping ague,' 'convulsionnaires', 'jumpers', 'rollers' and 'barkers'.

This dansomania is not a phenomenom limited to the Dark Ages. It is the result of superstition, libertinage and religious exaltation. It is spread through imitation, 'sympathy' and imposture. Most of these epidemics received the generic term of chorea from the Greek word meaning dance.

The first man to look more closely into the problem of the choreas was an erratic, unbalanced mystic, who was also a great reformer – Philippus Aureolus Theophrastus Paracelsus Bombastus von Hohenheim (1493–1541), better known as Paracelsus. The character of this man is exceptional. From the day of his inauguration, when he is said to have burned in public all the old textbooks, to the time of his death, he was a non-comformist. He always used the vernacular in contrast to the learned habit of his time, where Latin was the only scientific language. He even wrote, 'Since I saw that the doctrine accomplished nothing but the making of corpses, deaths, murder, deformity, cripples and decay, and had no foundation, I was compelled to pursue the truth in another way, to seek another basis which I have attained after hard labor[3]'. Arrogant and 'bombastic' in public, he became humane and charitable in the presence of the sick and was a keen observer of symptoms and signs.

Because of this respect for disease, he was the first to separate *chorea imaginata* and *chorea lascivia* from *chorea naturalis*. The dancing manias of the Middle Ages are classified among the chorea lascivia. Chorea naturalis to him is a milder form, where only anxiety, confusion and involuntary spasmodic laughter are present. He thought this form to be a natural cause and is confirmed in his belief by Shenckius of Graffenberg in 1607.

THOMAS SYDENHAM AND CHOREA

But the man who is universally recognized as the father of chorea is the 'English Hippocrates' Thomas Sydenham (1624–1689), a man who was never even elected to the Fellowship of the Royal College of Physicians, but whose name is remembered along with those of only two important contemporaries—William Harvey and John Locke.

Born in Wynford Eagle, England, he was baptized on 10th September, 1624. His family could boast of many important ancestors and it is believed that their financial position was more than satisfactory. He went to school at Magdalen Hall where he matriculated as a Fellow commoner on 20th May, 1642. He then went to Oxford, but his studies were soon interrupted by the political events of the time. In the Civil War of Britain the forces of the Parliamentary army (in which Thomas and his brothers served) opposed those of the King. After the war, a chance meeting with Dr Thomas Coxe led him to the study of medicine. Because the political affiliations of Oxford had now changed and because of the shortage of licensees, a number of degrees were then given 'by creation'. Through this strange process, Sydenham was created 'Bachelor of Medicine' on 14th April, 1648, by command of the Earl of Pembroke. At the most, he had served one year as a resident at the university, but again, through political influence, he replaced an expelled royalist as Fellow of All Soul's College in the same year. Luckily for the medical profession, he soon resigned this commission and started in practice around 1656. He moved to London and settled in Westminster, but only for a short time for it is believed that in 1659, he was at Montpellier studying under the then famous Charles Barbeyrac, whom his friend Locke had recommended. He was back in London by 1660 and obtained his license to practice from the Royal College in 1663 at 39 years of age.

By then, he had become interested in the study of fevers, the most prevalent diseases of his time and soon the city of London was visited by the famous Great Plague of 1664–1665, which killed close to 70 000 people. Unfortunately, and the fact is always deplored by his apologists, he fled the city to retire in the country, as he says, 'compelled by his friends'. During that year he published his first medical work of importance, *The Treatment of Fevers*. The method he prescribed caused quite some resentment amongst his contemporaries for he preconized the cooling method, in complete reversal to the accepted technics.

Sydenham was a scrupulous observer and an astute physician. He described in detail the gout, from which he suffered, and hysteria, which he found more common among women. His description of measles, chickenpox, dysentery and scarlet fever are classics. For them he never received distinctions, but he brushed this off with the statement, 'I have weighed on a nice scrupulous balance whether it be better to serve men or to be praised by them, and I prefer the former'. He had a profound disrespect for the knowledge of his time. One day, Dr Richard Blackmore asked him what books he should read to gain knowledge of medicine and he answered, 'Read Don Quixote. It is a very good book. I read it myself still'.

Despite, or because of this, he consigned his own observations in a book that is now famous; *Schedula Monitoria de Novae Febris Ingressa,* published in 1686. The book was dedicated to 'the most excellent and learned Charles Goodall, MD, Fellow of the College of Physicians in London'. The main part was called '*Processus Integri*' and contained the famous descriptions of Hysteria (Chapter 1) and *Chorea sancti viti* (Chapter 16).

The description of chorea is short but very concise and is worth citing here:

St Vitus Dance is a sort of convulsion which attacks boys and girls from the tenth year until they have done growing. At first it shows itself by a halting, or rather an unsteady movement of one of the legs, which the patient drags. Then it is seen in the hand of the same side. The patient cannot keep it a moment in its place, whether he lay it upon his breast or any part of his body. Do what he may, it will be jerked elsewhere convulsively. If any vessel filled with drink be put into his hand, before it reaches his mouth, he will exhibit a thousand gesticulations like a mountebank. He holds the cup straight, as if to move it to his mouth, but has his hand carried elsewhere by sudden jerks. Then, perhaps, he contrives to bring it to his mouth. If so, he will drink the liquid off at a gulp, just as if he were trying to amuse the spectators by his antics ... now this affection arises from some humor falling on the nerves, and such irritation causes the spasm[4].

At the close of his book Sydenham states, 'And this is about the sum of all I know respecting the cure of diseases, up to the day on which I write— namely, the 29th September, 1686'. From that day, Thomas Sydenham never wrote again and he died on 29th December, 1689, in Pall Mall. He was buried in St James Church, Westminster. Much later, in 1810, an epitaph was written on his tombstone, which qualified him as 'a physician famous for all time'. The disease he described so well is now known everywhere as Sydenham's chorea.

This original work was soon followed by the publications of theses on chorea, which added more details. Notable amongst these are the works of Richard Mead in 1751, Ewart in 1798 and Cullen in 1785. Most essays were published in German and until 1810 the knowledge of this disease had not reached France. The man responsible for popularizing chorea in France is Bouteille, who gives a very full and accurate historical study of the subject[5]. Besides a good clinical description of the disease, he also attempts a classification. He is probably the first man to have properly recognized the association of chorea with rheumatism, although the credit for this is often given to Germain Sée, whose memoir is a model of thoroughness. The great clinicians Charcot and Romberg and the school of Guy's Hospital in London contributed greatly to the better understanding of chorea and sealed its importance with their stamps. To conclude the early history of this disease, mention must be made of Roger, who, in 1866, first noticed the association of rheumatism, chorea and endocarditis.

Meanwhile, without much notice, Francis de la Böe, better known as Sylvius, had described tremor at rest and Gaubius in 1751 had demon- strated the possibility of propulsive movements. Hughes in 1846 and Sée in 1850 had separated the acute from the chronic forms of chorea. By this time the confusion over terms was complete. In the first edition of his *Practice of Medicine* in 1842, Dunglison gives 15 synonyms for the same disease.

In his *Leçons du Mardi* for the year 1888, Charcot makes a point to distinguish between chorea and tics. '*Entre le tic et la chorée, il y a un abîme ; ne l'oubliez pas, car il s'agit là d'affections auxquelles on donne quelquefois, bien à tort, le même nom et dont le pronostic est bien différent[6].*' The remark is of importance because there had been much confusion over some atypical forms of 'chorea'. As we have seen, Bouteille in 1810 had already described pseudochoreas and soon afterwards Itard reviewed the subject of abnormal convulsion of the face and limbs. Tics are, 'an abnormal and conscious convulsive movement, resulting in the contraction of one or more of the muscles of the body, reproducing, most frequently in an abrupt manner, some reflex or automatic action of common life and generally controlled by will' (Dictionnaire Encyclopédique Guinon). They can be simple and form the group of 'habit spasms', which Weir-Mitchell wrongly calls 'habit chorea' or they can be generalized with electric-like jerkings. Their name 'electric chorea' is unfortunately a misnomer for it should be used only to describe a peculiar disease reported in Lombardy in 1846 by Dubini and manifested by spasmodic movements and shock-like muscular contractions progressing rapidly to palsy and muscular wasting. It was thought to be due to some form of malaria.

GILLES DE LA TOURETTE

Chorea was also confused with the 'saltatoric spasms' of Bamberger, described in 1859, which were characterized by clonic spasms of the legs when the patient attempted to stand and caused springing or jumping movements. To be complete, one would have to include amongst the diseases leading to the confusion the coordinated tics of children: head nodding, head banging and Rubinowitch's 'Krouomania' which came to be recognized at about that time. But the most interesting study in differential diagnosis was done by Gilles de la Tourette in 1884, when he described a form of disease marked with explosive utterances of words or sounds and the existence of fixed ideas such as coprolalia, echolalia, arithomania and auditory hallucinations. In a historical 'tour d'horizon' he compared his 'maladie des tics convulsifs' to the 'jumping' seen in Maine by Beard[7], the Latah of Malaysia and the Myriachit of Siberia which Hammond had reported[8].

JAMES PARKINSON

While the limits of chorea were being fixed through a multitude of papers, a new disease was isolated by a humble practioner, perhaps better known to his contemporaries for his political pamphlets and his studhes of anthropology.

James Parkinson was born in Hoxton, England, on 11th April, 1755. His father, John, had practised medicine at No. 1 Hoxton Square for years and was amongst the first physicians to become a Diplomate of the Company of Surgeons after it had separated from the Company of Barber-Surgeons. He died in 1784 at the age of 59.

James was the eldest of three children and like them, was very religious. He studied his medicine as an apprentice to his father and was always interested in the mysteries of chemistry. In 1780, Dr Hugh Smith of Hatton Street had written, An Essay on Nerves, in which he stated that the nervous fluid was nothing more than air. The young Parkinson was prompt in answering with his first monograph, Observations of Dr Hugh Smit's philosophy of physics'. The urge for controversy and the absolute honesty of purpose which were to characterize every step of his life had already been apparent in this first essay. The next year he married Mary Dale by whom he had six children. In 1785, he went away to study under the great John Hunter and learned to observe the patient for the best clues to diagnosis.

His career has many aspects and shows the versatility of a great man. As a politician, James Parkinson was a fighter. He wrote constantly under the pseudonym of 'Old Hubert' on various subjects. During the French Revolution he was a pacifist and the titles of his pamphlets reveal his line of thought. In 1794, *Revolution without Bloodshed* created much controversy and he was even brought to trial for an alleged plot against the King. His feud with Edmund Burke is famous and still remembered. Parkinson advocated representation of the people in the House of Commons, he asked for annual parliaments and universal suffrage. He became a member or founder of the London Corresponding Society and the Society for Constitutional Information. As a social reformer, James Parkinson was also very active. He was a medical assistant in the Royal Humane Society and it was while working for this organization that he had the occasion of studying the methods of resuscitation of drowned children and the effect of lightning on men. He wrote a number of popular books to be used in the households: *Medical Admonitions for Families*, appeared in 1799, *The Villager's Friend and Physician*, in 1800 and *The Way to Health*, in 1802. He became very active in church work and asked for some reforms on the handling of trusses. After a sad experience in which he was accused of committing a sane person to the hospital to the benefit of her family, he asked for improvements in the laws for commitment of the insane. He was also a strong supporter of isolation for fever cases.

James Parkinson was probably best known to his contemporaries for his work on the *Fossils of England*. He was one of the founders of the Geological Society of London in 1807 and his towering work on the *Organic Remains of a Former World* which appeared in three volumes between 1804 and 1811 is considered a landmark in the history of British Paleontology. With his friend, Gideon Mantell, who later was to become famous in the same field, he travelled far and wide in the search for rare fossils.

As a physician, Parkinson was no less of an astute observer. In 1799 he published his *Medical Admonitions* and prepared his *Chemical Handbook*. Like others before him, Sydenham in particular, he suffered from and wrote on gout and was interested in many diseases. In 1812, he reported and described the postmortem of a case of perforated gangrenous appendicitis with peritonitis in a boy 5 years of age. This is believed by Shepherd to be the earliest reference to the disease in English medical literature.

The work for which he is best known in the medical world is the *Essay on the Shaking Palsy*[9] which he published in 1817. It is a remarkable rendering of concise information and an almost complete description of a hitherto unrecognized entity. He was 62 years of age at the time of this publication. It is of interest to note that he described the typical tremor, the festination, the masked facies, the classical gait, but he did not mention the rigidity so often found in this disease. He did not study the pathology of the malady but supposed that it was, 'in the medulla spinalis of the cervical region, its membrane or the containing Theca'.

Parkinson was rewarded with a few honours before his death. He was member of the London Medical and Chirurgical Society, a Fellow of the Medical Society of London and in 1822, he was the first physician to receive the honorary gold medal of the Royal College of Surgeons of England. When he returned to his Maker on 21st December, 1824, he had lived a full and rich life.

The story of the disease which bears the name of James Parkinson will be marked by many important contributions. In the years that follow, various types of familial and senile tremors will be described and the term 'Parkinsonism' will be applied to maladies closely related. We know of an idiopathic, a post-encephalitic and an 'arterio-sclerotic' form, thanks to the studies of von Economo, Critchley, and Keschner. In 1911, Willige postulated that there existed a juvenile form of paralysis agitans, quite different from the presenile type of Parkinson. The description of this disease and of its pathological entity was the work of Ramsay Hunt in 1917, who reported on a progressive atrophy of the globus pallidus and quoted both Willige and Oppenheim. Ludo van Bogaert helped later to understand the nature of this desease and to classify it amongst the other types of basal ganglia involvement. The role of the great Encephalitis Epidemic of 1918 to 1928 will be told later but it must now be stated that it constitutes the real landmark of the modern approach to the problem of *paralysis agitans*.

Meanwhile the New World was awakening to the fact of scientific medicine and the hardy pioneers took more time off from their overpowering practices to observe and record odd forms deseases. Piece after piece of the story of chronic familial chorea was told leading to the classical description by George Huntington in 1871. Dunglison in the first edition of his *Practice of Medicine*, published in 1842, is the first to call attention to this peculiar entity. He states that he had been consulted by a young medical friend in regard to the nature of a singular convulsive affection and he cites a letter dated 5th May, 1841, written by Dr C. O. Waters from Franklin, New York.

The Reverend Doctor Charles Oscar Waters was born in Franklin, Delaware County, in 1816. From his boyhood, he was a wanderer in search of health and religion. He studied at Williams College from 1834 to 1837 but received no degree and then decided to go to the Delaware Literary Institute as assistant teacher and then to Belvedere, New Jersey, as principal assistant to Rev. I. N. Candee.

Man of many talents, he studied for both the ministry and medicine. In 1839 he joined the medical department of Columbian University in Washington, sponsored by the Hon. Silas Wright. He then went to Philadelphia, where he graduated from Jefferson Medical College in 1841.

He must have sent his letter to Dunglison upon graduation from medical school and in all probability the cases he observed were from Westchester County, New York. He gives a fairly complete description of the common disease, 'in the south-eastern portion of this state (New York) and known among the common people as "the magrums". He notes the hereditary character and observes that it differs in several respects from ordinary chorea. 'First, it rarely occurs before adult age. Second, it never ceases spontaneously. Third, when fully developed, it wants the paroxysmal character.'

It is of interest to inquire into the origin of the word 'magrums'. Waters, himself, doubts that it is a corruption of megrim or migraine, for there is absolutely no relationship between the disease and any type of hemicrania. It probably derives from the Dutch and the term, not mentioned in the dictionary, is used to imply restlessness or nervousness and would be about equal to our own 'fidgets'.

After this claim to medical fame, which was never taken up, Dr Waters travelled to Iowa, where he practised for some 15 years in Muscatine. He married in 1848, was editor of the Muscatine paper for 1 year and a member of the Iowa Medical Society until he became a minister in the Presbyterian Church. He moved to Chicago to become trustee of the Chicago Theological Seminary in 1880. During the great fire of 1871, his home was completely burned. He died in 1892, having contributed to the world a model life, and to medical science, one letter.

In his third edition, published in 1848, Dunglison mentions another similiar report[10]:

> In an inaugural dissertation, presented before the faculty of Jefferson Medical College, of Philadelphia, by Charles R. Gorman of Luzerne County, Pa., the writer states that this affection prevails also in other portions of the country. According to him, it seems to be circumscribed by neighbourhood boundaries, and to be confined to sections of the country, the inhabitants of which are intimately connected in their social or business relations.

The original thesis of Dr Gorman was destroyed in the tearing down of the old Jefferson Medical College, where he had studied, and probably its details will never be known. Charles Rollin Gorman was born 4th August, 1817 at Barkhamstead, Connecticut. Before entering the profession of his father, he had taught school at Pittston, where he eventually settled to practice. It is interesting to note that like his predecessors, Parkinson and Waters, Gorman was a man of many fields. He was a member of the Odd Fellows and a Past Master in St. John's Masonic Lodge of Pittston. He became first president of Pittston Library Association and a vestryman in St Jame's Episcopal Church. The group of cases he reported would now be classified within the 'Wyoming branch' (Wyoming County, Pa.).

The next mention of the new disorder is to be found in the *American*

Medical Times of 1863 in an article under the name of Dr Irving W. Lyon, who was born at Bedford, Westchester County, N.Y., on 18th October, 1840. His father was ruling elder of the Presbyterian Church and the young Irving graduated from the University of Vermont in 1862 and from the College of Physicians and Surgeons in 1863. After a short stay as surgeon in the army, he became demonstrator in anatomy at Berkshire Medical School and soon was a member of the house staff of Bellevue Hospital in New York. It is probably from there that he sent his article on chorea in which he mentions [11] the chronic familial form which he had observed in Bedford and Connecticut, where he became medical director of the Hartford Life and Annuity Insurance Company until his death. His hobby was the collecting of antiques and he published a book on this subject, *The Colonial Furniture of New England*. He died on 4th March, 1896.

Someone once said that, 'genius is an infinite capacity for hard work' and this is probably the best qualification applied to the life of Dr George Huntington. But if he rose to fame and now has his name attached to a disease, it is the result of cumulative work by many others, particularly his father and grandfather. It is also, of course, the result of his own inquiry into the mysteries of medicine and of his sound judgement. George Huntington was born in East Hampton, Long Island, on 9th April, 1850. His father, George Lee, was a physician and so was his grandfather, Abel, who had settled in the same village in 1797. The grandfather, who probably was the first to observe the cases of adult chorea, but never reported them, was a well-known civic leader. He was New York State Senator in 1821 and he served 2 years as a congressman under President Andrew Jackson.

Huntington was only 8 when he saw the first cases of 'that disorder' as it was called by the natives. In 1909 before the New York Neurological Society he said:

> I recall it as vividly as though it had occurred but yesterday. It made a most enduring impression, every detail of which I recall today, an impression which was the very first impulse to my choosing chorea as my virgin contribution to medical lore. Driving with my father through a wooded road leading from East Hampton to Amagansett, we suddenly came upon two women, mother and daughter, both tall, thin, almost cadaverous, both bowing, twisting, grimacing. I stared in wonderment, almost in fear. What could it mean? My father paused to speak with them and we passed on. Then my Gamaliel-like instruction began; my medical education had its inception. From this point on, my interest in this disease has never wholly ceased [12].

This statement is true, for from the moment he finished his classical education, Huntington read books after books on medicine, worked with his father and graduated, then only 21, from the College of Physicians and Surgeons of Columbia University, with a thesis on opium. That summer he returned to East Hampton to study especially the cases of chorea in his father's practice and wrote a paper which his father corrected. In 1871, he went to Pomeroy, Ohio, to practise medicine and was invited by the 'Meigs and Mason Academy of Medicine' of Middleport, to give his paper on chorea. The text of the lecture appeared in the *Medical and Surgical Reporter of Philadelphia* on 13th April, 1872. At the end of what Osler calls an everyday paper on chorea, he states:

> 'And now I wish to draw your attention more particularly to a form of the disease which exists, as far as I know, almost exclusively on the East End of Long Island. It is peculiar in itself and seems to obey certain fixed laws. In the first place, let me remark that chorea, as it is commonly known to the profession and a description of which I have already given, is of exceedingly rare occurrence there. I do not remember a single instance occurring in my father's practice and I have often heard him say that it was a rare disease and seldom met with by him.
>
> The hereditary chorea, as I shall call it, is confined to certain and fortunately a few families, and has been transmitted to them, an heirloom from generations away back in the dim past. It is spoken of by those in whose veins the seed of the disease are known to exist, with a kind of horror, and not at all alluded to except through dire necessity, when it is mentioned as 'that disorder'. It is attended generally by all the symptoms of common chorea, only in an aggravated degree, hardly ever manifesting itself until adult or middle life, and then coming on gradually, but surely, increasing by degrees, and often occupying years in its development, until the hapless sufferer is but a quivering wreck of his former self.
>
> It is as common and is indeed, I believe, more common among men than among women, while I am not aware that season or complexion has any influence on the matter. There are marked peculiarities in this disease; (1) its hereditary nature, (2) a tendency to insanity and suicide, (3) its manifesting itself as a grave disease only in adult life.

He then goes on to prove each of the above points[13].

Very few descriptions of diseases ever appeared in such a concise and precise manner. And Huntington was only 22 when he wrote it! In 1884, he married Mary Elizabeth Hackard and returned to East Hampton, Long Island. Because of severe attacks of spasmodic asthma, he had to limit his practice and finally he moved to La Grangeville, New York. Mild-mannered, easy-going, a lover of fishing and hunting expeditions, he was the model of the devoted and generous country doctor. He moved successively to Asheville, N.C. and to Hopewell Junction. He became President of the Dutchess County Medical Society in 1888 and in 1898 honorary member of the Brooklyn Society for Neurology. He was to die in 1916, at the age of 66.

Despite the previous reports by Waters, Gorman, Lyon and Dunglison, Huntington's paper was the first complete description of the disease and it had the good fortune of being abstracted in German by Kussmaul and Nothnagel in 1872. Soon the disorder became recognized in various parts of the world and the name *Huntington's chorea* was found in articles by Perett in 1885 and Hubert in 1887. Osler stamped the final seal of approval in his monograph *On chorea and choreiform affections* in 1894.

By 1908 the disease had become so well known that a special issue of *Neurograph* was devoted to a bibliographical and biographical review. Smith Ely Jelliffe submitted a preliminary report of his investigations in which he recognized three groups of families: Group I or East Hampton Group, including the cases of Huntington; Group II or Bedford Group, with the cases of Browning and Waters and finally Group III or Wyoming Group, collecting the families of Sinkler (1889) and Gorman.

Frederick Tilney[14] made a special study of the Bedford Group and traced the disorder back to the 'P' family in 1777. This family was related through marriage to the Welles family, whose head was Governor Thomas Welles (1598–1660) who had married a certain Miss Hunt from England. But the classical description of the history of Huntington's chorea is told by P. R. Vessie in 1932 and traces the strain 300 years to the village of Bures in England in 1630.

In that year the famous John Winthrop fleet left England for America with about 700 passengers. Most of these came from towns and villages of Suffolk. It must be remembered that the popular sport of witch-hunting was prevalent in those days of Old England. Strangely enough, whole families of Bures and vicinity were branded as witches, tried or considered mad. Many were shunned by their neighbours and it is not surprising to find some of these miserable people amongst the passengers for the New World. The most famous of these were two brothers Wilkie and Nichols (fictitious names). Upon arrival into the colonies, Wilkie, a carpenter, was arrested for disorderly conduct and illegal actions. It is known that in 1643, his wife was mistress of a licensed 'house of entertainment' in Boston and that he himself died in 1658.

Their daughter, Priscilla, married a certain Mulfoot (or Mulford) and moved to East Hampton, Long Island. There is no doubt that they are at the origin of the cases described by Huntington.

Their granddaughter, Elizabeth, was tried, convicted and then pardoned as the celebrated Groton witch in 1671. In the transcript of her trial it is noted that she had, 'violent motions and agitations of her body'.

The other member of that family, Nichols (brother of Wilkie), brought his wife, Ellin, from Bures. She came from a family known to have this disorder and later was tried for witchcraft in 1653 and hanged. As if to prove the principle of heredity, the granddaughter of Ellin was also tried for witchcraft in 1692 but by this time the courts were more lenient and she was pardoned.

On the same ship that carried Wilkie and Nichols came a man named Jeffers, who was a magistrate of sorts and had married, despite the advice of his parents, a girl from a choreic family. His eldest son was sentenced on a charge of bestiality and was given two public whippings. The descendants of this man have many a choreic in their midst. The best known is probably Jefferson, one of the first settlers of Greenwich, Conn. This city was well known for its immorality and libertinage and it is not surprising to find Jefferson as one of the public officials. Unfortunately, he married the daughter of Nichols and Ellin, mixing in the same family the strains of two choreic sources. As we have just seen many of the descendents of the unfortunate passengers of the Winthrop fleet were tried and often convicted of witchcraft. It is hard for us to understand the state of mind that led to such orgies of execution in the early days of New England. Charles S. Potts in 1920 tried to analyse the witch craze in Salem in 1692 and could only ascribe it to hysteria, ignorance and Puritanism. One has only to remember the disgrace of Little Rock recently and the meetings of the Klu Klux Klan to realize that such an evil is not yet ready to disappear.

The victims of Huntington's chorea were, through the strange sight of their writhings and jumpings motions, well suited to be considered witches or sorcerers.

> Their contortions were interpreted as the presence of the devil changing him to animals . . . It was believed that the weaving motions, jerking backward and forward of the head, peculiar grimacing and twitching, puckering of the lips, squirming shoulders, spasmodic movements of the chest and diaphragm and the involuntary jerking of the hands, arms, feet and legs, represented the suffering of Christ during the Crucifixion; and that this was a curse inherited by these sad choreics from their forefathers for having dared to derisively pantomime the Saviour[15].

Huntington's chorea is becoming increasingly rare now, because of the ostracism attached to this disease and better awareness of its heredity pattern.

ATHETOSIS

We leave now the story of chorea to consider the work of another American physician, who described a new disease: athetosis.

William Alexander Hammond was born in 1828 in Maryland, the son of a physician. Upon graduation from Medical School, he entered the US Army as assistant surgeon. He served some 7 years and was a witness of many campaigns against the Indians in the south-west. Because of his health, he had to resign and then travelled to Europe studying the organization of military hospitals. Upon his return, he became interested in various experiments on questions of physiology and chemistry. With considerable courage, he carried out most of these experiments on himself, a habit which he kept for the rest of his life. His first paper on 'The nutritive value and physiological effects of albumen, starch and gum when singly and exclusively used as food' won him first place in a contest by the AMA and made him known to the medical profession. He was a friend of Silas Weir-Mitchell and with him, he made serious studies of poisons and snake venoms. In 1860, he accepted the chair of anatomy and physiology at the University of Maryland.

While at the University of Maryland he carried out important work on urea, ureamic intoxication and the excreta in urine. All these papers were published under the title *Physiological Memoirs* which he dedicated to Weir-Mitchell.

He returned to the army as assistant surgeon and, despite the fact that his name was far down the list for promotion, President Lincoln chose him, at 34, to become Surgeon-General. This was in 1862. The young Hammond, who had a very energetic character, did not lose any time. On 21st May, 1862, he announced his intention to establish an army medical museum and to this effect he asked for, and obtained, better reports on casualities, operations and statistics by his medical officers. In 1949 this museum became the Armed Forces Institute of Pathology, and holds a fabulous collection of pathological specimens.

In June of the same year he started the work that led to the *Medical and Surgical History of the Rebellion*, a treatise of great value to the scholars. Through tenacity and long arguments with Secretary Stanton, he obtained the formation of the Library of the Surgeon-General's Office. Later the Library started the publication of its famous *Catalogue* which has been discontinued only recently at the letter 'M' of the 4th Edition. The service rendered to medical science by this catalogue are impossible to measure.

His efforts also involved the establishment of an Army Ambulance Corps and a review of the system of medical supplies and laboratories in the army.

But, in 1863 his strong personality clashed with that of the Secretary of War, Stanton, and he was brought to court-martial. In a trial with a 'packed court' he was found guilty of irregularities in the purchase of medical supplies and dismissed from the army in 1864. Fourteen years later, an Act of Congress reversed the verdict and completely cleared him. He was again made a brigadier-general. During his stay in the army, Hammond published a *Treatise of Hygiene, Lectures on Venereal Diseases,* and *Military, Medical and Surgical Topics.*

The dismissal from the army did not stop Hammond's career: it only made it more active. Within 5 years he had established himself as a neurologist in New York and in 1871 published the first edition of his *Treatise of the Diseases of the Nervous System.* This book, written in an easy flowing style was so successful that it knew nine editions within a period of 25 years besides numerous translations in foreign languages.

Hammond became the editor of many journals among which were the *Quarterly Journal of Psychological Medicine and Medical Jurisprudence,* the *New York Medical Journal,* and the *Journal of Nervous and Mental Diseases.* He became interested in spiritualism on which subject he wrote a book, and in 1883 he published *A Treatise on Insanity* and *Sexual Impotence in the Male*.

At the age of 60, he decided to relinquish his practice and he moved to Washington. This last period of his life is not known for any particular scientific achievement except for some work on *Animal Extracts*. He was to die in 1900. He had been, besides his talents as an organizer and physician, a sound literateur and a superb teacher.

It is remembered that Parkinson, in1817, quoted Linnaeus on an affliction involving continued distortion of the limbs without affliction of the mind. It was known as hieranosos or 'Morbus Sacer'. He cites a report by Macbride in 1772. It had been observed for a long time that flaccid hemiplegia was often followed by spasticity. In young patients after a certain interval, the fingers could relax at the joints and the hands were seen to close and open at intervals. The fingers then wandered from over-extension to over-flexion. In a classical description of 'cortical hemiatrophy', in 1827, Cazanvieilh first mentioned these strange movements. They were known under the names of 'spasmoparalysis' or 'spastic-contracture' until 1871 when Hammond first applied to them the term athetosis, from the Greek 'Aθετοσ: without fixed position[8]. He described two cases, one of which belonged to Dr J. C. Hubbard of Ashtabula, Ohio, who had sent him his report on 11th January, 1870. The disorder, 'is mainly characterized by an inability to the fingers and toes in any position in which they may be placed, and by their continual motion'. With amazing foresight he predicted that the responsible lesion would be found in the striatum.

Unfortunately even his friend Weir-Mitchell did not recognize the importance of this contribution for, in 1874, he described some post-hemiplegic movements as 'hemichorea'. Two years later, Gowers referred to the same phenomenom as 'mobile spasm'. Gradually, however, Hammond accepted a wider use of the term and it became standard definition. Due credit to Hammond was finally given by Greidenberg in 1886. It was soon realized that some jerky movements were associated with the slower changes in posture and the term choreo-athethosis is now in more common use.

The movements recognized by Hammond, Weir-Mitchell and Gowers had also been described in *Cerebral Diplegia* by Little[16] in 1862. He definitely stated, 'In a few cases a distinct resemblance to severe chorea is perceptible' (p. 303). But the first adequate description of the condition now called 'athetose double' (or double athetosis) is given by Clay Shaw in 1873 under the title *On Athetosis, or Imbecility with Ataxia*[17]. He mentions difficulty in walking, movements of the hands and feet which he associates with athetosis, and movements of the muscles of the head, neck and face. The same year other reports by Allbutt and Purdon came to be known and a complete study was made by Oulmont in his thesis of 1878[18]. According to this author, athetosis can be found in all four limbs, but it is always present in the hands. In 1888, Déjerine and Sollier described the first case of infantile bilateral athetosis and a few years later, Audry collected some 79 cases from the literature. He already was able to isolate three forms; cerebral, medullar, and peripheral.

Early pathological studies

The next important step in the story of athetosis is the description by Anton of Graz in 1896 of the striatal lesion in this disease[9] which can be considered the first report on the pathology of the extra-pyramidal system. The tremendous work of Oppenheim and mainly of the Vogts will establish within a few years a very solid pathological basis of understanding for these diseases. The first breakthrough is the description in 1911 of the *Etat Marbré* or 'status marmoratus'[19] which led to the concept of a 'pure striatal syndrome'[20].

The life of the Vogts is interesting for it is another example of the close collaboration of a husband and wife team in the study of medicine. Cécile Mugnier was born in Annecy, France, on 27th March, 1875. She studied medicine, graduating when very young, for in 1898 she was with Pierre Marie at the Bicêtre. While there, she met her husband, Oskar Vogt-Dieckmann, who was studying neurology at La Salpétrière under Déjerine. Born on 6th April, 1870, he was the son of a Lutheran well respected for his liberal views. Oskar was already known in the medical world when he met Cécile. He had studied philosophy with Ferdinand Tonnier, medicine under Ernst Haeckel and Max Fürbringer, psychiatry under Otto Binswanger. Then he went to Zurich to work with August Forel and afterwards, in 1895, with Flechsig.

After one year in Paris, he left Déjerine and returned to Berlin to set up his own department of neurology. There Cécile came to write her thesis, fell in love and married him. In 1902, his department was incorporated into the University of Berlin. So successful was he that, in 1915, the Kaiser placed his laboratory under his protection and the *Kaiser Wilhelm-Institut* was born. Financial support came from the famous Krupp family. The growth of the Institute was such that a new one was built in 1931.

The scientific interests of the Vogts have covered many a field. From brain–psyche relationship to functional localization, they followed their pursuit in the new sciences of cytoarchitecture and myeloarchitecture. Their assistant, Brodmann, is now well known for his famous map of the cortex which appeared in 1907.

Cécile particularly became interested in the pathology of the striatum and published her description of 'athétose double' in 1911. The first case studied had been a patient of their friend Oppenheim. She was a 23-year-old girl with strange movements. The diagnosis of hereditary pseudo-bulbar palsy had been proposed because the mother was known to be similarly affected. The study of the brain revealed bilateral atrophy of the striatum. Her second case had been referred by Dr C. S. Freund of Breslow. In this brain, she found foci of myelinated fibres in the striatum which she described as *Etat Marbré*.

In 1924, Oskar Vogt was invited to Moscow to study Lenin's brain and to set up a Brain Research Institute. In 1929, he described the unusual features of that brain.

Unfortunately, in 1937 the Vogts, because of their political affiliations, had to resign from the Institute but they were permitted to name their successors. Hugo Spatz became director, with Hallervorden as chief of the Department of Neuropathology.

But the Vogt's love for research could not be stopped. With the help of the Krupp family, they built a private Institute for Brain Research at Neustadt and at 80 were still working every day.

MISCELLANEOUS DISEASES

With the impetus of such a wonderful team and improved methods, new varieties of chorea became known. In 1927, J.-P. Martin described hemichorea resulting from a focal lesion of the brain, which he called the 'Syndrome of the Body of Luys'[21]. This was not the first description and Martin himself found 21 studies of scientific value. Greiff, in 1883, Canfield and Putman in 1884, and others descibed cases in which the Body of Luys was destroyed. It was Marti's lot to isolate a syndrome from these observations. It usually consisted of violent chorea of the opposite side of the body, with unusual involvement of the shoulder and hip, and therefore with movements of very wide amplitude. The face was much less affected than one would expect and there was usually a mental disturbance. Death occurred in a few weeks.

Involuntary movements affecting the limbs unilaterally and sometimes both sides of the face have been described as Hemiballismus. The term is said to have been used by Kussmaul, but Whittier in 1947 has been completely unable to find any reference to it in his published words. Probably the first mention can be traced to an inaugural dissertation from the University of Vienna by Johann V. Pfefferkorn in 1833. The title of his thesis is *De Ballismo* but he calls the disorder chorea Sancti Viti and states, 'One does not come across traces of this disease in the writings of Hippocrates or in the early doctorate theses, unless one is willing to consider the condition scelotyrben as ballismus'[22]. Pfefferkorn, himself, states also that the word was used constantly by his master, Wilhelm Gottfried Plouequet (1744–1814) who also liked 'choreomania'.

Five years later, Langer also wrote a thesis on the subject and he used the term ballismus to mean, 'to jump, to dance and above all to throw, particularly to throw back and forth, especially the legs'. The disease must be particularly rare for in 1953, Malcolm B. Carpenter was able to review only 41 cases from the literature.

In advanced age, a condition known as 'senile chorea' had long been recognized. Huet in 1888 and Gowers were convinced this was a variant of Sydenham's chorea but following Osler most modern writers consider the condition a form of the hereditary chorea of Huntington.

The literature mentions numerous cases of choreic movements associated with toxemia of pregnancy, mental deficiency or other conditions but the name of no one particular author is associated with this.

Of interest, despite its rarity, is a form of familial paroxysmal choreo-athetosis reported by L. A. Mount and L. S. Reback in 1940 in which strange attacks of abnormal movements occur in otherwise healthy individuals[23]. In describing this disease the authors were able to show that the drinking of alcohol (definitely stated as 'Whiskey USP'!) could produce one of these attack. This same observation is true for other types of familial tremors where alcohol is known to have marked deleterious effecs.

'Double athetosis', as we have seen, can be found in cerebral diplegia and most frequently in association with the *Etat Marbré* of C. Vogt. But other syndromes have been described where the course is steadily progressive. These diseases are extremely rare but mention of their existence must be made in order to better understand the descriptions of dystonia musculorum deformans and of hepatolenticular degeneration.

The first of these bears a striking resemblance to the juvenile types of paralysis agitans mentioned above. It is the 'Status Dysmyelinisatus' described in 1919 and 1920 by Cécile and Oskar Vogt. The two cases they reported had athetosis in the early months of life which gradually changed to a more generalized rigidity. The first patient died at 10, the second at 13.

Two years later, the neurologists, who replaced the Vogts at the Kaiser-Wilhelm Institut, reported a progressive disorder characterized by rigidity, mental deterioration and athetoid movements in five sisters of a family of 12. Hallervorden and Spatz whose names were given to this syndrome were especially struck by the brownish coloration of the globus pallidus and substantia nigra without atrophy or softening[24]. Other such families have since been reported in the literature.

During a famine in China in 1925, Woods and Pendleton[25] had the occasion to observe a sudden epidemic of torsion spasm and rigidity which improved in some but which became progressive in others and eventually led to death. Fourteen people were affected with this strange disease that is probably related to the Hallervorden-Spatz syndrome.

To be thorough, one would have to mention the choreoathetosis encountered in the progressive rigidity described by Pelizaeus and Merzbacher but the other features of this disease, nystagmus, incoordination, ataxia and spasticity are much more important and would lead us to classify it elsewhere.

Finally, Creutzfeldt[26] and Jakob[27] described a syndrome characterized by cortico-striato-spinal degeneration and sometimes called 'spastic pseudo-sclerosis'. It included Parkinson-like slowness of movement with tremor and gradual development of weakness of limbs starting usually in middle life and accompanied by hesitating, dysarthric speech and mental symptoms of anxiety or depression.

Recently a new disease known as Kuru by the local inhabitants of New Guinea was described by Zigas and Gajdusek who observed some 154 cases in a total population of 16 000. It is limited to the natives of the Fore linguistic and cultural group of the eastern highlands of New Guinea. It is characterized by locomotor ataxia, malaise, fever, coryza and a Parkinson-like facies. There is little weaknesss or rigidity until the end which usually occurs within 6 to 9 months. Already studies have demonstrated a wide-spread neuronal degeneration and evidence of transmissibility. This led to the discovery and characterization of 'slow virus' diseases[28].

The history of myoclonus is not easy to recount because it may be present in a wide variety of disorders, each with its own story. It may be associated wth grand mal or petit mal seizures but also with degenerative diseases such as the Ramsay Hunt syndrome (dyssynergia cerebellaris myoclonica) or with post-anoxic encephalopathies (Lance–Adams syndrome).

Dystonia

Probably the most impressive of all the extra-pyramidal disorders is the one described as torsion-spasm or dystonia musculorum deformans. The spasmodic twisting and turning, the uncontrollable movements of face and limbs, the bizarre postions of the body represent the most frightening sight to the casual observer. The surprise of an epileptic attack or the antics of an hysterical woman are nothing compared to the gymnastics of the victim of this disease. It is true that no definite lesion has been found with consistency and that probably the syndrome is not entitled to a neurological independence. It is sometimes believed that it is closely related to hepatolenticular degeneration but until a better understanding is reached it will have to be considered separately.

The first man to report such a disease was probably Schwalbe in 1908[29]. In his inaugural dissertation in Berlin, he described a sister and two brothers with progressive involuntary movements who threw their hands behind their back and would bend in almost complete opisthotonos. Schwalbe worked in Ziehen's clinic and the next year the master himself reported two other cases before the Psychiatric Society of Berlin[30]. He called this disorder 'tonic torsion-neurosis'. It is very probable that many such cases had been previously decribed under the term 'tetanoid chorea' of Gowers, and Wilson states that he himself had seen some in London around 1904.

In 1911, the great Hermann Oppenheim who was already famous for his descriptions and diagnosis of brain tumours, tabes dorsalis, bulbar paralysis and neuritis, coined the term 'dystonia musculorum deformans' in reporting four cases of the disorder. He described the characteristic 'dromedary gait' due to lordosis. Since, much work has been done on this subject but, to date, it has only added to the confusion both on the pathology and the clinical independence of the disorder.

Wilson's disease

The period between 1900 and 1917 was extremely fertile in neurological discoveries. Great pathological studies were under way with new staining methods and improved instruments. Of all the publications which blessed the world of science, few deserve the praise and recognition that was given a doctoral thesis by a relatively young house physician of the National Hospital, London. In 1911, at 33 years of age, Kinnier Wilson described before the Neurological Society of London, 'Progressive lenticular degeneration: a familial nervous disease associated with cirrhosis of the liver'. His paper, a masterpeice of thoroughness and clairvoyance was published a year later and was a mere 200 pages long[87]!

Samuel Alexander Kinnier Wilson was born in New Jersey, but was brought up and educated in Scotland. His medical studies took him from the University of Edinburgh to Germany and France where he studied under Pierre Marie and Babinski. In 1904, he started in Queen Square one of the most brilliant careers in neurology which ranked him on a par with men like Gowers, Horsley and Jackson—most of them his friends and contemporaries.

After the publication of the famous paper on what is now known as Wilson's Disease, he devoted most of his energies to what he had himself christened the 'extra-pyramidal system'. His papers and lectures had an uncommon literary quality in which keen analytical powers and remarkable insight were evident. No neurologist can ever forget the reading of his volume *Modern Problems in Neurology* or of his posthumous textbook, *Neurology*.

A great teacher and a man devoted to truth, Wilson himself had to recognize the pioneer work of others in the description of the clinical syndrome of progressive lenticular degeneration. The disease, which is familial, is characterized by a coarsely nodular cirrhosis of the liver associated with the occurrence of progressive tremor and/or rigidity. The tremor is usually absent during complete rest but it is considerably increased in amplitude with movements. The rigidity is also variable but is in common with that found in many diseases of the basal ganglia.

The first effort to differentiate disorders of bodily posture from multiple sclerosis was attempted by Westphal in 1883[31] In two cases which he described, there was some tremor and disturbance of speech. He theorized that they could be attributed to, 'a neurosis which may, perhaps, though not very suitably, be described as *pseudo sclerosis*. Soon afterwards, in 1898, Strümpel revived the term in describing three cases with the same clinical appearance. The last of these, a young man of 24, had early hepatic cirrhosis[32].

The term 'pseudo sclorosis' or Westphal–Strümpel syndrome was vehemently attacked by Wilson and rejected from his syndrome, but despite this it must still be retained to qualify cases where tremor with little or no postural aberration is present.

We remember Gower's description in 1888 of 'tetanoid chorea', a familial, acute, progressive nervous illness. In his paper, he mentioned the presence of cirrhosis of the liver and similar reports appeared later under the name of Ormerod and Homen, both in 1890. Finally, in 1909, Fleischer[33] described a curious ring of golden corneal pigmentation in a case of pseudo sclerosis with cirrhosis of the liver. Seven years previously, Kayser had mentioned a similar finding and this sign was considered almost pathognomonic of Wilson's disease until recently when it was encountered in torsion-spasm. In the last few years as will be seen later a metabolic disorder of copper has been found in hepatolenticular degeneration, opening up a whole new field of studies[34]. The discovery of penicillamine[35] has now completely modified the prognosis of this disease.

Encephalitis lethargica

Just as the neuropathologists were beginning to describe the lesions of most of these disorders and as the physiologists, under the impulsion of Kinnier Wilson, were involved in understanding the functions of the extrapyramidal system, of the 'old and the new motor systems', there occurred in most of Europe a pandemic of encephalitis which was to creat the impetus for a tremendous amount of research. The epidemic of encephalitis lethargica, as it was known, came in the wake of a terrible pandemic of influenza which did considerable damage throughout the world.

The disease appeared in Rumania in the spring of 1915 and the first few cases were reported by Urechia who observed mainly the ophthalmoplegic and hyperkinetic forms. Some isolated cases were probably seen among soldiers near Verdun in the last few months of 1915 by Cruchet and again in Rumania by Marinesco, but the first real epidemic was reported during the winter 1916–17 in Vienna. The man who published the first account of this disease, and who is forever associated with it, is Constantin Baron Economo von San Serff. He was born in Braila, Rumania, in 1876, and lived in Trieste until he went to Vienna to study engineering (at his father's request) and then medicine. He worked with Nothnagel and then went to Paris to benefit from the teachings of Magnan and Pierre Marie. After a short stay with Bethe in Strassburg and Kraepelin in Munich, he returned to Vienna in the clinic of Wagner von Jauregg. It is interesting to note that he was passionately interested in aeronautics, became a balloon and then an aircraft pilot. His energy led him to organize the Vienna airports and the Austrian aeroclub, all the while studying the physiology and anatomy of the midbrain. He is mainly known for his studies in encephalitis lethargica but his best work is probably the atlas on the cytoarchitecture of the adult human cerebral cortex which he published in 1925. He was to die in 1931, shortly after becoming director of the brain research institute of the von Jauregg Clinic.

There has been some argument on the priority of von Economo's article over Cruchet's but it now appears certain that the Baron reached press at least 10 days before, and anyway, his account was much more complete and descriptive. It was dated 17th April, 1917. The mortality in Vienna of this epidemic was reported to be over 50%. The disease was soon recognized in Leipzig by Strümpel but it remained 'mysterious' in Queensland. The first few cases which appeared in 1918 in London were mistaken for botulism until in October it was identified as von Economo's disease. The epidemic reached France in March 1918 and was thoroughly described by Netter, Lhermitte, Claude, Pierre Marie, Vincent and Sicard. Towards the end of that year it had spread its damage to most of the world, including North America.

A recurrence took place in Italy at the end of 1919 and because of its violence rapidly spread along the Adriatic Coast to Austria. This time the hyperkinetic form was prevalent and became generalized to all Europe. 1920 and 1921 were considered pandemic years with an overall mortality of nearly 40%. Sporadic cases were still met with till 1928. By that time the great sequelae which make this disease so important in our study were beginning to appear. Parkinsonism in its new form became a common disorder and a multitude of reports appeared with the descriptions of various pathological involvement. This epidemic can truly be placed at the start of a renewed interest in the problem of involuntary movements, but it certainly was not the first of its kind in history.

The fact that influenza and encephalitis were prevalent at about the same time contributes to obscure the picture. It is quite probable that some of the tremors observed in the Middle Ages and mentioned earlier, were similar diseases. Von Economo and many others, among whom Riley stands out, have attempted to trace the history of encephalitis. Hippocrates mentioned a 'lethargus' accompanied by fever but its true nature is uncertain. In 1580 it is known that there was a bad influenza epidemic in Europe. In 1673 Sydenham reports a few cases of what he calls 'febris comatosa' while in 1695 Albrecht of Hildescheim definitely described a case of the sporadic somnolent-opthalmoplegic form of this disease. Many other similar epidemics are made mention of by Ozanam (1745), Lepecq de la Cloture (1763), Grand (1775), Pfendler (1830), but the one that is best remembered

is certainly the great epidemic of influenza of 1889 in Italy which was
followed the next year by a peculiar disease which the natives called 'nona'
and which since has received much attention.

TREAMENT OF MOVEMENT DISORDERS

Before reviewing the various steps of the history of medical treatments in
disorders of movement, it is important to establish the distinction between
akinesia and dyskinesia. Akinesia is the state of difficulty in initiating
movements, in changing from one motor pattern to the next, that one finds
generally in Parkinson's disease[36]. It is essentially a negative symptom. The
term dyskinesia, on the other hand, covers a variety of entities where
abnormal movements of many types are present. These movements, all
positive symptoms, include the varieties of tremor (rest, intention, postural), chorea, choreoathetosis, ballism, torsion-spasm, torticollis or dystonia, tics and myoclonias. For both these large categories of disorders,
empirical as well as rational approaches have been followed throughout the
years.

Empirical approaches

J. M. Charcot is credited with introducing the first effective treatment of
some forms of Parkinsonism. He would prescribe each day two or three
granules of hyoscyamine, a belladonna alkaloid. This approach remains the
basis for what is now called the 'conventional treatment'. It was later
recognized that the basis for the action of the alkaloids is their anticholinergic, mainly muscarinic, effect. Of all botanical preparations employed,
only those containing atropine or scopolamine achieved a degree of therapeutic success. The failure of quaternary analogues of atropine or scopolamine to influence Parkinson's disease indicates that an action in the central,
rather than the peripheral, nervous system is necessary. The beneficial
effects of atropine and scopolamine thus reflect a central anti-acetylcholine
action that is reversed by physostigmine.

The years following the Second World War were marked by the introduction of a number of synthetic drugs with simular properties to atropine.
The first class of drugs to be developed is one of a series of piperidyl
compounds first tested as antispasmodic drugs: trihexyphenidyl (Artane). It
was soon followed by a number of congeners: procyclidine (Kemadrin),
cycrimine (Pagitane) and biperiden (Akineton). Later a diphenyl ester of
tropanol, benztropine (Cogentin) became the most potent synthetic anticholinergic agent available. Soon afterward some antihistaminic drugs
received favour: diphenhydramine (Benadryl), orphenadrine (Disipal) and

chlorphenoxamine (Phenoxene). It is now known that the action of anti-histaminic agents is through this anticholinergic mechanism.

The above agents have proven, and still are, very useful in the management of early phases of Parkinson's disease. They are particularly successful against rigidity and tremor, but are to all intents and purposes useless against the incapacitating symptom of akinesia[37].

Rational approaches[38]

For a number of years it had been known that reserpine can produce a Parkinsonian syndrome. The reason for this was made clearer when many authors demonstrated a characteristic distribution within the brain of a newly identified substance. Dopamine was found mainly in the basal ganglia and substantia nigra while noradrenaline was mainly in the hypothalamus and brain stem. The brain could be depleted of both substances by reserpine[39]. This difference in localization, as well as some divergent peripheral effects, led to the postulate that dopamine could have independent physiological functions in the brain[39]. Initial experiments indicated that the precursor levodopa (L-Dopa) corrected some of the extra-pyramidal effects of reserpine, and that there was a correlation between the level of dopamine and increasing degrees of motor behaviour and aggressiveness in mice.

Following these studies two groups of authors reported on a deficit in dopamine in Parkinson's disease. Ehringer and Hornykiewicz[40] found low levels of dopamine in the striatum of patients with both the postencephalitic and the idiopathic form of the disease and Barbeau et al.[41] reported low urinary excretion of dopamine in that disease. The same two groups then launched the new era of specific and rational therapy by introducing the use of levodopa, orally or intravenously, for the management of Parkinson's disease[42,43]. In 7 years these results were confirmed by over 30 authors, but the availability and cost of the compound limited proper therapeutic studies. Most authors agreed that levodopa could modify akinesia and rigidity. It was up to Cotzias and his collaborators[44] to show that this approach could become an effective treatment, even if a variety of side-effects were soon recognized[39,45]. In the experience of all authors there has been partial improvement in almost all symptoms of Parkinson's disease in the majority of patients. Levodopa is now recognized as the best available treatment for most Parkinsonian patients. However, two groups of complications had to be contended with: peripheral side-effects of nausea, vomiting, hypotension and cardiac arrythmias; and central side-efects of oscillations in performance, confusion, hallucinations and abnormal involuntary movements[45]. The introduction of peripheral dopa-decarboxylase inhibitors which do not cross the blood–brain barrier[46] has permitted correction of most of the peripheral side-effects, while the addition of dopamine analogues (apomorphine, bromocriptine, pergolide, lisuride) to levodopa has reduced some of the oscillations in performance[47]. The most recent approach is the utilization of peptides (such as proline-leucine-glycine amide, PLG or MIF-1) as potentiators of levodopa.

In 1962, Barbeau[48] proposed—after a suggestion by McGeer—that the extrapyramidal nuclei were controlled pharmacologically through a sort of balance between dopaminergic and cholinergic systems. In Parkinson's disease, the dopamine deficit previously described, and which is corrected by levodopa, is associated with a cholinergic preponderance. Anticholinergic drugs which block this hyperstimulation of cholinergic receptors have been proved to be useful. By analogy, Barbeau and others[49], also proposed that the inverse relationship existed in hyperkinetic disorders, such as Huntington's chorea. This concept has now been extended to Gilles de la Tourette's syndrome, dystonia musculorum deformans, and tardive dyskinesia. In such entities, a postulated dopaminergic predominance can be counteracted by dopamine receptor blockers like Haloperidol or, more recently, by modifications of acetylcholine (physostigmine, choline or phosphatidycholine). Further developments will follow the seminal observation of Perry[50] of a deficit in γ-amino-butyric acid (GABA) in Huntington's chorea; the identification of new pathways in the basal ganglia with substance P, enkephalin or angiotensin as postulated neurotransmitters and should increase our understanding of the pharmaclogy of hyperkinetic disorders.

It would not be fair to end this historical review without mentioning the important contribution of surgery to the understanding and treatment of movement disorders. From Horsley's excision of the precentral cortex in 1890 in a case of athetosis, one can really say that all levels of the pyramidal and extrapyramidal tracts have been assaulted. Cortical excision was attempted by Bucy and Klemme (1937) and internal capsule lesion by Browder (1948). The peduncles were cut by Walker (1949), the spinal cord by Putnam (1938), Olivier (1949) and Ebin (1949). Posterior nerve root separations were done by Pollock (1929) and sympathectomy by Gardner (1949). Finally, the basal ganglia were attacked by Meyers (1940), Spiegel and Wycis (1951), Fenelon (1950), Guiot (1952) and Bertrand (1954). Cooper (1953) introduced ligation of the anterior choroidal artery, chemopallidectomy and a variety of other procedures.

But what of the results of all these approaches? Many patients are improved that a few years ago would have been miserable, many are permitted a more active life and forever grateful . . . but none are cured! The cause and exact pathology of the various diseases grouped under the extrapyramidal system remain mysteries almost as deep as in the days of Sydenham and Parkinson. However, as the chapters of the present volume will attest, great strides have been made in the pharmacological approach to extrapyramidal diseases.

References

1 Barbeau, A. (1958). The understanding of involuntary movements. *J. Nerv. Ment. Dis.*, **127**, 469

2 Hecker, J. F. C. (1844). *The Epidemics of the Middle Ages*, pp. 87–150. (London)

3 von Hohenheim, (1658). Opera omnia medico-chimico-chirurgica. *Ed. Novissima*, pp. 1–110. (Genoa: J. Antonii & S. De Tournes)

4 Sydenham, T. (1848–1850). *The Entire Works of Thomas Sydenham*, 2 vols. (London: Sydenham Society)

5 Bouteille, E. M. (1810). *Traité de la Chorée ou danse de St-Guy*, pp. 1–362. (Paris: Vincard)

6 Charcot, J. M. (1888–9). *Lecons du Mardi à la Salpêtrière*, p. 464. (Paris: Delahaye et Lecrosnier)

7 Beard, G. M. (1880). The Maine Jumpers. *J. Nerv. Ment. Dis.*, **7**, 487

8 Hammond, W. A. (1871). *A Treatise of the Diseases of the Nervous System*. 1st Edn., pp. 1–876. (New York: Appleton-Century-Croft)

9 Parkinson, J. (1817). *An Essay of the Shaking Palsy*, pp. 1–66. (London: Sherwood, Neely and Jones)

10 Dunglison, A. (1848). *The Practice of Medicine, or a Treatise on Special Pathology and Therapeutics*. 3rd Edn., p. 218. (Philadelphia: Lea and Blanchard)

11 Lyon, E. W. (1863). A peculiar form of chorea. *Am. Med. Times*, pp. 120–122

12 Huntington, G. (1910). Recollections of Huntington's Chorea as I saw it at East Hampton, Long Island, during my boyhood. *J. Nerv. Ment. Dis.*, **37**, 255

13 Huntington, G. (1872). On chorea. *Med. Surg. Reporter*, **26**, 317

14 Tilney, F. A. (1908). A family in which the choreic strain may be traced to colonial Connecticut. *Neurographs*, **1**, 124

15 Vessie, P. R. (1932). On the transmission of Huntington's chorea for 300 years—The Bures family Group. *J. Nerv. Ment. Dis.*, **76**, 533

16 Little, W. J. (1862). On the influence of abnormal parturition, difficult labours, premature birth, and asphyxia neonatorum on the mental and physical condition of the child, especially in relation to deformities. *Trans. Obstet. Soc.*, **3**, 293

17 Shaw, T. C. (1873). On athetosis, or imbecility with ataxia. *St Barth. Hosp. Rep.*, **9**, 130

18 Oulmont, P. (1878). *Etude Clinique sur l'Athétose*, pp. 1–38. (Paris: Delahaye)

19 Oppenheim, H. and Vogt, C. (1911). Nature et localisation de la paralysie pseudo-bulbaire congénitale et infantile. *J. F. Psychol. Neurol.*, **18**, 293

20 Vogt, C. (1911). Quelques considérations générales à propos du Syndrome du Corps Strié, *J. F. Psychol. Neurol.*, **18**, 479

21 Martin, M. P. (1927). Hemichorea resulting from a local lesion of the brain (Syndrome of the Body of Luys). *Brain*, **50**, 637

22 Pfefferkorn, J. W. (1833). *De Ballismo*. pp. 1–34. *Inaug. Dissert*. (Vindobonae: Antonii Strauss)

23 Mount, L. A. and Reback, L. S. (1940). Familial Paroxysmal Choreoathetosis. *Arch. Neurol. Psychiatry*, **44**, 841

24 Hallervorden, J. and Spatz, H. (1922). Die extrapyramidalen Erkrankungen. *Z. Gesamte Neurol. Psychiatr.*, **79**, 254

25 Woods, A. M. and Pendleton, L. (1925). Fourteen simultaneous cases of an acute degenerative striatal disease: necropsy of one case revealing gross necrosis of the globus pallidus (Symmetrical) and substantia nigra. *Arch. Neurol. Psychiatry*, **13**, 549

26 Creutzfeldt, H. G. (1920). Uber eine eigenartige herdförmige Erkrankung des Zentralnervensystems. *Z. Gesamte Neurol. Psychiatry*, **57**, 120

27 Jakob, A. (1921). Uber eigenartige Erkrankungen des Zentralnervensystems mit blerkenswertem anatomischen Befunde. Spastiche Pseudo-sklerose. *Z. Gestante Neurol. Psychiatry*, **64**, 112

28 Gajdusek, D. C. (1967). Slow virus infections of the nervous system. *N. Engl. J. Med.*, **276**, 392

29 Schwalbe, B. (1908). A peculiar tonic form of spasm with hysterical symptoms. pp. 1–88. *Inaug. Diss., Berlin.*

30 Ziehen, H. (1911). Demonstrat. eines Patienten mit Tonishes Torsionsneurose. *Neurol. Zentralb.*, **30**, 109

31 Westphal, C., (1883). Ueber sine dem Bilde des cerebrospinalen granen Degeneration ähnliche Erkrankung des centralen Nervensystems ohne anatomischen Befund nebst einigen Bemerkungen über paradoxe Contraction. *Arch. Psychiatry*, **14**, 87

32 Strümpell, A. (1898). Ueber die Westphal'sche Pesudosklerose und über diffuse Hirnsklerose, insbesondere bei Kindern. *Deutsche Zentralbl. Nervenheilk.*, **12**, 115

33 Fleischer, B. (1909). Die periphere braun-grünliche Hornhaut-verfärbung, als Symptom einer eigenartigen allgermeinerkrankung. *München. Med. Wochenschr.*, **56**, 1120

34 Cummings, S. N. (1948). The copper and iron content of brain and liver in the normal and in hepatolenticular degeneration. *Brain*, **71**, 410

35 Walshe, J. M. (1956). Penicellamine, a new oral therapy for Wilson's disease. *Am. J. Med.*, **21**, 487

36 Barbeau, A. (1972). Contributions of levodopa therapy to the neuropharmacology of akinesia. In Siegfried, J. (ed.) *Parkinson's Disease : Rigidity, Akinesia, Behavior.* Vol. 1. pp. 151–174. (Bern: Hans Haber)

37 Yahr, M. D. and Duvoisin, R. C. (1968). Medical therapy of parkinsonism. In *Modern Treatment*, pp. 283–300. (New York: Hoeber)

38 Barbeau, A. (1969). L-DOPA therapy in Parkinson's disease: a critical review of nine years' experience. *Can. Med. Assoc. J.*, **101**, 791

39 Carlsson, A. (1959). The occurrence, distribution and physiological role of catecholamines in the nervous system. *Pharmacol. Rev.*, **11**, 490

40 Ehringer, H. and Hornykiewicz, O. (1960). Verteilung von noradrenalin und Dopamin (3-hydroxytyramin) in Gehirm des Menschen und ihr Verhalten bei Erkrankungen des extrapyramidalen system. *Klin. Wochenschr.*, **38**, 1236

41 Barbeau, A., Murphy, D. F. and Sourkes, T. L. (1961). Excretion of dopamine in diseases of basal ganglia. *Science*, **133**, 1706

42 Barbeau, A. (1961). Biochemistry of Parkinson's disease. In *Proceedings of the Seventh International Congress of Neurology*, Rome, September 10, 1961. (Societa Grafica Romana)

43 Birkmayer, W. and Hornykiewicz, O. (1961). Der L-3-4-dihydroxy-phenylalanine (DOPA) effekt bei der Parkinson-akinese. *Wien Klin. Wochenschr.*, **45**, 787

44 Cotzias, G. C.; Van Woert, M. H. and Schiffer, L. M. (1967). Aromatic amino-acids and modification of parkinsonism. *N. Engl. J. Med.*, **276**, 374

45 Barbeau, A.; Mars, H. and Gillo-Joffroy, L. (1971). Adverse clinical side-effects of levodopa therapy. In McDowell, F. H. and Markham, C. H. (eds.) *Recent Advances in Parkinson's disease.* pp. 203–237. (Philadelphia: Davis)

46 Birkmayer, W. and Mentasti, M. (1967). Weitere experimentelle Untersuchungen über den catecholaminstoffwechsel bein extrapyramidalen erkrankungen Parkinson und chorea syndrome. *Arch. Psychiatry*, **210**, 29

47 Barbeau, A. (1978). The last 10 years of progress in the clinical pharmacology of extrapyramidal symptoms. In Lipton, M. A., Mascio, A. D. and Killam, K. F. (eds.) *Psychopharmacology: A generation of progress.* (New York: Raven Press) pp. 771–776

48 Barbeau, A. (1962). The pathogenesis of Parkinson's disease: a new hypothesis. *Can. Med. Assoc. J.*, **87**, 802

49 Barbeau, A. (1973). Biochemistry of Huntington's chorea. *Adv. Neurol.*, **1**, 473

50 Perry, T. L., Hansen, S., Lesk, D. and Kloster, M. (1973). Amino acids in plasma, cerebrospinal fluid, and brain of patients with Huntington's chorea. *Adv. Neurol.*, **1**, 609

2

Treatment of the choreas

C. G. Goetz, W. J. Weiner and H. L. Klawans

INTRODUCTION

In a discussion of the treatment of choreatic disorders, the distinction between pathogenesis and pathophysiology must be clearly delineated. While there are multiple aetiologies or pathogenic factors that are associated with the development of chorea, all choreatic movement disorders appear to

Table 1 Classification of choreas

CHOREAS WITH PREFERENTIAL STRIATAL PATHOLOGY
   Huntington's disease
   Senile chorea
   Acquired hepatocerebral degeneration

CHOREAS WITH DIFFUSE NEUROPATHOLOGY
   Sydenham's chorea
   Systemic lupus erythematosis

CHOREA WITHOUT KNOWN PATHOLOGY
   Hyperthyroid chorea

DRUG-INDUCED CHOREAS
   Levodopa
   Amphetamine and methylphenidate
   Birth control pills
   Phenytoin (Dilantin ®)
   Others, especially Tardive dyskinesia (not discussed).

share a common pathophysiology in terms of neurotransmitter balance. Regardless of cause, chorea appears to relate anatomically to the striatum (caudate and putamen). Evidence suggests that enhanced activity of the dopaminergic system relative to the antagonistic cholinergic and possibly gabaergic systems is important to the development of all types of chorea. This enhanced dopaminergic function can theoretically occur from a variety of mechanisms including increased dopamine concentrations presynaptically, altered neurotransmitter degradation or enhanced sensitivity of dopaminergic receptor sites. These different factors may play different roles depending on the specific type of chorea. In summary, if a movement disorder is choreatic in nature, its pathophysiology always includes increased activity of the striatal dopaminergic system. Clarification of the pathogenesis of the chorea requires further evaluation for each such disorder. In those forms of chorea where the pathogenesis is understood, therapy can be directed to the cause. Therapy that modifies the pathophysiology of the chorea is reserved for those choreatic disorders where the cause is unknown, or where there is no effective means of reversing that cause.

The naturally occurring choreatic disorders can be divided conveniently into three groups according to the degree of proven striatal pathology (Table 1). The first group of syndromes are ones in which there is definite striatal alteration (Huntington's chorea, senile chorea, acquired hepatocerebral degeneration); the second group demonstrates less specific striatal pathology (Sydenham's chorea, systemic lupus erythematosus); the third group shows no known anatomic alteration of the striatum (chorea associated with hyperthyroidism). Each of these groups will be discussed separately. A final section discusses a variety of drug-induced choreas and their treatment.

CHOREAS WITH PREFERENTIAL STRIATAL CHANGES

Huntington's chorea

Huntington's disease is a chronic degenerative disease of the central nervous system, characterized by choreiform movements and progressive mental deterioration[1,2]. It commonly begins during adult life and is inherited in an autosomal dominant pattern. At autopsy there is degeneration of the small cells of the caudate nucleus and diffuse cortical atrophy[2]. As already discussed, the pathophysiology of the disorder is felt to relate to the striatum where there is a functional overactivity of dopaminergic influences relative to cholinergic and possibly gabaergic systems[3]. The pathogenesis relates to a presumed biochemical defect, transmitted genetically. Since the details of the pathogenesis are not clearly understood, no therapy can arrest the progress of striatal cell loss. The management of Huntington's disease has focused instead on abatement of the pathophysiology with pharmacological

logical advances have prompted the introduction of numerous new agents to complement traditional pharmacological treatment.
manipulation of the involved neurotransmitter systems. Recent pharmaco-

Dopaminergic antagonists

Since the basic pathophysiology of this disorder is related to relative striatal dopaminergic overactivity, the mainstay of therapy remains the dopamine receptor site antagonists. Phenothiazine derivatives and the butyrophenones share the property of dopaminergic receptor blockage and are the accepted mode of therapy in Huntington's disease[4,5]. In a recent survey, haloperidol and chlorpromazine were the two specific neuroleptic agents most widely employed[6]. The amelioration of chorea is felt to relate directly to blockade of striatal dopamine receptor sites, while the amelioration of the often severe psychotic behaviour may relate to dopamine receptor antagonism in the limbic system[7].

Other agents that decrease striatal dopaminergic activity include reserpine and α-methyl-*para*-tyrosine. Historically, reserpine was the first agent reported to be of use in the treatment of chorea. A rauwolfia alkaloid, reserpine acts to block intravesicular neurotransmitter reuptake and thereby depletes the brain of dopamine[8]. Because it also acts to deplete central norepinephrine and serotonin stores, reserpine's activity is not specific, and it has now become generally obsolete in the treatment of Huntington's disease. α-Methyl-*para*-tyrosine inhibits tyrosine hydroxylase and thereby prevents the synthesis of dopamine and norepinephrine[9]. Birkmayer reported amelioration of choreatic movements in patients with Huntington's disease after intravenous administration of the agent[10]. Since α-methyl-*para*-tyrosine acts on two neurotransmitter systems and necessitates parenteral usage, it has not gained wide clinical acceptance.

Recent identification of dopamine receptors on the cell bodies of dopaminergic neurons has prompted interest in their function relative to extrapyramidal disease. It has been suggested that when dopaminergic agonists activate these presynaptic receptors, dopamine synthesis and release are inhibited[11]. Accordingly, dopamine receptor agonists that preferentially affect presynaptic receptors sites may inhibit, not facilitate, dopamine-mediated transmission[12]. Apomorphine is a dopaminergic agonist which acts as a direct dopamine receptor site stimulant on both presynaptic and postsynaptic receptors. When administered in low doses, it appears to influence primarily presynaptic receptors[13]. Using this premise, beneficial rather than deleterious effects might be expected to occur in patients with Huntington's disease treated with low dose apomorphine. Tolosa and Sparber reported that apomorphine reduced involuntary movements in both Huntington's chorea and chorea caused by other factors[14]. Apomorphine's paradoxical response in terms of chorea emphasizes the complexity of drug–receptor site interactions. The possibility that apomorphine is a weak or partial dopaminergic agonist and ameliorates chorea by blocking the effects of dopamine itself has yet to be delineated.

Cholinergic agonists

As discussed, a competitive balance exists in the striatum between two major neurotransmitters, dopamine and acetylcholine. Viewed from the perspective of this chemical balance, Parkinson's disease and Huntington's chorea have opposite pathophysiologies. In parkinsonism, a decreased influence of the dopaminergic system is the primary pathophysiological lesion so that there is a functional predominance of cholinergic activity. Therapy is aimed at increasing dopaminergic and decreasing cholinergic influences[15]. In contrast, in Huntington's disease, the primary pathophysiological lesion appears to relate to a functional predominance of the dopaminergic system. Anticholinergic agents, therapeutic in Parkinson's disease, would be expected to aggravate Huntington's disease, and cholinergic agents, contraindicated in parkinsonism, might be therapeutic in the treatment of Huntington's disease. Physostigmine and other centrally active cholinesterase inhibitors have been shown to ameliorate the choreatic movements of patients with Huntington's disease[16, 17]. Because of their rapid metabolism, however, these agents are therapeutically impractical. Recently, choline chloride and lecithin, presumed dietary precursors of central acetylcholine have been administered to choreatic patients with Huntington's disease with reported improvement in the involuntary movements[18, 19].

Gabaergic interactions

The influence of a third putative neurotransmitter, γ-amino-butyric acid, (GABA) has been of recent interest in the study of Huntington's disease. High levels of GABA and the enzyme responsible for its synthesis have been identified in the normal globus pallidus and substantia nigra, suggesting a possible role in extrapyramidal movement disorders[20]. Perry and colleagues demonstrated depressed levels of GABA in the brain and cerebrospinal fluid of patients with Huntington's disease and replacement therapy with GABA or GABA anolgues has been attempted[21]. Sodium valproate, felt to act as a GABA transaminase inhibitor, has been tried alone and with GABA supplementation, although no amelioration of chorea was noted[22, 23]. Isoniazid when given with pyridoxine also acts as a GABA transaminase inhibitor and in preliminary studies, has been reported to lessen involuntary movements in patients with Huntington's disease[24]. Since the depressed levels of GABA are neither consistent nor specific for the disorder, the role of this neurotransmitter relative to Huntington's disease remains speculative.

Psychiatric therapy

While the foundation of therapy in Huntington's disease remains pharmacological, psychiatric research has yielded a number of therapeutically pertinent observations. Psychiatric care is naturally important to the management of the behavioural problems implicit to the disease, whether they relate to psychotic behaviour or dementia. The management of these problems, from a behavioural viewpoint, is not specific to Huntington's disease and the same environmental restrictions and general supportive care administered to other psychotic or demented patients are required. It has been suggested that psychotherapy aimed specifically at allaying anxiety and reducing stress may improve cerebral blood flow and thereby abate chorea[25]. Huntington's disease, however, appears to be a primary neurodegenerative disorder and there is little evidence to support a hypothesis for vascular insufficiency in the striatum[26].

Aspects of Huntington's chorea that present unique psychological dilemmas appear to stem from the special genetic character of the disorder. The disease affects 50% of family offspring, but usually does not manifest itself until middle-age. These facts mean that all medically aware members of a given family must spend their childhood, adolescence and early adult life under the stress of possibly developing the devastating condition. Pearson has studied offspring of parents with Huntington's disease with attention to emotional attitudes and family planning[27]. He was perplexed by the seeming paradox that even with well-educated adults and sound counselling on the genetic consequences of bearing children, the fertility rate remained 2.15 per person at risk. The emotional evolution of these adults provides insight into their psychological dilemma and allows for earlier intervention in anticipated psychiatric complications. Pearson describes four states which adults at risk encounter; *first*, shocked disbelief—a brief reaction occurring when confronted with the genetic reality of Huntington's chorea; *second*, a stage of depression merging into a *third*, angry stage, that can be handled with a variety of psychological adjustments ranging from sublimation to projection. Denial forms the *final* state when the patient may intellectually still recognize the disorder but emotionally dissociates himself from it. With the disease psychologically compartmentalized, child bearing and future planning become issues emotionally unrelated to the disease. Whether these stages are unique or consistent in Huntington's disease has not been confirmed. The dynamics, however, may serve the physician in anticipating possible dilemmas in patients at risk and attempting to intervene with a reasonable perspective. It is important to realize that the supportive intervention needed may additionally involve relatives, spouses and neighbours within the nuclear family grouping[28].

Future perspectives

The eventual therapy of Huntington's disease will depend on accurate identification of the primary responsible pathogenic defect. This identification may suggest specific therapy, and additionally may serve as a biochemical marker of the disease. The fact that the disease is genetic suggests that, while patients may remain asymptomatic until adult life, they, must carry the biochemical defect even *in utero*. Identification of this defect offers a potential means of presymptomatic detection in Huntington's disease. Unfortunately, while multiple detection parameters have been suggested, none has yet proven altogether reliable or accurate[29, 30]. Primary questions that remain to be answered include when the degenerative process actually begins and whether there are environmental stimuli, external or internal, that initiate it. Until earlier means of detection are available, therapy in Huntington's disease cannot be aimed at cure but instead towards better pharmacological homeostasis within the context of a progressive degenerative disease.

Senile chorea

The syndrome of spontaneous lingual–facial–buccal movements in the elderly consists of repetitive, uncontrolled, unintentional movements of the tongue, lower facial (oral or buccal) muscles, and the jaw or masticatory muscles. Other descriptive terms include oral–masticatory movements and mouthing. Phenomenologically, such movements are indistinguishable from choreatic movements of Huntington's disease.

In senile chorea there is marked degeneration of the cells of the caudate and putamen, with a reduction in the striatal neuronal population, an alteration in the structure of the remaining neurons, and a proliferation of astrocytes. Both the large and small neurons of the caudate are affected to an equal degree, but the total degeneration in the striatum, while considerable, is not as extensive as that seen in Huntington's disease[31].

Like Huntington's chorea, senile chorea appears to be a neurodegenerative disorder without a specifically known cause, other than ageing. Therapy has therefore focused on modifying the pathophysiology of the striatal disorder primarily with dopaminergic blocking agents. These agents should be given in low doses initially, either haloperidol 1 mg twice daily or chlorpromazine 25 mg twice daily; the dosage is gradually increased until the symptoms are alleviated. Treatment should be undertaken only if the movements are disabling, since long-term use of these drugs can elicit analogous disorders[32].

Acquired hepatocerebral degeneration

Acquired hepatocerebral degeneration is the term used to describe the appearance of several chronic neurological syndromes in association with chronic liver disease. This syndrome usually consists of progressive symptoms including dementia, ataxia, rigidity, tremor, and choreathetotic movements.

The choreathetotic movements, especially of the tongue, face and mouth, have been described frequently and bear no constant relationship to the presence of frank hepatic coma or to the degree of hepatic encephalopathy (as mirrored by the level of consciousness). Once they occur, these movements are usually identical to the dyskinesias seen in Huntington's disease and other choreatic disorders.

The fact that in these other syndromes decreasing striatal dopaminergic activity or increasing striatal cholinergic activity has resulted in some amelioration of the movements, suggests that the lingual–facial–buccal dyskinesia of acquired hepatocerebral degeneration could also be influenced in the same way. We have reported a series of four patients with acquired hepatocerebral degeneration secondary to advanced post-necrotic cirrhosis whose lingual facial–buccal dyskinesias were successfully treated with the dopamine blocking agent, haloperidol[33]. Three of these four patients had cerebrospinal fluid homovanillic acid analysis prior to the initiation of haloperidol treatment and the cerebrospinal fluid concentration of homovanillic acid was normal. This implies that central dopamine turnover is normal. The clinical observation that a dopamine blocking agent ameliorates the dyskinesias in a situation in which the central dopamine turnover is normal suggests that altered dopamine receptor sites within the striatum are again involved in the pathogenesis of this particular aspect of the acquired hepatocerebral degeneration syndrome.

No data exists on the use of cholinergic agents in this disorder. We have, however, observed anticholinergic worsening and would predict that cholinergic agents would have some efficacy.

CHOREAS WITH DIFFUSE AND FOCAL NEUROPATHOLOGIC CHANGES

Sydenham's chorea and systemic lupus erythematosus

Chorea seen in association with systemic lupus erythematosus and Sydenham's chorea represent transitional syndromes in terms of their neuropathology. Although the clinical appearance of the movements is similar to the previously discussed syndromes, the neuropathologic alterations in the striatum are not entirely clear[34]. Because of the favourable prognosis of Sydenham's chorea, there have been relatively few postmortem studies. The central nervous system lesions are usually widespread and nonspecific. They include acute and chronic neuronal degenerative changes as well as vascular and inflammatory lesions[35]. The brain is often diffusely involved in this process but most early reports noted a predilection for the striatum. Similarly, patients dying from systemic lupus erythematosus with neurological involvement have both diffuse and focal cerebral degenerative lesions which are secondary to the necrotizing arteritis characteristic of the disease. These lesions usually involve the grey matter, and one reported patient with systemic lupus erythematosus and associated chorea had such a lesion in the striatum[36]. Although specific pathological changes in the striatum have not been demonstrated in every case of Sydenham's chorea or chorea associated with systemic lupus erythematosus, the widespread central nervous system pathology in these syndromes often includes the striatam. It is our belief that striatal dysfunction in these disorders underlies the abnormal movements.

Support for this concept is derived from the favourable influences that dopamine blocking agents have in these syndromes. Several investigators have reported single patients with systemic lupus erythematosus and recurrent severe chorea. In these patients haloperidol therapy has resulted in a marked improvement of abnormal involuntary movements. The cessation of haloperidol therapy resulted in the resumption of chorea[37].

Sydenham's chorea has been treated over the years with various agents including cortisone, ACTH, salicylate, bromides, and barbiturates, with variable and mainly unsatisfactorily results. The first specific, successful form of symptomatic therapy in Sydenham's chorea was the use of chlorpromazine. Other phenothiazines, such as thioproperazine, have also been used successfully, and haloperidol has also been used for symptomatic relief of both acute and residual chorea[33,37]. Dopamine depleting agents (reserpine) have been shown to produce amelioration in this disorder while dopamine agonists tend to worsen or exacerbate the disorder.

CHOREAS WITHOUT KNOWN PATHOLOGICAL CHANGES

Hyperthyroid chorea

Chorea associated with hyperthyroidism is a rare clinical entity but is the first choreatic disorder in this chapter where treatment of the pathogenesis is significant. Clearly, hyperthyroid chorea responds to treatment with antithyroid medication, so that as hyperthyroidism abates there is a parallel amelioration of chorea[38]. The fact that dopamine blocking agents also will ameliorate the chorea of hyperthyroidism underscores the probable common pathophysiology of this and all choreas.

We have reported a case of severe thyrotoxicosis and severe chorea whose choreiform movements were controlled with haloperidol. The improvement in chorea following treatment with a dopamine blocking agent alone suggests that dopamine is involved in the production of this movement disorder. After one week of haloperidol therapy this neuroleptic was stopped and chorea returned. After treatment of hyperthyroidism with radioactive iodine and the achievement of a euthyroid state the haloperidol was discontinued without a recurrence of the abnormal involuntary movements[33].

Preclinical studies with laboratory animals demonstrate that thyroid homone potentiates dopaminergic behaviours[39]. In hyperthyroid humans, dopamine turnover rates as assessed by levels of cerebrospinal fluid homovanillic acid, appear to be depressed. Their decreased turnover suggests that the heightened dopaminergic behaviour seen with hyperthyroidism may reflect a hypersensitive phenomenon at the level of the dopaminergic receptor site. The changes in dopamine metabolism responsible for hyperthyroid chorea appear to be entirely reversible, implying functional rather than structural alterations in striatal neurones. Treatment of hyperthyroid chorea focuses on arresting both the pathogenesis and pathophysiology of the disorder.

DRUG-INDUCED CHOREAS

Levodopa-induced dyskinesias

Among the most common side-effects of long-term levodopa therapy are levodopa-induced dyskinesias. The continued occurrence of these abnormal movements ofter necessitates a decrease in levodopa dosage, which prevents maximal therapeutic efficacy. While it is generally agreed that the chorea is related to increased activity of the dopaminergic striatal system, it remains controversial whether denervation hypersensivity or chronic agonist hypersensitivity best explains the choreatic phenomenon.

Treatment of levodopa-induced dyskinesias has focused on three different therapies. Since the abnormal movements are choreatic and felt to relate to increased activity of a dopaminergic striatal system, the easiest method would be to stop or decrease the levodopa. This method of 'drug holiday' has gained increasing acceptance in clinical practice of the control and possible prevention of this long-term complication of dopaminergic therapy[40]. The drug holiday involves cessation of anti-parkinsonian medications for 5–7 days usually in the controlled setting of the hospital. Medication is reinstituted slowly over the subsequent 2 weeks to achieve maximal efficacy without side-effects. In our experience all patients show abatement of dyskinesia with cessation of levodopa and after drug holiday, approximately one-third show diminished dyskinesias after reinstitution of their anti-Parkinsonian medication[40].

The biochemical basis of levodopa induced dyskinesias is not entirely clear, although animal studies suggest that chronic drug exposure by itself can alter striatal dopaminergic receptor sites. Normal animals treated with chronic levodopa demonstrate hypersensitive dopaminergic behaviour which correlates biochemically with an increase in the number and affinity of dopamine receptor sites in the strial homogenates[41].

A second therapeutic approach would be to diminish dopaminergic activity with dopaminergic blocking agents, analogous to the other choreas discussed. Although the administration of phenothiazines or butyrophenones can effectively stop levodopa-induced dyskinesias, the use of these neuroleptics in large doses will also block all dopaminergic activity and result in loss of the therapeutic effects of the levodopa, possibly even exacerbating the clinical findings of parkinsonism.

Klawans and Weiner attempted to use haloperidol, a butyrophenone, in the treatment of levodopa-induced dyskinesias[42]. Unfortunately, although haloperidol led to decreased dyskinesia this was accompanied by a simultaneous increase in parkinsonian symptoms in two-thirds of their population. In the remaining one-third, haloperidol resulted initially in decreased dyskinesia and no increased parkinsonian disability, but after 6 weeks of continued haloperidol, all patients demonstrated increased parkinsonism. Thus, as a practical therapeutic manoeuvre, the use of haloperidol is not a successful approach to treating levodopa-induced dyskinesia.

A third way to attempt treatment of levodopa-induced dyskinesia is with cholinergic agonists. As discussed with Huntington's disease, anti-cholinergic agents tend to exacerbate choreatic disorder and cholinesterase inhibitors, at least transiently, tend to ameliorate chorea. Choline chloride and lecithin, potentially dietary precursors of acetylcholine, have abated the levodopa-induced dyskinesias, but tend to aggravate parkinsonism (Barbeau, personal communication). The use of gabaergic agents remains experimental.

Amphetamine- and methylphenidate-induced chorea

Amphetamine is a sympathomimetic amine that acts primarily as an indirect dopaminergic agonist. Its mechanism of action is felt to relate to its ability to release endogenous presynaptic catecholamine stores, into the synaptic cleft[43]. The drug is used in the treatment of narcolepsy, parkinsonism, depression, obesity and orthostatic hypotension. Amphetamine is also a major drug of abuse.

Amphetamine psychosis and amphetamine-induced chorea represent two striking results of chronic amphetamine administration. Amphetamine-induced dyskinesias are abnormal involuntary movements most often observed in the facial and masticatory muscles, producing chewing, licking, teeth grinding, and protrusion of the tongue[44]. These abnormal movements are strikingly similar and in fact often indistinguishable from the movements seen with levodopa-induced dyskinesias and Huntington's disease. As already discussed, these latter movement disorders are felt to relate to heightened response of dopaminergic receptors to dopamine in the striatum[33]. The similarity of amphetamine-induced dyskinesias to movement disorders whose pathophysiology is better understood, suggests that amphetamine-induced dyskinesias may also relate to an altered sensitivity of the striatal dopaminergic system.

Additionally, the fact that amphetamine usually does not cause dyskinesias early, but only after chronic exposure, supports the hypothesis that chronic amphetamine administration induces dopaminergic hypersensitivity. This appears to be the case clinically in both adult amphetamine abusers and young children being treated with amphetamine for hyperkinesis[45]. Furthermore, while the dyskinetic movements have been reported to disappear after withdrawal of the drug, they can return with a single dose of amphetamine even after several weeks of abstinence. The fact that the suprasensitivity remains after the chronic drug exposure has ceased, supports the hypothesis that altered receptor site sensitivity, and not drug accumulation, underlies the pathophysiology of chronic amphetamine-induced dyskinesias. Treatment involves cessation of the drug and caution with future use since hypersensivity appears clinically to remain for prolonged periods.

Methylphenidate (Ritalin) is another central stimulant that acts to alter the catecholaminergic system, and specifically dopamine. Like amphetamine, methylphenidate when administered chronically is associated with the gradual development of dyskinetic movements. Pharmacologically this phenomenon may relate to altered dopaminergic receptor site sensitivity induced by chronic agonism[46]. Treatment involves cessation of the causative agent.

Birth control pill induced chorea

Most patients with this form of chorea have a past history of Sydenham's chorea. It appears that female sex hormones (like thyroid hormones) increase striatal dopamine receptor responsiveness and can cause chorea in patients with previous striatal dysfunction. Treatment involves prompt cessation of the oral contraceptives and in almost all cases, chorea abates within several days[47].

Phenytoin-induced chorea

Phenytoin can induce chorea in two settings. The first is a part of a clear encephalopathy due to toxicity. The second is as an isolated syndrome with therapeutic phenytoin levels. The latter is seen in patients with pre-existing striatal dysfunction. Again, treatment focuses on modifying the pathogenesis by withdrawing the causitive agent.

References

1 Huntington, G. (1872). On chorea. *Med. Surg. Rep.*, **26**, 317

2 Wilson, S. A. K. (1940). In Bruce, A. N. (ed.) *Neurology* (Baltimore: Williams & Wilkins)

3 Klawans, H. L. (1970). A pharmacological analysis of Huntington's chorea. *Eur. Neurol.*, **4**, 148

4 Van Rossum, J. M. (1966). Significance of dopamine-receptor blockade for mechanism of action of neuroleptic drugs. *Arch. Int. Pharmacodyn. Ther.*, **160**, 492

5 Barbeau, A. (1973). Biochemistry of Huntington's chorea. In Barbeau, A., Chase, T. N. and Paulson, G. W. (eds.) Huntington's Chorea: 1872–1972. (New York: Raven Press)

6 Ringel, S. P., Guthrie, M. and Klawans, H. L. (1973). Current treatment of Huntington's chorea. *Advances in Neurology*. Vol. 1, p. 797. (New York: Raven Press)

7 Klawans, H. L. and Weiner, W. J. (1976). The pharmacology of choretic movement disorders. *Prog. Neurol.*, **6**, 49

8 Berti, F. and Shore, P. A. (1967). Interaction of reserpine and ouabain on amine concentration mechanisms in the adrenergic neuron. *Biochem. Pharmacol.*, **16**, 2271

9 Spector, S., Sjoerdsma, A. and Undenfriend, U. (1965). The blockade of endogenous norepinephrine synthesis by alpha-methyl-tyrosine. *J. Pharmacol.*, **147**, 86

10 Birkmayer, W. (1969). Alpha-methyl-*p*-tyrosine effect in extrapyramidal disorders. *Wien. Klin. Wochenschr.*, **81**, 10

11 Aghajanian, G. K. and Bunney, B. S. (1973). In Usdin, E. and Snyder, S. (eds.) *Frontiers in Catecholamine Research*, pp. 643. (New York: Pergamon)

12 Kehr, W., Carlson, A., Lindquist, M., Magnusson, T. and Atack, C. (1972). Evidence for a receptor-mediated feedback control of striatal tyrosine hydroxylase activity. *J. Pharm. Pharmacol.*, **24**, 744

13 Walters, J. R., Bunney, B. S. and Roth, R. H. (1975). Piribedil and apomorphine pre and post synaptic effects. *Adv. Neurol.*, **9**, 273

14 Tolosa, E. S. and Sparber, S. B. (1974). Apomorphine in Huntington's chorea: Clinical observation and theoretical considerations. *Life Sci.*, **15**, 1371

15 Calne, D. B. (1970). *Parkinsonism: Physiology, Pharmacology and Treatment*, p. 1–136. (London: E. J. Arnold)

16 Klawans, H. L. and Rubovits, R. (1972). Cholinergic-anticholinergic antagonism in Huntington's chorea. *Neurology (Minneap.)*, **22**, 107

17 Hirsch, M. J., Growdon, J. H. and Wurtman, R. J. (1977). Oral choline chloride administration to patients with tardive dyskinesia. *Neurology*, **27**, 391

18 Davis, K. L., Hollister, L. E., Barchas, J. D. and Berger, P. A. (1976). Choline in tardive dyskinesia and Huntington's disease. *Life Sci.*, **19**, 1507

19 Barbeau, A. (1978). Phosphatidyl choline (Lecithin) in neurologic disorders. *Neurology*, **28**, 358

20 Feltz, P. (1971). Gamma-aminobutyric acid and caudatonigral inhibition. *Can. J. Physiol. Pharmacol.*, **49**, 1113

21 Perry, T. L., Hansen, S. and Klodter, M. (1973). Huntington's chorea: Deficiency of gamma aminobutyric acid in brain. *N. Engl. J. Med.*, **288**, 337

22 Shoulson, I., Kartzinel, R. and Chase, T. N. (1976). Huntington's disease: Treatment with dipropylacetic acid and gamma-aminobutyric adic. *Neurology*, **26**, 61

23 Pearce, I., Heathfield, K. W. G. and Pearce, J. M. S. (1977). Valproate sodium in Huntington's chorea. *Arch. Neurol.*, **34**, 308

24 Perry, T. L., MacLead, P. M. and Hansen, S. (1977). Treatment of Huntington's chorea with isoniazid. *N. Engl. J. Med.*, **297**, 840

25 Walsh, A. C. and Melaney, C. (1978). Huntington's Disease: Improvement with an anticoagulant-psycho-therapy regimen. *J. Am. Geriatr. Soc.*, **26**, 127

26 Bruyn, G. W. (1968). Huntington's chorea: historical, clinical and laboratory synopsis. In

Vinken, P. J., Bruyn, G. W. (eds.) *Handbook of Clinical Neurology*,Vol. 6, pp. 298–377. (North-Holland: Amsterdam)

27 Pearson, J. S. (1973). Behavioral aspects of Huntington's chorea. *Advances in Neurology*. Vol. 1, p. 701. (New York: Raven Press)

28 Wise, T. N. (1975). Psychiatric involvement in Huntington's chorea. *Psychosomatics*, **16**, 135

29 Chandler, J. H. (1966). EEG in prediction of Huntington's chorea. An 18-year follow-up. *Electroencephalogr. Clin. Neurophys.*, **21**, 79

30 Klawans, H. L., Paulson, G. W., Ringel, S. P. and Barbeau, A. (1972). Use of L-dopa in the detection of presymptomatic Huntington chorea. *N. Engl. J. Med.*, **286**, 1332

31 Alcock, N. S. (1936). Note on the pathology of senile chorea. *Brain*, **59**, 376

32 Weiner, W. J. and Klawans, H. L. (1973). Lingual-facial-buccal movements in the elderly. *J. Am. Geriatr. Soc.*, **21**, 314

33 Klawans, H. L. (1973). Pharmacology of extrapyramidal movement disorders. *Monographs in Neural Science*. (Basel: S. Karger)

34 Johnson, R. T. and Richardson, E. P. (1968). The neurological manifestations of systemic lupus erythematosus. *Medicine*, (Balt.), **47**, 337

35 Thiebaut, F. (1968). Sydenham's chorea. In Vinken, P. and Bruyn, G. (eds.), *Handbook of Clinical Neurology*, **6**, pp. 409–433. (Amsterdam: North-Holland)

36 Bauer, F. K., Riley, W. C. and Cohen, F. B. (1950). Disseminated lupus erythematosus with Sydenham's chorea and rheumatic heart disease. *Ann. Intern. Med.*, **33**, 1042

37 Nick, J. and Nicolle, M. H. (1964). Une médication spécifique du mouvement choréique. *Bull. Soc. Méd. Hop. (Paris)*, **115**, 275

38 Heffron, W. and Eaton, R. P. (1970). Thyrotoxicosis presenting as choreathetosis. *Ann. Intern. Med.*, **73**, 425

39 Klawans, H. L., Goetz, C. G. and Weiner, W. J. (1973). Dopamine receptor site sensitivity in hyperthyroid guinea pigs. *J. Neurotransmission*, **34**, 189

40 Weiner, W. J., Perlik, S., Koller, W. J., Nausieda, P. A. and Klawans, H. L. (1979). Role of "Drug Holiday" in the management of Parkinson disease. *Neurology*, **29**, 553

41 Klawans, H. L., Hitri, A., Nausieda, P. A. and Weiner, W. J. (1978). Studies on the pathophysiology of levodopa induced hypersensitivity. *Neurology*, **28**, 343

42 Klawans, H. L. and Weiner, W. J. (1974). Attempted use of haloperidol in treatment of levodopa induced dyskinesias. *J. Neurol. Neurosurg. Psychiatry*, **37**, 427

43 Hanson, L. C. F. (1966). Evidence that the central action of amphetamine is mediated via catecholamines. *Psychopharmacol.*, **9**, 78

44 Ellinwood, E. H. (1967). Amphetamine psychosis. *J. Nerv. Ment. Dis.*, **144**, 273

45 Case, Q. and McAndrew, J. B. (1974). Dexedrine dyskinesia. *Clin, Pediatr.*, **13**, 69

46 Weiner, W. J., Nausieda, P. A. and Klawans, H. L. (1978). Methyphenidate-induced chorea. *Neurology*, **28**, 1041

47 Koller, W. C., Weiner, W. J., Klawans, H. L. and Nausieda, P. A. (1980). Oral contraceptive-induced chorea. *Neurology*. (In Press)

3

The pharmacology of athetosis

R. D. Sweet

INTRODUCTION

Athetosis is a movement disorder in which wormlike, complex, irregular movements occur randomly[1,2]. The movements are slightly slower than those of chorea and confluent rather than rapid and discrete. They are accompanied by erratic fluctuations in tone. The irregular contraction of agonists and antagonists leads to abnormal postures which Wilson called 'caricatures of movement'[3]. These include spreading and hyperextension of the fingers with wrist flexion, hyperextension of the great toe, plantar flexion of the feet, and hyperextension of the neck and trunk. 'Overflow'—abnormal movements of a limb or axial muscles—often accompany purposeful movements of another body part. Dysarthria, poor modulation of voice volume and dysphagia are common.

The phenomenon of athetosis is generally associated with acquired lesions of the basal ganglia, 'cerebral palsy' in children and vascular events in adults. Perinatal hypoxia, venous thrombosis, or hyperbilirubinaemia and 'kernicterus' with striatal and/or pallidal neuronal loss, gliosis, and hypermyelination are typical in 'cerebral palsy'. The infant is usually hypotonic until the second year of life when athetosis begins. Spasticity or mental retardation may also be found. Impairment of upward gaze and of hearing is common in kernicterus.

The appearance of athetosis after vascular events is often delayed by several weeks or months. Lesions usually involve the striatum and internal capsule, producing a spastic hemiparesis which is resolving as athetosis becomes apparent. Less often, mass lesions or trauma affecting the same areas of the brain cause athetosis.

Paroxysmal choreoathetosis[4,5] is a familial disorder with onset in childhood or early adulthood in which episodes of choreoathetoid movement are

precipitated by voluntary movement. It is unique among athetoid conditions in its good response to phenytoin. Athetosis is also seen as one of the
phenomena in familial or metabolic conditions such as Lesch–Nyhan syndrome, ataxia telangiectasia, phenylketonuria, hepatolenticular degeneration, and Hallervorden–Spatz syndrome.

METHODS OF MEASURING ATHETOSIS

Pharmacotherapy has not been nearly as helpful for athetosis as it has been
for other extrapyramidal disorders such as parkinsonism or chorea. The
relatively minor effects of medicines as well as the inherent variability of
athetoid movements make the assessment of pharmacotherapy difficult.
Objective criteria, such as tone, accuracy of movements, or the amount of
overflow movement do not always correlate with a patient's functional
ability.

Denoff and Holden[6] outline their rating scheme for drug trials in children
with cerebral palsy at the Meeting Street School in Providence, R. I.
'Neuromotor function' was assessed with the standard neurological examination, ratings of motor skill and adeptness of performance, and ratings of
accuracy and speed of fine motor performance. 'Behaviour' was rated by a
series of standardized puzzles testing visual–motor skills and attention span.
Therapists or teachers rated activity, socialization, fantasy, group inte-
gration, anxiety, distractibility, dependency, aggression, and mood. However, Denhoff and Holden considered 'body anxiety' to be 'a more realistic
evaluation of performance than the other items'. They assessed each child's
reaction while he/she was suspended by the hands from a pair of gymnastic
rings and while he/she was blindfolded and rotated 10 times on a revolving
see-saw. The child was also rated while walking on a six-inch-wide plank
elevated 45° from the floor. Walking rate and balance were noted. 'Body
anxiety' in these three activities was assessed as follows: 0—no anxiety,
1—stiffening, 2—trembling, 3—sweating, 4—crying, 5—screaming, 6—uncontrolled kicking.

Baird and his colleagues attempted to rate athetosis by objective measurements of tone[7] but he eventually concluded that this correlated poorly with
ability to use the muscles[8].

Heggarty and Wright[9] used tests of hand function; the number of hand-
taps in 10 seconds, the number of pegs put into a cup, of pegs inserted into
a peg-board, of beads threaded, and of draughtsmen turned over in 30
seconds. A timed sample of handwriting or typing was also obtained.
Patients who could not perform intricate hand tasks were timed while
placing tennis balls in a bucket.

Olson devised a set of criteria to rate the movement disorder of adults with
athetoid cerebral palsy (Table 1). Mood, functional abilities, dyskinesias,

and tone were assessed. Dyskinesias were divided into athetosis, dystonia, tremor, and chorea. These dyskinesias, tension, and spasticity were rated in all extremities, head (neck), and trunk, while the patients were lying, sitting, and standing, during rest and activity.

Phelps[10] employed observations by physical, occupational, and speech therapists, nurses, and teachers in evaluating the effect of diazepam on cerebral palsy athetoids. Subjective evaluations were made of emotional status and physical skills with a scale of excellent, good, fair, no response or poor. Objective measurements included the duration of independent standing and or sitting balance, of holding the head upright, and of phonation of 'ah' (longest of three attempts). The distance a wheel-chair was pushed in 1 minute and arm control and the ability to reach were also noted. Dr Phelps commented that, 'while these tables give a generalized summary of changes in the group as a whole, it must be pointed out that no two children reacted in the same pattern, and only the individual case records tell the complete story'.

It should also be pointed out that no one criterion appeared to change independently in any of these studies and that global assessments of posture, limb function, and attitude by concerned rehabilitation therapists provide the bulk of data in most studies.

PLACEBO EFFECT

Since detection of change in patients with athetosis is so difficult, placebo effect must be considered in evaluating any therapy. Denhoff and Holden[6] compared the results of treatment with various medications to the results of using placebo in the same children. Neuromotor improvement during treatment with medications ranged from 9% to 56% (mean 38.7%). Favourable behavioural effects of medicine were 8% to 53% (mean 37.1%) and of placebo were 17% to 80% (mean 46.2%). Therefore, the results of placebo treatment were equal to or better than those with medication.

In addition, Denoff and Holden[6] reported that medication trials in office practice yielded an average improvement of 51.4% compared to the average improvement of 38.5% in their controlled experimental studies. The difference could reflect a healthier population seen in office practice, a greater placebo effect in the single practioner's observations, or random variation in gross observations.

Denhoff and Holden's[6] experience suggests that a new therapy for athetosis must produce a better than 50% improvement to qualify as even possibly effective.

Pharmacotherapy

The pharmacotherapy of athetosis has included sedatives and muscle

Table 1 Evaluation of athetoid cerebral palsy. (M. E. Olson—unpublished)

	Grade					
	0	*1*	*2*	*3*	*4*	
Speech	No speech	Speech unintelligible	Somewhat intelligible	Generally intelligible	Normal	
Sialorrhoea	Severe	Marked	Moderate	Mild	Normal or absent	
Gait						
Station						
Sitting						
supported						
unsupported	Total inability to perform or totally incapacitated	Poor ability to perform. Greatly interferes with function.	Noticeable impairment. Some interference with function.	Slight impairment. Barely noticeable.	Normal	
Head control						
Trunk control						
Finger to nose (R and L)						
Heel-knee-shin (R and L)						
	RUE	LUE	RLE	LLE	Head	Trunk

Dyskinesias
(Grade 0–4 for each body part)
FACIAL GRIMACING
ATHETOSIS
  lying
  at rest
  in activity
  standing
DYSTONIA
  At rest
  In activity

Table 1—*continued* Evaluation of athetoid cerebral palsy. (M. E. Olson—unpublished)

	Grade					
	0	*1*	*2*	*3*	*4*	
	RUE	LUE	RLE	LLE	Head	Trunk
TREMOR						
At rest						
In activity						
CHOREA						
Tension	Hypotonic	Normal	Mildly increased	Moderately increased	Severe or rigid	
Spasticity						
Present or absent						
Mood						
Normal						
Elated						
Depressed						
Contractures						
Location						
Degree						
Tone						

relaxants, medication to modify behaviour, and substances which affect neurotransmitters.

Initial attempts to modify cerebral palsy pharmacologically focused on the relief of spasticity by agents which affect the neuromuscular junction. Denhoff and Bradley[11] treated six children with spastic cerebral palsy with intramuscular curare and produced temporary relaxation which was helpful in physical therapy. Higher doses produced shallow respirations and confusion which attributed to 'possible shock'. One hopes that the absence of reports of respiratory arrests in the subsequent literature means that curare was abandoned before this complication could occur.

Perlstein and Barnett[12] used neostygmine, which potentiates cholinergic transmission by inhibiting acetylcholinesterase. They reasoned that potentiation of cholinergic inhibitory internuncial neurons in the spinal cord might be beneficial. Two of 31 athetoid patients were improved, with reduced tension and better speech and hand function. One of 22 spastic patients was better. The authors attributed these three instances to chance variation or placebo effect and concluded that neostygmine is not helpful in cerebral palsy.

Denhoff and Holden[6] studied eight 'relaxant' drugs from 1949–1960. Two of these drugs, chlorpromazine and reserpine, are catecholamine antagonists and are discussed below. The other six were mephenesin, mephenesin and glycerol α-ethyl-γ-isopropyl ether (Lissephen), zoxazolamine, α-ethyl-β-methylvaleramine, carisoprodol, and emylcamate. None of the six 'relaxant' medicines produced more neuromotor or behavioural improvement than the placebo.

Baird[8] compared Meprospan, a slow release form of meprobamate, with zoxazolamine, reserpine, and promazine in 210 children with cerebral palsy, including 13 athetoids. Seven of the 13 athetoid children were best on Meprospan while four were better on promazine, and two had no effect from any medicine. Of the larger group of 210 children, 109 were best on Meprospan, 59 were better with another medicine, and 42 did not improve with any medicine. Charash and Cooper's[13] results with meprobamate were not as good. They studied 40 patients with cerebral palsy, 28 of whom had generalized athetosis. There was early improvement in 13 of the 28 patients. However, sustained subjective improvement was found in only four patients and there was no sustained objective improvement in any patient. Deterioration of function related to sedation or hyperarousal on withdrawal was noted in eight of the 28 athetoid patients.

The meprobamate congener carisoprodol was evaluated in three separate studies by double-blind comparison with placebo in both athetoid and spastic cerebral palsy[6,14,15]. No difference in improvement was found for athetoids or spastics in any study.

Diazepam produced good results in two evaluations soon after its introduction. Phelps[10] tested diazepam in 19 cerebral palsy patients of whom 16 were athetoids. Thirteen of the group had previously been on meprobamate or carisprodol. The dose of diazepam ranged from 2–20 mg and most children were evaluated for 6 months. Reports by therapists and teachers on the 16 athetoid patients' 'handicap' were: excellent, 16; good, 23; fair, 16; no change, 14; and worse, 4 (total of 72 reports). Changes in emotional status were not as favourable; only 25 of 73 reports were excellent or good. Balance and control of arms, head, and lips were improved and opisthotonus reduced. Children with athetosis responded much better than those with spasticity.

Marsh[16] also reported a favourable effect of diazepam on athetoid but not spastic cerebral palsy. Diazepam at an average dose of 2.5 mg three times a day was compared with placebo in a single-blind crossover design for a total period averaging 5 months. Although nine of 14 athetoid quadriplegics showed an excellent or good response during treatment with diazepam, Marsh accepted only six of them as being truly improved when he compared the results of diazepam and placebo treatments. He was especially impressed with diazepam's production of general relaxation and suppression of startle reflexes.

Denhoff[17] reported that diazepam produced improvement in nine of 25 children with cerebral palsy. The best results were in those with rigidity (six of ten improved). One of six athetoid and two of five spastic children also improved, but four athetoids, three spastics, and three of four children with ataxia worsened. These results may reflect dose (2.5–5.0 mg three times a day), age (2–6 years old) and concomitant medication (often anticonvulsants). Thirty-six per cent (9/25) of patients improved during a 'controlled' study of the type discussed above, but 48% of these patients improved with placebo![18] Nevertheless, Denoff maintains that in disabled non-ambulatory cases of cerebral palsy rigidity, '... it is a very helpful adjunct when used properly'.

Three more recently developed relaxant medicines have also been evaluated for athetosis. Chayette and colleagues[19] tested dantrolene against placebo, in a double-blind protocol, in 17 patients with athetoid cerebral palsy. Dantrolene, 20–400 mg/day, and placebo were each given for 4 weeks. Twelve of 17 patients elected to continue dantrolene, although four of the 12 dropped therapy after several more months. Eight patients continued dantrolene for more than a year with 'substantial relief of involuntary movement and spasm'. Best results were found in patients with increased tone ('tension').

Spinnler[20] tested two young women with post encephalitic athetosis and dementia with clonazepam, using the large dose of 12 mg/day for 15 days. Both patients were severely drowsy. Athetosis, grimacing, torsion spasms, and dystonia disappeared almost completely in one patient but there was only slight improvement of grimacing and spasms in the other.

Milla and Jackson[21] studied Baclofen (chlorphenylgaba), 60 mg/day in 20 children with cerebral palsy and found that one of the three athetoid patients improved.

Behavioural medicines

Emotions have a strong influence on motor performance in athetoid patients. Phelps[10] cited an 'emotional paralysis, a profound passivity'. Sedation produced by the relaxant medicines discussed above is said to decrease anxiety and increase co-operation with rehabilitation. Denhoff and Holden[6,22] tested for the behavioural effects of all the relaxants they examined and found that only zoxazolamine and chlorpromazine did better than placebo. Despite zoxazolamine's behavioural effect, its 'neuromotor effect was identical to that of placebo'. The authors tested chlorpromazine 'solely on behavioural rating, since we did not expect neuromotor effects'. They noted that 'neuromotor effectiveness was achieved secondarily after the children were relaxed and happy'. One wonders how much bias about mechanism of action influenced this conclusion.

Medicines which affect neurotransmitters

There has been relatively little study of the role of putative neurotransmitters in athetosis. The several causes and complex pathology of athetosis have discouraged investigators of movement disorders. As noted above, the beneficial effects of chlorpromazine, a dopamine antagonist, have been attributed to tranquilization. Denhoff and Holden[6] found no benefit from reserpine, which depletes granular stores of bioamines, mainly because the children who were treated became excessively drowsy.

Heggarty and Wright[9] administered tetrabenazine to 30 athetoid cerebral palsy patients whose ages ranged from 3–19 years, the majority being 8–12 years. Tetrabenazine is a benzoquinolizine derivative which interferes with intraneuronal granular storage of catecholamines and serotonin in a manner similar to reserpine but with more specificity for brain than the periphery. Patients younger than 10 years were given 25 mg/day and those 10 years or older were given 50 mg/day for 3 weeks in a double-blind crossover with placebo. Tetrabenazine produced statistically significant improvement over placebo in three of five tests of hand function. However, 'the overall clinical improvement in the patients receiving tetrabenazine was barely noticeable ..., and the drug would have been judged ineffective without statistical analysis of the tests given'.

Rosenthal and colleagues[23] published a preliminary study of levodopa treatment for athetoid cerebral palsy. Nine teenage or adult patients (15–46 years old) of normal intelligence were included. Five patients had generalized tension athetosis, three had unilateral tension athetosis, and one had generalized athetosis due to kernicterus. Levodopa was gradually increased

Table 2   Results of evaluations after levodopa treatment[23]

	Number of patients improved			
Function	No change	Slight	Moderate	Marked
Handwriting	2	1	3	1
Motor tests	1	3	1	2
Walking	—	4	2	—
Standing	—	5	1	—
Sitting posture	3	5	1	—
Head balance	3	3	3	—
	(Normal)			
A.D.L.	4	2	2	3
Speech	—	2	4	—
Muscle pain and tension	2	2	3	1
Tremor	3	3	3	—
Grimace, drool, swallow	4	4	1	—
	(Normal)			
Subject's feelings and parents' report	1	4	4	—
Mood	3	5	1	—

to a mean maximum dose of 4.5 g/day (range 4.0–6.0) and then reduced to a mean maintenance dose of 3.3 g/day (range 2.0–4.0). Changes in the patients' function are shown in Table 2. Although only seven of 113 ratings indicated marked improvement, moderate and functionally significant changes were found in many functions, especially in those of the upper extremities. One patient did much better in writing and in activities of daily living because her hand posture changed from a clenched fist to a functional grasp and pinch. Another patient did moderately or markedly better in 10 of the 13 rating categories. Improvement was spotty among the other patients. Six patients went on to a 2–6-week long double-blind placebo crossover trial in which five were better on levodopa than on placebo.

Spinnler[20] reported the results of drug trials in two young women with postencephalitic athetosis and dementia. Diazepam, 15 mg/day, was not helpful. When haloperidol, 3 mg/day, was added to diazepam, there was slight improvement of athetosis and almost complete recovery from torsion spasms in both cases. Despite this benefit from the catecholamine antagonist, haloperidol, Spinnler then used the dopamine agonists, amantadine and levodopa. Amantadine, 300 mg/day for 10 days, produced 'remarkable improvement' of athetosis in one case and of rigidity in both. Levodopa changed rigidity to upper limb hypotonia in both patients. One patient's athetosis, torsion spasm, dystonia and grimacing, were much worse and she became drowsy on 2.25 g/day. The other patient demonstrated 'severe excitement' and minimal reduction of athetosis on 1.25 g/day. This second patient was then given levodopa, 600 mg/day, and benserazide (an extra-cerebral inhibitor of dopa decarboxylase), 150 mg/day for 13 days. Athetosis, grimacing, torsion spasms and rigidity, disappeared almost completely but the patient became excited and aggressive after 5 days of treatment. This behaviour was reversed by the addition of diazepam, 15 mg/day. The regime was continued for 3 months with good results.

Olson and McDowell[24] administered levodopa for 5–11 months to 11 children (7–14 years old) with athetoid cerebral palsy. The initial dose of 5 mg/kg/24 h was increased by 2–5 mg/kg every 2–3 days. Gradually, athetosis, dystonia, and oral dyskinesias decreased and tremor disappeared. Control of sitting, standing and walking improved and parents noted the children to be more relaxed. Speech improved in six patients. However, the condition of all children deteriorated when higher doses (45–100 mg/kg/24 h) were reached. Dyskinesias and muscular tension recurred, speech became more dysarthric and sialorrhea more prominent.

Six children were lethargic and irritable and 10 had anorexia and nausea. Three children stopped levodopa and reverted to their pretreatment state. The other eight children gradually improved again when maintained on doses of 22–41 mg/kg/24 h.

Jaffe and Browning[25] treated two patients with kernicterus related choreoathetosis with methylphenidate, 20 and 30 mg/day. Choreoathetosis was reduced to minimal levels and motor performance improved. This effect lasted 18 months and disappeared when methylphenidate was stopped. The investigators attributed methylphenidate's success to its amphetamine-like adrenergic effects but a dopaminergic mechanism seems equally plausible.

Table 3   The effect of apomorphine on athetoid cerebral palsy

Patient	Dose mg	Change from baseline*			
		Oral dyskinesias	Limb athetosis	Muscle tone	Reduced overflow
1	1.0	1	1	1	0
	1.5	0	1	1	0
2	1.0	1	1	1	0
	1.5	0	1	1	0
3	0.5	1	1	1	0
	1.0	0	2	1	0
4	0.5	0	3	2	3
5	1.0	1	2	0	0
6	0.5	0	0	0	0
	1.5	1	1	1	3
7	0.5	0	0	0	0
	1.0	3	2	1	0
8	0.5	0	3	2	2
9	1.0	0	2	2	0

*Change based on 0–4 scale. Number indicates point improvement from baseline minus the point improvement after double-blind saline injection.

Dopamine agonists were further assessed in athetoid cerebral palsy by Olson and Sweet (unpublished). Nine adult patients with generalized tension athetoid cerebral palsy were studied in the hospital. Five patients were independent, one patient ambulated with Kenny sticks and three patients required complete care. The dopamine agonists apomorphine, 0.5–1.5 mg subcutaneously, and piribedil, 2–3 mg i.v. over 20 min, were given on separate days. Then 50 mg levodopa and 20 mg carbidopa per day orally were started and gradually increased.

The salutary effects of apomorphine could be distinguished from normal saline in all nine cases whether or not side-effects were apparent (Table 3). Mild to moderate reduction of muscle tone was noted on examination. Two patients reported a sensation of extreme relaxation even while vomiting forcefully. Athetosis, including the slower dystonic component, was relieved. For example, the patient's hand, normally fisted and flexed at the wrist, became open and relaxed and could be manipulated voluntarily. Six of nine patients demonstrated moderate to marked improvement of athetosis and three showed a great reduction in overflow movements when attempting a voluntary act. Only one patient showed marked improvement of oral dyskinesia, but five others had mild improvement. Two of these patients exhibited lip smacking and chewing movements on higher doses of apomorphine. The overall effect was most prominent during the first 10 min and gradually disappeared over 30–45 min.

Side-effects

Side-effects were dose related. These included hypotension in four patients, mild tachycardia in four, nausea in seven, vomiting in six, diaphoresis in five and mild drowsiness in six. Nausea, vomiting and diaphoresis occurred within 5 min after the injection and disappeared after a few minutes.

Only one of six patients demonstrated moderate reduction in athetosis and mild reduction in tension during intravenous administration of piribedil. The other five failed to show a significant change. Three patients became very drowsy. Three became nauseated, but only one vomited. All effects were related to the speed of infusion and ceased when it was completed.

Levodopa and carbidopa were advanced to 750/150 mg/day in eight patients, but were then reduced to 300–600/90–120 mg/day because of dyskinesia and increased tone at higher doses. All three severely affected patients had moderate relief of tension, athetosis and overflow movements but had no improvement in function. One self-sufficient patient had smoother control of movements, faster performance times, and a feeling of general relaxation and better control in climbing stairs, carrying a cafeteria tray and eating. Speech improved in this patient and two others. More stable posture or smoother gait was noticed in six patients. However, overall improvement was mild or not apparent in five patients.

Improvement with apomorphine did not predict improvement with levodopa and carbidopa. Nevertheless, we concluded that the changes seen in this study suggest that dopamine modulates coordination in athetoid cerebral palsy. Since carbidopa, which inhibits the conversion of levodopa, to dopamine outside the central nervous system, did not prevent the pattern of changes previously seen with levodopa alone, the dopamine effect is probably located within the C.N.S.

The results of the treatment of athetoid cerebral palsy defy straight-forward interpretation. With the background of Denhoff and Holden's[6] work, the subtle improvement seen in patients given levodopa or dopamine agonists may be interpreted as placebo effect. Even if it reflects changes in brain chemistry, the effect of levodopa and therefore of dopamine, is clearly only modulating rather than primary. The improvement of some patients by chlorpromazine and tetrabenazine, dopamine antagonists, must also be considered. One might postulate a dopaminergic modulating mechanism with several types of receptors, one more sensitive than the other to dopamine and its agonists or to blockage by antagonists. However, the data are too incomplete to permit further speculation.

Non–pharmacological treatment

Biofeedback

Biofeedback training of six athetoid cerebral palsy patients was reported by Finley and colleagues[26]. Surface frontalis EMG activity was fed back to patients as auditory clicks and as a graphic summation of total EMG activity. After a 6 week trial of two sessions per week, peak to peak EMG activity decreased from 29 to 13 µV. Four mildly or moderately affected patients improved by clinical criteria while two severely affected patients did not. Speech improved in four, fine motor performance in three, and gross performance in five of six patients. No long term data were presented.

Surgery

Stereotaxic techniques have enabled surgeons to place lesions in specific locations within the brain and such lesions have been used to interrupt abnormal movements as disparate as parkinsonian tremor and dystonia.

Hassler[27] devised a sagittal thalatomy which produced coagulation lesions 2 mm apart in a sagittal row at the base of the ventral thalamic nuclei and found it to be especially effective against the combination of athetosis and spasticity in 31 cases. Athetotic hyperkinesias were 'regularly alleviated or reduced by 80%'. Athetotic postures 'nearly disappeared at first ... but many partly reappeared after some months. Lasting partial improvement against spastic symptoms is present in 50% of the patients'. The results were not as encouraging when the status of stereotaxic surgery in cerebral palsy was reviewed in a symposium edited by Gillingham and Hitchcock[22]. Narabayashi (pp.1–10, Ref. 22) reported that thalamotomy (ventral border of VL and VIM nuclei) produced slightly better speed and extended activities in 12 athetoid patients. Guidette and Fraioli (pp. 27–39, Ref. 22) performed bilateral dentatolysis on 16 patients with dystonic–athetoid syndromes and found improvement in all of them, marked in four. Three patients could open and close hands they had not used before. However, the athetoid component alone improved in only two of five choreoathetoid patients. Galanda and colleagues (pp. 21–26, Ref. 22) combined transentorial dentatomy with pulvinarotomy in 45 cerebral palsy patients, 18 athetoid and three dystonic. Dentatomy alone did not control involuntary movements but the combined procedure did. Significantly, the authors commented that 'late results are much more dependent on rehabilitation, in which it is necessary to train new movement patterns ...'

Other authors reported long term results of dentate operations. Four of 13 patients with hemi- or double athetosis and three of four with choreoathetosis remained improved in Siegfried and Verdie's series (pp. 41–48, Ref. 22) while three of six of Zervas' patients with dyskinesia (pp. 49–51, Ref. 22) were still improved.

Chronic electrical stimulation of the cerebellum by an electrode grill surgically implanted over the dorsal superior surface has been used in attempts to ameliorate seizure disorders, spasticity, and cerebral palsy. Davis and colleagues[29] treated 142 patients with cerebral palsy. Twenty-eight per cent of the athetoids were improved at 1 week and 'almost all' were improved at 6 months. Independent mobility improved in 56% of patients and hand control in 92% of patients in whom it was impaired. Speech, drooling, feeding and dressing were all better. Ratusnik and colleagues[30] found that speech was better in three but worse in two of eight cerebral palsy patients treated with chronic cerebellar stimulation.

Cooper and colleagues[31,32] reported that 68 of 100 cerebral palsy patients were judged to be significantly improved by an evaluating team and their families after 13 months of cerebellar stimulation. Athetosis benefited less than spasticity, but was more improved after 13 months than 1 month. Eleven per cent of patients were totally dependent after treatment as compared with 33% before. Cooper and Upton[32] postulate that cerebellar stimulation acts on the reticular formation of the brain stem rather than on the Purkinje cells to produce thalamic inhibition.

CONCLUSION

The abundance of medicines and methods for the treatment of athetosis demonstrates the inadequacy of current therapy. The lack of clear understanding of the neuronal and pharmacological interactions of athetosis has led to trials of each new type of medicine without any unifying hypothesis or plan of investigation.

Within the limits of current knowledge, there are several questions which might be asked:

1. What is the pharmacological anatomy of athetosis? One might expect profuse neuronal sprouting after injury to the basal ganglia. Histochemical examination of the brains of athetoid patients might demonstrate sprouting and suggest which neurotransmitters are missing or in excess.

2. What is the effect at several doses of agonists and antagonists of dopamine (bromocriptine, haloperidol), serotonin (L-5-hydroxytryptophan and carbidopa, methysergide), norepinephrine (clonidine), acetyl choline (lecithin, benztropine), GABA (γ-hydroxybutyrate, isonicotinic acid), and endogenous opioids (naloxone)?

Without the answers to these naive, inclusive questions, treatment for early-athetosis today is limited to rehabilitation therapy, orthopedic correction and low doses of relaxants.

Acknowledgements

Partially supported by grant RR47, General Clinical Research Center Program, Division of Research Resources, National Institute of Health, and by grants from the United Cerebral Palsy Association and the American Parkinson's Disease Association. I thank Mrs. Carmen James for preparing the manuscript.

References

1 Carpenter, M. B. (1950). Athetosis and the basal ganglia. Review of the literature and study of forty-two cases. *Arch. Neurol. Psychiatry*, **63**, 875

2 Spiegel, E. A. and Baird, H. W. (1968). Athetotic Syndromes. In Vinken, P. J. and Bruyn, G. W. (eds.) *Handbook of Clinical Neurology, Diseases of the Basal Ganglia*. Vol. 6, pp. 440–475. (Amsterdam: North-Holland)

3 Wilson, S. A. K. (1925). Disorders of motility and muscle tone with special reference to the corpus striatum (Croonian Lectures). *Lancet*, **2**, 215

4 Mount, L. A. and Reback, S. (1940). Familial paroxysmal choreoathetosis. Preliminary report on a hitherto undescribed clinical syndrome. *Arch. Neurol. Psychiatry*, **44**, 841

5 Stevens, H. (1966). Paroxysmal choreoathetosis *Arch. Neurol.*, **14**, 415

6 Denhoff, E. and Holden, R. H. (1961). Relaxant drugs in cerebral palsy: 1949–1960. *N. Eng. J. Med.*, **264**, 475

7 Spiegel, E. A., Wycis, H. T., Baird, H. W. III, Rovner, D. and Thur, C. (1956). Pallidum and muscle tone. *Neurology*, **6**, 350

8 Baird, H. W. III (1959). A comparison of Meprospan with other tranquilizing and relaxing agents in children. *J. Pediatr.*, **54**, 170

9 Heggarty, H. and Wright, T. (1974). Tetrabenazine in athetoid cerebral palsy. *Devel. Med. Child. Neurol.*, **16**, 137

10 Phelps, W. M. (1963). Observation of a new drug in cerebral palsy athetoids. *Western Med.*, **4**, 5

11 Denhoff, E. and Bradley, C. (1942). Curare treatment of spastic children. *N. Eng. J. Med.*, **226**, 411

12 Perlstein, M. A. and Barnett, H. E. (1950). Neostigmine therapy in cerebral palsy. *J. Am. Med. Assoc.*, **142**, 403

13 Charash, L. I. and Cooper, W. (1958). Experiences with meprobamate in cerebral palsy. *Pediatrics*, **21**, 605

14 Woods, G. E. (1962). Double-blind trial of carisoprodol. *Devel. Med. Child Neurol.*, **4**, 499

15 Gooch, J. M. (1963). Carisoprodol in cerebral palsy. A controlled trial. *Devel. Med. Child. Neurol.*, **5**, 603

16 Marsh, H. O. (1965). Diazepam in incapacitated cerebral-palsied children. *J. Am. Med. Assoc.*, **191**, 93

17 Denhoff, E. (1964). Cerebral palsy—a pharmacologic approach. *Clin. Pharmacol. Ther.*, **5**, 947

18 Denhoff, E. (1976). Medical aspects of cerebral palsy. In Cruikshank, W. (ed.) *Cerebral Palsy*, pp. 65–71. (Syracuse University Press)

19 Chayette, S. B., Birdsong, J. H. and Roberson, D. L. (1973). Dantrolene sodium in athetoid cerebral palsy. *Arch. Phys. Med. Rehabil.*, **54**, 365

20 Spinnler, H. (1972). New pharmacologic approaches to double athetosis. *N. Engl. J. Med.*, **286**, 610

21 Milla, P. J. and Jackson, A. D. M. (1977). A controlled trial of Baclofen in children with cerebral palsy. *J. Int. Med. Res.*, **5**, 398

22 Denhoff, E. and Holden, R. H. (1955). The effectiveness of chlorpromazine with cerebral palsied children. *J. Pediatr.*, **47**, 328

23 Rosenthal, R. K., McDowell, F. H. and Cooper, W. (1972). Levodopa therapy in athetoid cerebral palsy. A preliminary report. *Neurology*, **22**, 1

24 Olson, M. E. and McDowell, F. H. (1973). L-DOPA administration in children with athetoid cerebral palsy. *Neurology*, **23**, 416

25 Jaffe, S. C. and Browning, R. A. (1974). Methylphenidate in the treatment of kernicterus-related choreoathetosis. *Neurology*, **24**, 368

26 Finley, W. W., Niman, C., Standley, J. and Ender, P. (1976). Frontalis EMG-biofeedback training of athetoid cerebral palsy patients. *Biofeedback and Self-Regulation*, **1**, 169

27 Hassler, R. (1972). Sagittal thalamotomy for relief of motor disorders in cases of double athetosis and cerebral palsy. *Confin. Neurol.*, **34**, 18

28 Gillingham, F. J. and Hitchcock, E. R. (eds.) (1977). Advances in Stereotactic and Functional Neurosurgery (2). *Acta Neurochirugica*, (Suppl. 29)

29 Davis, R. M., Cullen, R. F. Jr., Flitter, M. A., Duenas, D., Engle, H. and Ennis, B. (1977). Control of spasticity and involuntary movements, *Neurosurgery*, **1**, 205

30 Ratusnik, D. L., Wolfe, V. I., Penn, R. D. and Schweitz, S. (1978). Effects on speech of chronic cerebellar stimulation in cerebral palsy. *J. Neurosurg.*, **48**, 876

31 Cooper, I. S., Amin, I., Upton, A., Riklan, M., Watkins, S. and McLellan, L. (1977). Safety and efficacy of chronic cerebellar stimulation. *Neurosurgery*, **1**, 203

32 Cooper, I. S. and Upton, A. R. M. (1978). Use of chronic cerebellar stimulation for disorders of disinhibition. *Lancet*, **1**, 595

4

Treatment of myoclonus

M. H. van Woert and E. Chung Hwang

INTRODUCTION

Myoclonus may be present as a major or minor symptom in a wide variety of neurological disorders. The clinical characteristics of myoclonus may vary with different aetiologies. Myoclonus may be arrhythmic or rhythmical, generalized or focal, synchronous or asynchronous, spontaneous or stimulus sensitive. As will become evident in the subsequent discussion, the characteristics of the myoclonus and its aetiology can be important in determining the optimum therapeutic regime.

Intention or action myoclonus is a common form of this disorder and is characterized by sudden unpredictable, irregular skeletal muscle contractions which are either precipitated or aggravated by volitional action. The myoclonic movements are typically aggravated by visual, auditory or tactile stimuli and may disappear during sleep. Characteristically the muscle jerks are worse on awakening in the morning and premenstrually. Intention myoclonus is commonly seen in progressive myoclonus epilepsy, post-anoxic encephalopathy, hereditary essential myoclonus and dyssynergia cerebellaris myoclonica (Ramsay Hunt syndrome).

Myoclonus may occur as in isolated phenomenon without any epileptic manifestations or EEG abnormalities. However, myoclonus is also commonly associated with both grand mal and petit mal seizures.

Another major type of myoclonus is called segmental or rhythmical myoclonus which is characterized by synchronous rhythmical jerking movements of muscles innervated by one or several contiguous segments of the spinal cord or brain stem. Segmental myoclonus may continue during sleep and is usually unaffected by sensory stimulation or voluntary activities. This form of myoclonous may be seen after localized damage to the central nervous system (CNS) such as may occur with viral infections and vascular, neoplastic or traumatic lesions of the spinal cord or brain stem.

Palatal myoclonus is a well-known type of rhythmical myoclonus which is characterized by muscle contractions, usually at a steady rate of 60–200 per minute, involving the soft palate and sometimes other muscles, particularly those of the pharynx, larynx, eyes, face and diaphragm.

PATHOPHYSIOLOGICAL AND NEUROCHEMICAL MECHANISMS IN MYOCLONUS

Myoclonus, like seizures, may be due to a paroxysmal neuronal discharge from an excitable focus[1-3]. An alternate hypothesis is that myoclonus may result from loss of higher centre controls which modify the effects of sensory input to the reticular formation of the brain[4-5]. A loss of higher centre inhibitory regulation could produce a hyperexcitability of the CNS resulting in involuntary muscle contractions that occur in response to visual, tactile or auditory stimuli or develop during willed motor activity. At the present time, no pathological lesion has been identified as the cause of myoclonus. In the case of patients with hereditary essential myoclonus, the brains have been reported to be normal at autopsy, suggesting the presence of only a biochemical lesion. On the other hand, diffuse pathological changes have been found at autopsy in conditions such as post-anoxic intention myoclonus, progressive myoclonic epilepsy and Ramsay Hunt syndrome[6-9]. The cerebellum has been the region of the brain in which microscopic changes at autopsy have been most consistently observed[6-9] and cerebellar symptoms frequently accompany myoclonus. In animals ablation of the cerebellum has been shown to enhance stimulus-sensitive myoclonus[4]. If myoclonus follows a suppression or loss of inhibition, the cerebellum may be the site of some or all of these inhibitory circuits.

Recently a possible causal relationship between certain types of myoclonus and a deficiency of serotonin in the brain has been suggested. Patients with post-anoxic intention myoclonus and progressive myoclonus epilepsy have been found to consistently have a low concentration of 5-hydroxy-indoleacetic acid (5HIAA), a metabolite of serotonin, in their cerebrospinal fluid (CSF) suggesting a reduced concentration of brain serotonin[10-16]. The concentration of CSF 5HIAA is decreased both before and after treatment with probenecid which blocks the transport of 5HIAA from the brain. This suggests that brain serotonin synthesis is impaired in these patients with myoclonus. In support of this hypothesis numerous studies have shown that serotonin precursors dramatically improve certain types of myoclonus. L-5-hydroxytryptophan (L-5HTP) administered in conjunction with the peripheral decarboxylase inhibitor, carbidopa, and L-tryptophan plus a monamine oxidase (MAO) inhibitor both alleviate myoclonus of several different aetiologies[10-24]. L-5HTP and L-tryptophan are precursors of serotonin and have been shown to elevate brain serotonin and 5HIAA and

CSF 5HIAA (Figure 1). Methysergide, a serotonin receptor blocker, counteracts the antimyoclonic action of L-5HTP and carbidopa[18]. Furthermore, chronic treatment with levodopa, which decreases brain serotonin, aggravates post-anoxic intention myoclonus[11].

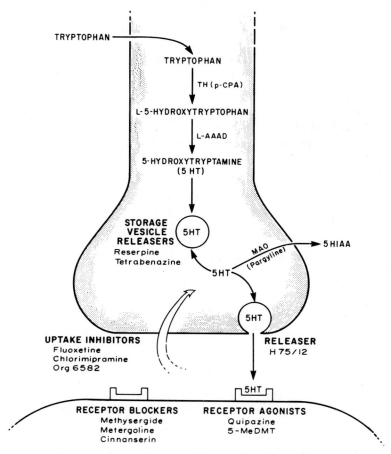

Figure 1 Serotonergic synapse; TH = tryptophan hydroxylase, p-CPA = p-chlorophenyl-alanine, L-AAAD = L-aromatic amino acid decarboxylase, MAO = monoamine oxidase, 5HIAA = 5-hydroxyindoleacetic acid, 5-MeDMT = 5-methoxy N,N-dimethyl-tryptamine

A number of experimental animal models have demonstrated that brain serotonin may influence stimulus-sensitivity and seizure threshold. In the photosensitive baboon, *Papio papio*, decreasing brain serotonin lowers seizure threshold, while raising brain serotonin decreases the susceptibility to seizures[25-26]. In animals with chemically or electrically induced epilepsy, inhibition of serotonin synthesis by p-chlorophenylalanine or depletion of

brain serotonin by reserpine or tetrabenazine lower the threshold to
seizures[27-29] and antagonize the anticonvulsant action of benzodiazepine
compounds[30]. These effects are reversed by L-5HTP[26-28, 30].

De la Torre *et al.*[31] have reported that L-5HTP in combination with the
peripheral decarboxylase inhibitor benserazide, markedly protected rats
from metrazol-induced seizures. Decreasing brain serotonin by *p*-chloro-
phenylalanine (*p*-CPA) exacerbates metrazol-provoked seizures[31]. We have
confirmed these results and observed that subconvulsant doses of metrazol
(60 mg/kg i.p.) produces stimulus-sensitive myoclonic jerks and a startle
response which can be prevented by pretreatment with L-5HTP (200 mg/kg)
in combination with alpha-methyl-dopa hydrazine (carbidopa) and aggravated by decreasing brain serotonin with *p*-CPA (400 mg/kg 24 h prior to
metrazol). It is of interest that intravenously injected metrazol combined
with intermittent photic stimulation produced precentral and frontal poly-
spikes and myoclonic jerks, particularly in the upper extremities in normal
human subjects[32].

Another animal model of myoclonus which has many similarities to
patients with myoclonus who respond to L-5HTP and carbidopa therapy
can be produced in rodents with the organochlorine insecticide, *p,p'*-DDT[33].
Two to three hours after the intragastric injection of *p,p'*-DDT (600 mg/kg
in olive oil) mice and rats develop generalized arrhythmic myoclonus which
is aggravated by noise and tactile stimuli. The myoclonus in these rodents is
similar to the action myoclonus seen in patients after toxic brain damage or
oxygen deprivation. Intracisternal injection of serotonin produced dramatic
remission of the myoclonic jerking for 5 to 7 minutes suggesting that a
deficiency of serotonergic activity in the brain might be responsible for *p,p'*-
DDT-induced myoclonus. Drugs which increase the action of serotonin in
the brain, i.e. the serotonin precursor, L-5HTP, the serotonin releaser
H75/12 (4-methyl-α-ethyl-*m*-tyramine), the serotonin agonists quipazine
and 5-methoxy-*N,N*-dimethyltryptamine (5MeDmt) and the serotonin
uptake blockers fluoxetine, Org 6582, chlorimipramine, all decreased *p,p'*-
DDT-induced myoclonic movements[33] (Table 1). Chlorimipramine potentiated the antimyoclonic action of L-5HTP. Drugs which block serotonin
receptor sites (methysergide, metergoline, cinnanserin) increased the intensity of *p,p'*-DDT-induced myoclonus. *p,p'*-DDT-induced myoclonus
decreased in intensity after treatment with clonazepam, another effective
antimyoclonic agent in patients. The antimyoclonic action of clonazepam
was blocked by methysergide. Sodium valproate (dipropylacetate) also
reduced *p,p'*-DDT-induced myoclonus when co-administered with chlorimipramine. Pharmacological agents which modify dopamine, GABA, and
acetylcholine metabolism in the brain had no significant effect on this animal
model of myoclonus. Although beta receptor blockers also had no effect on
p,p'-DDT-induced myoclonus an alpha noradrenergic receptor blocker,
phenoxybenzamine, significantly reduced *p,p'*-DDT-induced myoclonus.

Seven other alpha receptor blockers potentiated the antimyoclonic action of L-5HTP in this animal model[34]. In addition, reducing brain norepinephrine by pretreatment with the tyrosine hydroxylase inhibitor α-methyl-*p*-tyrosine (α-MPT) also potentiated the antimyoclonic activity of L-5HTP (Table 1).

Table 1 Effect of pharmacological agents on myoclonic activity in *p,p'*-DDT (600 mg/kg) treated mice. Each value is the mean of 4–9 determinations. (−) = decreased myoclonus; (+) = increased myoclonus. Alpha-methyl-*p*-tyrosine (200 mg/kg) was injected 2 h prior to the administration of *p,p'*-DDT.

	Dosage mg/kg	% Change from control
Serotonin precursor		
L-5HTP	200	− 32
L-5HTP	100	− 14
Serotonin releaser		
H75/12	25	− 57
Serotonin agonist		
Quipazine	10	− 34
Serotonin uptake blocker		
Chlorimipramine	25	− 34
Chlorimipramine	10	− 9
L-5HTP + Chlorimipramine	100 + 10	− 72
Serotonin receptor blocker		
Methysergide	5	+ 32
Anticonvulsants		
Clonazepam	2	− 50
Clonazepam + methysergide	2 + 5	− 4
Dipropylacetate	400	− 12
Dipropylacetate + chlorimipramine	400 + 10	− 68
Phenytoin	50	+ 34
Alpha-receptor blocker		
Phenoxybenzamine	5	− 74
Tyrosine hydroxylase inhibitor		
α-methyl-*p*-tyrosine + L-5HTP	200 + 100	− 32

The data obtained from this animal model suggests that a deficiency of serotonergic activity in the brain might be causally related to the myoclonic movements induced by *p,p'*-DDT. Furthermore, the antimyoclonic action of L-5HTP, clonazepam and sodium valproate may be due to the restoration of brain serotonergic activity toward normal. An alpha noradrenergic inhibitory synapse may be located in the neural circuit connecting a serotonergic neuron to the final motor response (*p,p'*-DDT-induced myoclonus). Since norepinephrine inhibits the firing of serotonergic raphe neurons[35], phenoxybenzamine could improve myoclonus by reducing the inhibitory effect of norepinephrine on serotonergic neurons.

THERAPY OF MYOCLONUS

When Muskens[36] published his classic work on epilepsy he insisted that myoclonus should be regarded as an epileptic phenomenon. Myoclonus is a common occurrence in idiopathic epilepsy and is frequently associated with other seizure disorders. Neurotoxic agents such as p,p'-DDT, mono-bromide of camphor and metrazol which produce only myoclonus at low doses will produce both myoclonus and seizures at higher doses. However, myoclonus may occur alone, without major or minor seizures or EEG abnormalities such as in hereditary essential myoclonus. The relationship of myoclonus to seizures is still not resolved. Nevertheless, anticonvulsant drugs are the most frequently used therapeutic agents for myoclonus. Ethosuximide and phenobarbital have been of limited value in treating myoclonic epilepsy. Only three classes of drugs have demonstrated consistent impressive antimyoclonic action; benzodiazepine derivatives, dipropyl-acetate (sodium valproate) and the investigational drug, L-5HTP, in combination with carbidopa. The remaining anticonvulsants have produced minimal or no significant improvement.

Benzodiazepine drugs

Benzodiazepine derivatives that have antimyoclonic activity include chlordiazepoxide hydroxide (Librium), flurazepam (Dalmane), diazepam (Valium), nitrazepam (Mogadon), and clonazepam (Clonopin). The most recently developed and most effective of these drugs is clonazepam. Clonazepam has a broad spectrum of activity against various types of epilepsy and its chief uses are in; petit mal absences, the Lennox–Gastaut syndrome, infantile spasms and myoclonic epilepsies.

Myoclonic seizures

Clonazepam has been reported to alleviate 'myoclonic epilepsy' in a number of reports which have not specifically identified the aetiology or specific type of myoclonus. In general, the therapeutic response has been quite favourable. Rett[37] reported a series of 44 patients with myoclonic epilepsy in which 25 had a 50% or greater reduction in myoclonic attacks with clonazepam, and 13 had complete control of myoclonic attacks. Hanson and Menkes[38] observed that clonazepam completely controlled myoclonic seizures in three out of nine patients and reduced the frequency of attacks by 50% or more in every case. Similar favourable results have been reported in six smaller series of patients[39–44]. More specifically, clonazepam has effectively controlled bilateral massive epileptic myoclonus (juvenile myoclonic epilepsy)[37,45–48] and myoclonic seizures associated with generalized epilepsy[49].

In patients with photosensitive myoclonic seizures, clonazepam can abolish the EEG and clinical paroxysmal activity produced by photic stimulation[40]. Clonazepam also has been found to be effective in treating Unverricht-Lundborg's progressive myoclonus epilepsy[50-52], Ramsay Hunt syndrome[40,53,54], postencephalitic myoclonus[55], and epilepsia partialis continua[56,57].

Clonazepam also appears to be effective in the Lennox-Gastaut syndrome (Myoclonic-astatic epilepsy), even in those patients resistant to other drugs. In a therapeutic trial of 37 patients with Lennox-Gastaut syndrome[58], clonazepam was effective in abolishing seizures in 35% and reducing their frequency by greater than 50% in 37% of the cases.

Post-anoxic intention myoclonus

Boudouresques et al.[59] reported that clonazepam was therapeutically effective in post-anoxic intention myoclonus. These results have been confirmed by others[14,15,60].

Infantile spasms

Fifty per cent or greater reduction in seizure frequency has been reported in 21–75% of patients with infantile spasms and hypsarrhythmia and complete control in 12–36% [56,58,61,62]. Hypsarrhythmic activity disappeared in some but not in others and the EEG did not always correlate with clinical improvement. However, some investigators have reported that clonazepam was ineffective in this disorder[38,42]. Nitrazepam (Mogodon), which is structurally similar but somewhat less potent than clonazepam, is also effective in the treatment of infantile spasms and some cases of myoclonic epilepsy[63-65].

Status myoclonus

Intravenous clonazepam is perhaps the most effective drug available for controlling status myoclonus[66-68]. As yet intravenous clonazepam is not available in the United States; intravenous diazepam is a less satisfactory substitute. The response to intravenous clonazepam is usually rapid, within a minute, and the effects of a single dose may last for over 24 hours.

Clinical pharmacology

The initial dose of clonazepam for infants and children should be 0.01 to 0.03 mg/kg per day given in two to three divided doses. Dosage should be increased by no more than 0.25–0.5 mg every third day until a daily maintenance dose of 0.1–0.2 mg/kg has been reached, unless myoclonus is controlled with tolerable side-effects at a lower dose. The initial dose for adults should not exceed 1.5 mg/day in divided doses which can be increased by

0.5–1.0 mg every third day up to a maximum of 20 mg daily. Single intravenous doses of 1–4 mg of clonazepam or 2.5–10 mg of diazepam are usually sufficient to control status myoclonus or status epilepticus.

The biological half life of clonazepam varies from 18.7 to 39.0 h (mean 26.4 h) and peak plasma concentrations generally occur 2–4 h after oral administration[69,70]. The correlation between serum concentrations of clonazepam and clinical response or side-effects has been poor; therapeutic serum concentrations varied from 5 to 50 ng/ml[41,70].

Tolerance may develop to the antimyoclonic and anticonvulsant actions of clonazepam after 1–6 months of administration. Kruse and Blankenhorn[71] found that the percentage of patients with a positive response to clonazepam fell from 63% in the first month to less than 30% after 12 months. Bergamini et al.[53] reported spectacular initial success followed within 6 months by deterioration in patients with Lennox–Gastaut and Ramsay Hunt syndrome treated with clonazepam. Temporary interruption and re-institution of treatment may overcome this tolerance in some patients.

The most common side-effects of clonazepam are drowsiness, ataxia, lethargy, behavioural changes, dizziness, hypotonia and hypersalivation. A tolerance to these side-effects may develop with chronic administration. Withdrawal of clonazepam must be gradual in order to avoid the risk of precipitating status epilepticus or status myoclonus.

Mechanism of action of clonazepam

Benzodiazepine drugs alter the CNS metabolism of several neurotransmitters including glycine, GABA (γ-aminobutyric acid) and serotonin. However, whether these or other undiscovered pharmacological actions are responsible for the antimyoclonic or anticonvulsant action of clonazepam is not known.

Glycine

Glycine is a putative inhibitory neurotransmitter in the spinal cord and brain stem[72]; glycinergic nerve terminals may account for approximately 25% of all synapses in these tissues[73]. The interaction of glycine with its receptor site is blocked by strychnine. Presumably the convulsive actions of strychnine are due to blockade of glycine receptors[74]. Glycine receptors can be labelled biochemically with [^{3}H]strychnine[75]. Young et al.[76] suggested that the benzodiazepine anticonvulsants may act by mimicking the action of glycine at receptor sites, since they found that benzodiazepine drugs displaced [^{3}H]strychnine binding to glycine receptors in rat brain in vitro. The order of potency for binding to glycine receptors of 21 benzodiazepines correlated with their order of potency in preventing pentylenetrazol seizures and electroshock seizures[76]. The relatively large concentrations of benzodiazepines necessary for interaction with the glycine receptor[77] and the failure of *in vivo* electrophysiological experiments to detect any glycineergic actions on the part of diazepam[78] or flurazepam[79] has made this proposed mechanism of action less attractive.

GABA

GABA is another inhibitory neurotransmitter in the CNS. Recently pharmacological[80-82] and neurophysiological[79,80,83] evidence has accumulated which suggests that benzodiazepine compounds enhance GABAergic neurotransmission and that the anticonvulsant action of benzodiazepines may be mediated through GABA. Levels of GABA are decreased in patients with myoclonus and seizure disorders[84]. Drugs which interfere with GABA synthesis produce epileptic seizures in animals and man. Benzodiazepine drugs antagonize the seizures elicited by picrotoxin and bicuculline, blockers of GABA receptors, and by isoniazid, thiosemicarbazide, and 3-mercaptopropionic acid, drugs which reduce the synthesis of GABA[77,82].

In at least one synapse, benzodiazepine drugs have been demonstrated to enhance GABAergic neurotransmission. Purkinje cells in the cerebellum are under the influence of basket cells whose transmitter is GABA. Intraperitoneal administration of chlordiazepoxide[80], diazepam[79] and bromazepam[79] and microiontophoretic administration of flurazepam[80] reduce the firing of the single Purkinje cells in a dose-dependent manner, presumably secondary to enhanced GABAergic influence from basket cells[85]. This interpretation is further supported by the observation that diazepam prolongs basket-cell induced inhibition of Purkinje cells[86]. Furthermore, increased activity of Purkinje cells is associated with increased cyclic GMP content[87]. Benzodiazepines decrease cyclic GMP in the cerebellum[77,88]. Cerebellar cyclic GMP has been reported to be elevated in several experimental seizure disorders[89] and after administration of p,p'-DDT[90]. At the present time it has not been determined whether the anticonvulsant or antimyoclonic actions of benzodiazepines are due to a restoration of cerebellar cyclic GMP to normal, but it remains an attractive hypothesis.

The cerebellum is generally regarded as being inhibitory to the motor cortex. Purkinje cells in the cerebellar cortex inhibit the neurons of the deep cerebellar nuclei which send inhibitory projections to the cerebral cortex. Therefore, inhibition of Purkinje cells should disinhibit (i.e. facilitate) the deep cerebellar nuclei which inhibit the motor cortex. This could be one mechanism by which benzodiazepine drugs counteract epileptic and myoclonic activity. Benzodiazepines also facilitate GABAergic presynaptic inhibition on nerve terminals of primary sensory efferent fibres in the dorsal gray matter of the spinal cord[91]. This presynaptic inhibition may modulate or reduce the amount of incoming sensory information which could conceivably reduce stimulus sensitive intention myoclonus.

The molecular mechanisms by which benzodiazepines enhance GABA-ergic inhibition is not clear. [^{3}H]diazepam has been demonstrated to bind specifically to saturable binding sites[92] which correlated with the localization of GABA receptors[93]. However, GABA does not interact with benzodiazepine receptors. Recently, it has been reported that an endogenous protein inhibitor reduces the affinity of GABA for its receptor sites[94]. Benzodiazepine compounds have been found to react with this protein inhibitor and thereby reduce the inhibition of GABA binding to its own receptor sites[95] which could explain benzodiazepine-induced enhancement of GABA transmission. Mitchell and Martin[96] have suggested an alternate mechanism by which benzodiazepines stimulate GABA transmission. They observed that diazepam and flurazepam in concentrations of 10^{-6} ml/l facilitated potassium-induced release of [^{3}H]GABA in rat cortical tissue *in vitro*.

Serotonin

Clonazepam, like previously reported serotonin agonists[33,34], reduces stimulus sensitive myoclonus induced in mice by p,p'-DDT; this action was blocked by the serotonin receptor blockers, methysergide, metergoline and cinnanserin[97]. This suggests that the antimyoclonic action of clonazepam could be due to enhancement of serotonergic transmission in the CNS. Drugs which stimulate the central serotonergic system also produced head twitching and a pinna response in mice[98]. Chadwick et al.[99] and Nakamura and Fukushima[100] have reported that clonazepam produces head twitching and a pinna response in mice which they attribute to stimulation of serotonin neuronal pathways. Fludiazepam and diazepam have been reported to potentiate head twitches in mice induced by intracerebrally injected serotonin and intraperitoneally injected 5-methoxytryptamine, potent serotonin receptor agonists; cyproheptadine, a serotonin receptor blocker, counteracted this potentiating action of benzodiazepines[101,102]. The mechanism by which benzodiazepine drugs potentiate serotonergic systems in these behavioural models is not known. Clonazepam has no effect on whole mouse brain serotonin or 5HIAA levels or serotonin synthesis rate[97]. Clonazepam (10^{-5} mol/l) did inhibit the uptake of [^{3}H]serotonin into brain synaptosomes and enhanced the release of previously accumulated [^{3}H]serotonin[97]. These actions would enhance serotonergic function in the CNS by increasing serotonin concentrations in the synaptic-cleft, however, it is questionable whether the concentration of 10^{-5} mol/l clonazepam would be found *in vivo* in nerve terminals of clonazepam-treated animals. Although clonazepam did not alter [^{3}H]serotonin receptor binding, it is possible that clonazepam might activate serotonin receptor coupled reactions without having a direct affinity for the serotonin receptor.

Dipropylacetate (Depakene, sodium valproate)

Dipropylacetate also has a broad spectrum of anticonvulsant activity; it has been effective in the treatment of grand mal, petit mal, temporal lobe epilepsy, and myoclonic epilepsy. Most of the clinical studies have failed to differentiate between the various types of myoclonus in their patient trials. In a summary of eight separate studies comprising a total of 101 patients with various types of myoclonic epilepsy, dipropylacetate reduced seizure frequency by over 75% in 73 patients[103]. Dipropylacetate has been particularly effective in the long-term therapy of progressive myoclonus epilepsy[104]. Recently, Fahn[105] reported that two patients with postanoxic intention myoclonus derived substantial benefit from dipropylacetate therapy. Infantile spasms and the Lennox–Gastaut syndrome respond somewhat better to the benzodiazepines than dipropylacetate.

Clinical pharmacology

The initial dose of dipropylacetate is 15 mg/kg per day in divided doses with increases by 5–10 mg/kg per day at one week intervals until myoclonus and seizures are controlled or side-effects preclude further increases. The maximum recommended dosage is 60 mg/kg per day. The peak plasma level generally occurs 1–4 h after oral administration of dipropylacetate and the plasma half life is 8–12 h[106,107]. The therapeutic blood levels are 50–100 µg/ml in most patients, associated with a daily dose of 1200–1500 mg.

Dipropylacetate produces relatively few side-effects. Nausea, vomiting, diarrhoea and abdominal pain are the most common adverse effects but they are usually very transient. Gastrointestinal side-effects can be decreased by administering dipropylacetate with meals or slowly increasing the dose from an initial low level. Temporary loss of hair and prolonged bleeding time caused by inhibition of platelet aggregation also have been reported.

Mechanism of action of dipropylacetate

GABA. Animal studies indicate that dipropylacetate can increase brain levels of GABA by inhibiting GABA transaminase[108] and perhaps also by inhibiting GABA uptake into the presynaptic nerve terminal[109]. It has been proposed that the effect of dipropylacetate on brain GABA is related to its anticonvulsant activity. However, the changes in GABA metabolism produced by dipropylacetate in animals only occur at levels of the drug much higher than those likely to be achieved in patients. Therefore the mechanism of action of dipropylacetate in patients with myoclonus and seizures is still undetermined.

Serotonin. The effect of dipropylacetate on serotonin has been examined. Dipropylacetate alone does not have significant antimyoclonic activity in the *p,p'*-DDT animal model. However, when dipropylacetate is combined with a subthreshold dose of chlorimipramine, the intensity of myoclonus is reduced by 68% in *p,p'*-DDT-treated mice (Table 1). Dipropylacetate was found to decrease total serum tryptophan and increase brain tryptophan and 5HIAA[110]. Recently dipropylacetate has been reported to increase 5HIAA in the CSF of a patient with post-anoxic intention myoclonus[105]. Perhaps the increase in CSF 5HIAA and the antimyoclonic action of dipropylacetate in patients might be due to enhancement of brain serotonin synthesis.

Serotonin precursors

L-Tryptophan and L-5HTP are precursors of serotonin (Figure 1). L-Tryptophan is converted to L-5HTP by the enzyme tryptophan hydroxylase. This enzyme is not saturated by normal levels of brain tryptophan, therefore the rate of serotonin synthesis is influenced by changes in brain tryptophan concentrations[111]. L-Tryptophan administration in animals can elevate brain serotonin to about 20–50% above normal[112,113]. This increase in brain serotonin synthesis is localized exclusively to serotonergic neurons. L-Tryptophan has been used in combination with a monoamine oxidase inhibitor, which blocks the degradation of newly synthesized serotonin, to treat intention myoclonus. Much larger increases in brain serotonin levels can be obtained by the administration of L-5HTP since the enzyme (L-aromatic amino acid decarboxylase) which decarboxylates L–5HTP (Figure 1) is present in high activity throughout the brain.

L-5HTP is administered in combination with carbidopa, a peripheral decarboxylase inhibitor, which prevents the conversion of L-5HTP to serotonin outside the brain, thereby decreasing peripheral side-effects and increasing the fraction of L-5HTP reaching the brain and being converted to serotonin. Both L-5HTP in combination with carbidopa[11,13–24] and L-tryptophan in combination with a monoamine oxidase inhibitor[11,13,15,18,22] have been shown to have a dramatic therapeutic effect in various types of intention myoclonus. L-5HTP and carbidopa have produced the most consistent results and the majority of clinical trials have been performed with this drug combination. All of the clinicial trials of L-5HTP and carbidopa have shown that patients with the postanoxic form of intention myoclonus have the greatest degree of symptomatic improvement. Patients with intention myoclonus associated with head trauma, methyl bromide toxicity, probable encephalitis, progressive myoclonus epilepsy, familial cerebellar degeneration, essential myoclonus and palatal myoclonus also have improved during L-5HTP and carbidopa therapy. In our series of 26 patients with intention myoclonus, 65% derived more than 50% overall improvement during treatment with L-5HTP in combination with carbidopa[16]. Four patients with progressive myoclonus epilepsy derived 25–49% improvement and two cases greater than 75% overall improvement in their myoclonic symptoms[16]. Single case reports of patients with myoclonus associated with infantile spasms[14], olivoponto-cerebellar degeneration[24], Ramsay Hunt syndrome[12], congenital encephalopathy[23], nonprogressive childhood myoclonus[23], and lipid storage disease[23] have shown no therapeutic response in these disorders. Although L-5HTP and carbidopa reduced major motor seizure frequency in patients whose seizures were preceded by progressively increasing myoclonus, the drug combination had no anticonvulsant action in other types of seizure disorders[14].

The therapeutic effect of L–5HTP and carbidopa in postanoxic intention myoclonus has been blocked by methysergide (12 mg/day) suggesting that the mechanism of action of this drug combination was enhancement of serotonergic function[18].

Clinical pharmacology

The starting dose of L-5HTP is 25 mg four times a day which is increased by 25 mg four times a day every 2–3 days depending upon the severity of side-effects. The optimal daily dose of L-5HTP may range from 400 to 2800 mg in four to six divided doses. The optimal dose of carbidopa can range from 25 to 75 mg four times a day depending upon gastrointestinal side-effects. Magnussen and Engbaek[114] investigated the accumulation and elimination of L-5HTP in plasma in the presence or absence of carbidopa. They observed that the presence of carbidopa increases the plasma concentration of L-5HTP by about ten-fold. The plasma half-life of L-5HTP was 2.3–3.0 h following oral administration of a single dose of L-5HTP with or without pretreatment with a single dose of carbidopa. The half-life of L-5HTP in plasma increased to 5.5 h during long-term therapy with carbidopa. Despite the co-administration of carbidopa (200 mg/day) which should inhibit the conversion of L-5HTP to serotonin outside the brain, serum levels of serotonin and urinary 5HIAA increase directly proportional to the dose of L-5HTP[14]. The inhibition of peripheral decarboxylation of L-5HTP by carbidopa is not complete. L-5HTP and carbidopa therapy also increases CSF 5HIAA and decreases CSF homovanillic acid (HVA) levels, suggesting that dopamine synthesis may be reduced by this therapy[14].

The most common side-effects of L-HTP with carbidopa are anorexia, nausea and diarrhoea which can be counteracted by prochlorperazine (Compazine), trimethobenzamide (Tigan), antacids and diphenoxylate hydrochloride (Lomotil). These side-effects usually disappear or diminish after several months of therapy and prochlorperazine, trimethobenzamide, antacids and diphenoxylate can be discontinued. Other side-effects include mydriasis, vomiting, lightheadedness, euphoria, hypomanic behaviour, and dyspnea. The only change in routine laboratory tests after chronic administration is an approximately 20% decrease in plasma cholesterol[14].

Table 2 Suggested therapeutic approach to myoclonus

Type of myoclonus	First choice	Second choice	Third choice
Post-anoxic intention myoclonus	L-5HTP	Clonazepam	Dipropylacetate
Myoclonic epilepsy	Dipropylacetate Clonazepam	L-5HTP	
Progressive myoclonus epilepsy	Dipropylacetate	Clonazepam	L-5HTP
Palatal myoclonus	L-5HTP		
Essential myoclonus	Clonazepam Dipropylacetate L-5HTP	Lioresal (?)	
Infantile spasms	ACTH Prednisone	Clonazepam	Dipropylacetate
Respiratory myoclonus	Phenytoin (?)		

APPROACH TO THERAPY

Table 2 lists some diseases associated with myoclonus and the relative effectiveness of various therapeutic agents. The rating of choices is based on therapeutic effectiveness and side-effects according to both the authors' experience and reports in the literature. For example, the benefit/side-effect ratio of L-5HTP and carbidopa may be low initially because of gastrointestinal symptoms, however with time higher therapeutic doses can be tolerated with minimal or no side-effects. In comparison, clonazepam is usually better tolerated initially but at therapeutic levels sedation and ataxia may decrease the benefit/side-effect ratio. The combination of L–5HTP with clonazepam or dipropylacetate may produce the optimal therapeutic benefit with minimal side-effects in some cases. Preliminary experience with the combination of L-5HTP with carbidopa and valproate suggests some potentiation of therapeutic effect in patients as has been observed in the p,p'-DDT animal model of myoclonus. Dipropylacetate should not be given with clonazepam since the use of these two drugs together has resulted in absence status.

ACTH (adrenocorticotropic hormone) and prednisone have been used to treat infantile myoclonic spasms[115,116] and polymyoclonia and opsoclonus associated with neuroblastoma and myoclonic encephalopathy of infants[117,118]. The mechanisms responsible for the therapeutic effects of adrenocorticosteroids in these conditions are not known, but it has been suggested that they may counteract the adverse effects of auto-immune phenomena or viral infections in some cases. Jeavons and Bower[116] recommended a dose of 20–30 U ACTH gel daily divided into two doses or prednisone 2 mg/kg per day orally every 6 h for patients with infantile spasms. Both the myoclonus and EEG abnormalities may be decreased by the use of ACTH or adrenal cortical steroids in infantile spasms, however, the mental retardation persists. Dumermuth and Kovacs[58] reported complete control of infantile spasms with corticotropin or hydrocortisone in nine of 31 patients whose myoclonic spasms were not controlled by clonazepam.

4B-phenyl-γ-aminobutyric acid (Lioresal, Baclofen), 65 to 80 mg/day has been reported to reduce myoclonus in patients with hereditary essential myoclonus[119].

Respiratory myoclonus has been treated by phrenicectomy when the diaphragmatic contractions become very uncomfortable. A recent encouraging report indicates that phenytoin may be an effective pharmacologic mode of therapy for some patients with this disorder[120].

CONCLUSION

One might argue whether or not the present data indicates that certain types of intention myoclonus are brain serotonin deficiency disorders. For example, anoxic brain damage may cause preferential degeneration of serotonergic neurons thereby reducing brain serotonin synthesis. The decrease in CSF 5HIAA and the dramatic response to the serotonin precursor L-5HTP when combined with carbidopa in these patients are strong arguments for this hypothesis. The aggravation of post-anoxic intention myoclonus by large doses of levodopa which depress brain serotonin synthesis, adds further support for this hypothesis. Several possible mechanisms by which L-5HTP might be having an antimyoclonic action have been suggested in this chapter. CNS serotonin may act as an inhibitory modulator of sensory input preventing excessive and erratic motor responses. Serotonergic neurons have been shown to suppress hypersensitivity to auditory, visual and nociceptive stimuli. The pharmacologic studies in the p,p'-DDT animal model of stimulus sensitive myoclonus confirms the antimyoclonic action of brain serotonin and indicates that blockade of α-noradrenergic receptors may enhance this effect. The localization in the brain of the abnormal neuronal circuits which produce myoclonus is not known, but efferent cerebellar pathways have been implicated in pathological and experimental investigations.

The three drugs which are most effective in the therapy of myoclonus, clonazepam, dipropylacetate and L-5HTP have all been shown to enhance brain serotonergic activity. Although an attractive hypothesis, it would be premature to conclude that this is the basis for the antimyoclonic action of these drugs. Certainly, further studies on the mechanism of action of anti-myoclonic drugs should enhance our understanding of the pathophysiology of myoclonus.

Acknowledgement

This work was supported by USPHS grants NS 12341 and NS 05802, the Clinical Center for Research on Parkinson's and Allied Diseases NS-71631 and RR 00071 from the Division of Research Resources, General Clinical Research Center Branch.

References

1 Gastaut, H. and Remond, A. (1952). Etude électroencephalo-graphique des myoclonies. *Rev. Neurol.*, **86**, 596

2 Gastaut, H. and Hunter, I. (1950). An experimental study of the mechanism of photic activation in idiopathic epilepsy. *Electroencephalogr. Clin. Neurophysiol.*, **2**, 263

3 Halliday, A. M. (1975). The neurophysiology of myoclonic jerking—a reappraisal. In Charlton, M. H. (eds.) *Myoclonic Seizures*, pp. 1–29. (Amsterdam: Excerpta Medica)

4 Denny-Brown, D. (1968). Quelques aspects physiologiques des myoclonies. In Bonduelle, M. and Gastaut, H. (eds.) *Les Myoclonies*, pp. 121–129. (Paris: Mason et Cie)

5 Milhorat, T. H. (1967). Experimental myoclonus of thalamic origin. *Arch. Neurol.*, **17**, 365

6 Farrell, D. F. and Swanson, P. D. (1975). Infectious diseases associated with myoclonus. In Charlton, M. H. (ed.) *Myoclonic Seizures*, pp. 77–110. (Amsterdam: Excerpta Medica)

7 Koskiniemi, M., Donner, M., Majuri, H. and Norio, R. (1974). Progressive myoclonus epilepsy. *Acta Neurol. Scand.*, **50**, 307

8 Greenfield, J. G. (1965). *The Spinocerebellar Degenerations*, p. 79. (Oxford: Blackwell Scientific Publications)

9 Castaigne, P., Cambier, J., Escourolle, R., Cathala, H. P. and Lecasble, R. (1964). Observation anatomo-clinique d'un syndrome myoclonique post-anoxique. *Rev. Neurol.*, **111**, 60

10 Lhermitte, F., Marteau, R. and Degos, C. F. (1972). Analyse pharmacologique d'un nouveau cas de myoclonies d'intention et d'action post-anoxiques. *Rev. Neurol. (Paris)*, **128**, 107

11 Van Woert, M. H. and Sethy, V. H. (1975). Therapy of intention myoclonus with L-5-hydroxytryptophan and a peripheral decarboxylase inhibitor, MK 486. *Neurology*, **25**, 135

12 Guilleminault, C., Tharp, B. R. and Cousin, D. (1973). HVA and 5HIAA measurements and 5HTP trials in some patients with involuntary movements. *J. Neurol. Sci.*, **18**, 435

13 Chadwick, D., Harris, R., Jenner, P. and Marsden, C. D. (1975). Manipulation of brain serotonin in the treatment of myoclonus. *Lancet*, **2**, 434

14 Van Woert, M. H., Rosenbaum, D., Howieson, J. and Bowers, M. B. Jr. (1977). Long-term therapy of myoclonus and other neurological disorders with L-5-hydroxytryptophan and carbidopa. *N. Engl. J. Med.*, **296**, 70

15 Chadwick, D., Hallett, M., Harris, R., Jenner, P., Reynolds, E. H. and Marsden, C. D.

(1977). Clinical, biochemical and physiological features distinguishing myoclonus responsive to 5-hydroxytryptophan and a monoamine oxidase inhibitor and clonazepam. *Brain*, **100**, 455

16 Van Woert, M. H. and Rosenbaum, D. (1980). L-5-hydroxytryptophan therapy in myoclonus. In Fahn, S. (ed.) *Cerebral Hypoxia and its Consequences*, pp. 107–122. (New York: Raven Press)

17 Lhermitte, F., Degos, C. F. and Marteau, R. (1975). Association d'un inhibiteur de la dopadécarboxylase aux traitments par le 5-hydroxytryptophane. *Nouv. Press Med. (Paris)*, **4**, 31

18 Magnussen, I., Dupont, E., Engbaek, F. and Olivarius, B. de Fine. (1978). Post-hypoxic intention myoclonus treated with 5-hydroxytryptophan and an extracerebral decarboxylase inhibitor. *Acta Neurol. Scand.*, **57**, 289

19 Magnussen, I., Dupont, E., Prange-Hansen, Aa. and Olivarius, B. de Fine (1977). Palatal myoclonus treated with 5-hydroxytryptophan and a decarboxylase inhibitor. *Acta Neurol. Scand.*, **55**, 251

20 Thal, L., Sharpless, N., Wolfson, L., Engel, J. and Katzman, R. (1976). Clinical and metabolic observations on the treatment of myoclonus with L-5HTP and carbidopa. *Trans. Am. Neurol. Assoc.*, **101**, 48

21 Williams, A., Goodenberger, D. and Calne, D. (1978). Palatal myoclonus following herpes zoster ameliorated by 5-hydroxytryptophan and carbidopa. *Neurology*, **28**, 358

22 DeLean, J., Richardson, J. C. and Hornykiewicz, O. (1976). Beneficial effects of serotonin precursors in postanoxic action myoclonus. *Neurology*, **26**, 863

23 Growdon, J. H., Young, R. R. and Shahani, B. T. (1976). L-5-Hydroxytryptophan in treatment of several different syndromes in which myoclonus is prominent. *Neurology*, **26**, 1135

24 van Woert, M. H. and Chung Hwang, E. (1978). Biochemistry and pharmacology of myoclonus. In Klawans, H. L. (ed.) *Clin. Neuropharmacol*, Vol. 3, pp. 167–184. (New York: Raven Press)

25 Meldrum, B. S., Balzamo, E., Wada, J. A. and Vuillon-Cacciuttolo, G. (1972). Effects of L-tryptophan, L-3,4-dihydroxyphenylalanine and tranylcypromine on the electro-encephalogram and on photically induced epilepsy in the baboon, Papio papio. *Physiol. Behav.*, **9**, 615

26 Wada, J. A., Balzamo, E., Meldrum, B. S. and Naquet, R. (1972). Behavioral and electro-encephalographic effects of L-5-hydroxytryptophan and D, L-para-chlorophenylalanine on the epileptic Sengalese baboon (Papio papio). *Electroencephalogr. Clin. Neurophysiol.*, **33**, 520

27 Prockop, D. J., Shore, P. A. and Brodie, B. B. (1959). Anticonvulsant properties of monoamine oxidase inhibitors. *Ann. N.Y. Acad. Sci.*, **80**, 643

28 Chen, G., Ensor, C. R. and Bohner, B. (1968). Studies on drug effects on electrically induced extensor seizures and clinical implications. *Arch. Int. Pharmacodyn. Ther.*, **172**, 182

29 Gray, W. D., Rauk, C. E. and Shanahan, W. S. (1963). The mechanism of the antagonistic action of reserpine on the anticonvulsant effect of inhibitors of carbonic anhydrase. *J. Pharmacol. Exp. Ther.*, **139**, 350

30 Mennear, J. H. and Rudzik, A. D. (1966). Mechanism of action of anticonvulsant drugs. 3. Chlordiazepoxide. *J. Pharmacol. Sci.*, **55**, 640

31 de la Torre, J. C., Kawanga, H. M. and Mullan, S. (1970). Seizure susceptibility after manipulation of brain serotonin. *Arch. Int. Pharmacodyn. Ther.*, **188**, 298

32 Gastaut, H. (1950). Combined photic and metrazol activation of the brain. *Electroencephalogr. Clin. Neurophysiol.*, **2**, 249

33 Chung Hwang, E. and van Woert, M. H. (1978). p,p′-DDT-induced neurotoxic syndrome: experimental myoclonus. *Neurology*, **28**, 1020

34 Chung Hwang, E. and van Woert, M. H. (1980). p,p'-DDT-induced myoclonus: serotonin and alpha noradrenergic interaction. *Res. Comm. Chem. Pathol. Pharmacol.*, **23**, 257

35 Couch, J. R. (1970). Response of neurons in the raphe nuclei to serotonin, norepinephrine and acetylcholine and their correlation with an excitatory synaptic input. *Brain Res.*, **19**, 137

36 Muskens, L. J. J. (1928). *Epilepsy, Comparative Pathogenesis, Symptoms, Treatment.* (London: Baillère, Tindall and Cox)

37 Rett, A. (1973). Zwei Jahre erfarungen mit clonazepam bei zerabralen krampfanfallen im Kindesalter. *Acta Neurol. Scand.*, **49** (Suppl. 53), 109

38 Hanson, R. A. and Menkes, J. H. (1972). A new anticonvulsant in the management of minor motor seizures. *Devel. Med. Child. Neurol.*, **14**, 3

39 Turner, M., Fejerman, N., Schugurensky, E., Cordero Funes, B., Cantlon, R., Aspinwall, R. and Lon, J. C. (1970). Evaluation clinicoelectroencefalografica de al accion antiepileptica de una nueva derivados benzodiazepinicos. *Acta. Neurol. Latin Am.*, **16**, 97

40 Lison, M. P. and Fassoni, F. L. (1970). Estudio Clinicoelectrencefalografico longitude em pacientes epilepticos tratados com RO5-4023. *Arq. Neuropsyquiatr.*, **28**, 25

41 Huang, C. Y., McLeod, J. O., Sampson, D. and Hensley, W. J. (1973). Clonazepam in the treatment of epilepsy. *Proc. Aust. Assoc. Neurol.*, **10**, 67

42 Barnett, A. M. (1973). Treatment of epilepsy with clonazepam. *S. Afr. Med. J.*, **47**, 1683

43 Boudin, G., Guillard, A., Pepin, B. and Fabiani, J. M. (1972). Notre expérience d'un nouvel anti-épileptique: le clonazepam (RO5-4023). A propos de 71 observations. *Ann. Med. Intern.*, **123**, 617

44 Edwards, V. E. and Eadie, M. J. (1973). Clonazepam: a clinical study of its effectiveness as an anticonvulsant. *Proc. Aust. Assoc. Neurol.*, **10**, 61

45 Mikkelsen, R., Birket-Smith, E., Brandt, S., Holm, P., Lund, M. Thorm, I., Vestermark, S. and Zander Olsen, P. (1976). Clonazepam in the treatment of epilepsy. A controlled clinical trial in simple absences, bilateral massive epileptic myoclonus, and atonic seizures. *Arch. Neurol.*, **33**, 322

46 Rett, A. (1971). Moglichkeiteb und Grenzen der Clonazepam – Therapie in Kindesalter. *Wein. Klin. Wochenschr.*, **83**, 725

47 Munthe-Kass, A. W. and Strandjord, R. E. (1973). Clonzepam in the treatment of epileptic seizures. *Acta Neurol. Scand.*, **49** (Suppl. 53), 97

48 Lund, M. and Trolle, E. (1973). Clonazepam in the treatment of epilepsy. *Acta Neurol. Scand.*, **49** (Suppl. 53), 82

49 Edwards, V. E. and Eadie, M. J. (1973). Clonazepam—a clinical study of its effectiveness as an anticonvulsant. *Proc. Austr. Assoc. Neurol.*, **10**, 61

50 Fazio, C., Manfredini, M. and Piccinelli, A. (1975). Treatment of epileptic seizures with clonazepam. *Arch. Neurol.*, **32**, 304

51 Laitinen, L. and Toivakka, L. (1973). Clonazepam (RO5-4023) in the treatment of myoclonus epilepsy. *Acta Neurol. Scand.*, **49** (Suppl. 53), 72

52 Lope, E. S., Junguera, S. R. C. and Berenquel, A. B. (1974). Progressive myoclonic epilepsy with Lafora's bodies—a clinicopathological study. *Acta Neurol. Scand.*, **50**, 537

53 Bergamini, L., Mutani, L., Fariello, R. and Liboni, W. (1970). Elektroencephalographische und klinische Bewertung des neuen Benzodiazepin RO5-4023. *Z. EEG-EMG*, **1**, 182

54 Mutani, R., Fariello, R., Liboni, W. and Quattrocolo, G. (1971). Utilizzazione terrapeutics della nueva benzodiazepina RO5-4023 nella sindrome di Ramsay Hunt. *Riev. Neurol.*, **41**, 283

55 Guldenpfennig, W. M. (1973). Clinical experience with a new benzodiazepine in the treatment of epilepsy. *S. Afr. Med. J.*, **47**, 998

56 Rebollo, M. A. (1971). El RO5-4023 en el tratamiento de la epilepsia en el nino. *Arch. Pediatr. Urug.*, **42**, 147

57 Rett, A. (1973). Zwei jahre Erfahrungen mit Clonazepam bei zerabialen Krampfanfallen im Kindesalter. *Acta Neurol. Scand.*, **49** (Suppl. 53), 109

58 Dumermuth, G. and Kovacs, E. (1974). Wirkung von Clonazepam der peroralen Langzeittherapie schwerer Epleprieformen des Kindenalters. *Schweiz Med. Wochenschr.*, **104**, 608

59 Boudouresques, J., Roger, J., Khaili, R., Vigouroux, A., Grosset, A. Pellissier, J. F. and Tassinari, C. A. (1971). A propos de deux observations de syndrôme de Lance et Adams. Effect thérapeutique du RO5-4023. *Rev. Neurol.*, **125**, 306

60 Goldberg, M. A. and Dorman, J. E. (1976). Intention myoclonus: successful treatment with clonazepam. *Neurology*, **26**, 24

61 Martin, A. and Hirt, H. R. (1973). Clinical experience with clonazepam (Rivotril) in the treatment of epilepsies in infancy and childhood. *Neuropaediatrie*, **4**, 245

62 Dreifuss, F. E., Penry, J. K., Rose, S. K., Kupferberg, H. J., Dyken, P. and Sate, S. (1975). Serum clonazepam concentrations in children with absence seizures. *Neurology*, **25**, 255

63 Killian, J. M. and Fromm, G. H. (1971). A double-blind comparison of nitrazepam versus diazepam in myoclonic seizure disorders. *Devel. Med. Child Neurol.*, **13**, 32

64 Millichap, J. G. and Ortiz, W. R. (1966). Nitrazepam in myoclonic epilepsies. *Am. J. Dis. Child.*, **112**, 242

65 Volzke, E., Doose, H. and Stephan, E. (1967). The treatment of infantile spasms and hysparrhythmia with Mogadon. *Epilepsia*, **8**, 64

66 Gastaut, H., Courjon, J., Poire, R. and Weber, M. (1971). Treatment of status epilepticus with a new benzodiazepine more active than diazepam. *Epilepsia*, **12**, 197

67 Gimenez Roldan, S., Peraita, P., Lopez Agerada, J. M. *et al.* (1972). Un nuevo medicamento eficaz en el tratamiento del 'status' epileptico (RO5-4023). *Med. Clin.*, **58**, 133

68 Papini, M. (1971). The treatment of epilepsy in childhood and of status epilepticus with RO5-4023. *Electroencephalogr. Clin. Neurophysiol.*, **31**, 532

69 Kaplan, S. A., Alexander, K., Jack, M. L., Puglisi, C. V., de Silva, J. A. F., Lee, T. L. and Weinfeld, R. E. (1974). Pharmacokinetic profiles of clonazepam in dog and humans and of flunitrazepam in dog. *J. Pharmacol. Sci.*, **63**, 527

70 Naestoft, J. and Larsen, N. E. (1974). Quantative determination of clonazepam and its metabolites in human plasma by gas chromatography. *J. Chromatogr.*, **93**, 113

71 Kruse, R. and Blankenhorn, V. (1973). Zuzammenfassender Erfahrunze-beright uber die klinische Anwendung und Wirksamkeit von RO5-4023 (Clonazepam) auf verachiedene Fromer epileptischer Anfalle. *Acta Neurol. Scand.*, **49** (Suppl. 53), 60

72 Aprison, M. H., Davidoff, R. A. and Werman, R. (1970). Glycine: Its metabolic and possible transmitter roles in nervous tissue. In Lajtha, A. (ed.) *Handbook of Neurochemistry*. Vol. 3. (New York: Plenum Press)

73 Iversen, L. L. and Bloom, F. E. (1972). Studies of the uptake of (^{3}H)-GABA and (^{3}H) glycine in slices and homogenates of rat brain and spinal cord by electron microscopic autoradiography. *Brain Res.*, **41**, 131

74 Curtis, D. R., Duggan, A. W. and Johnston, G. A. R. (1971). The specificity of strychnine as a glycine antagonist in the mammalian spinal cord. *Exp. Brain Res.*, **12**, 547

75 Young, A. B. and Snyder, S. H. (1973). Strychnine binding associated with glycine receptors of the central nervous system. *Proc. Natl. Acad. Sci. USA*, **70**, 2832

76 Young, A. B., Zurkin, S. R. and Snyder, S. H. (1974). Interaction of benzodiazepines with central nervous glycine receptors: possible mechanism of action. *Proc. Natl. Acad. Sci. USA*, **71**, 2246

77 Costa, E., Guidotti, A., Mao, C. C. and Suria, A. (1975). New concepts on the mechanism of action of benzodiazepines. *Life Sci.*, **17**, 167

78 Curtis, D. R., Game, C. J. A. and Lodge, D. (1976). Benzodiazepines and central glycine receptors. *Br. J. Pharmacol.*, **56**, 307

79 Dray, A. and Straughan, D. W. (1976). Benzodiazepines: GABA and glycine receptors on single neurons in the rat medulla. *J. Pharm. Phamacol.*, **28**, 314

80 Lippa, A. S., Greenblatt, E. N. and Pelham, R. W. (1977). The use of animal models for delineating the mechanisms of action of anxiolytic agents. In Hanin, I. and Usdin, E. (eds.) *Animal Models in Psychiatry and Neurology*, pp. 279–292. (New York: Raven Press)

81 Costa, E., Guidotti, A. and Mao, C. C. (1975). Evidence for involvement of GABA in the action of benzodiazepines: studies on rat cerebellum. In Costa, E. and Greengard, P. (eds.) *Advances in Biochemical Pharmacology*. Vol. 14, pp. 113–130. (New York: Raven Press)

82 Haefely, W., Kulcsar, W. A., Mohler, H., Pieri, L., Polc, P. and Schaffner, R. (1975). Possible involvement of GABA in the central action of benzodiazepines. In Costa, E. and Greengard, P. (eds.) *Adventures in Biochemical Pharmacology*. Vol. 14, pp. 131–151. (New York: Raven Press)

83 Polc, P., Mohler, H. and Haefely, W. (1974). The effect of diazepam on spinal cord activities: possible sites and mechanisms of action. *Naunyn-Schmiedeberg's Arch. Pharmacol.*, **284**, 319

84 Enna, S. J., Ferkany, J. W., van Woert, M. H. and Butler, I. J. (1979). Measurement of GABA transaminase inhibitors. In Chase, T., Wexler, N. and Barbeau, A. (eds.). *Huntington's Disease, Advances in Neurology*. Vol. 23, pp. 741–750. (New York: Raven Press)

85 Pieri, L. and Haefely, W. (1976). The effect of diphenylhydantoin, diazepam and clonazepam on the activity of Purkinje cells in the rat cerebellum. *Naunyn-Schmiedeberg's Arch. Pharmacol.*, **29**, 61

86 Curtis, D. R., Lodge, D., Johnston, G. A. R. and Brand, S. J. (1976). Central actions of benzodiazepines. *Brain Res.*, **118**, 344

87 Mao, C. C., Guidotti, A. and Costa, E. (1974). Interaction between gamma-aminobutyric acid and guanosine cyclic 3', 5'-monophosphate in rat cerebellum. *Mol. Pharmacol.*, **10**, 736

88 Mao, C. C., Guidotti, A. and Costa, E. (1975). Evidence for an involvement of GABA in the mediation of the cerebellar cGMP decrease and the anticonvulsant action of diazepam. *Naunyn Schmiedeberg's Arch. Pharmacol.*, **289**, 369

89 Ferrendelli, J. A., Steiner, A. L., McDougal, D. B. and Kipnis, D. M. (1970). The effect of oxotremorine and atropine on cGMP and cAMP levels in mouse cerebal cortex and cerebellum. *Biochem. Biophys. Res. Commun.*, **41**, 1061

90 Aldridge, W. N., Clothier, B., Forshaw, P., Johnson, M. K., Parker, V. H., Price, R. J., Shilleter, D. N., Verschoyle, R. D. and Stevens, C. (1978). The effect of DDT and the pyrethroids cismethrin and decamethrin on the acetylcholine and cyclic nucleotide content of rat brain. *Biochem. Pharmacol.*, **27**, 1703

91 Schmidt, R. F. (1971). Presynaptic inhibition in the vertebrate central nervous system. *Ergeb. Physiol. Exp. Pharmacol.*, **63**, 20

92 Braestrup, C. and Squires, R. F. (1977). Specific benzodiazepine receptors in rat brain characterized by high affinity [³H]diazepam binding. *Proc. Natl. Acad. Sci. USA*, **74**, 3805

93 Mackerer, C. R., Kochmna, R. L., Bierschenk, B. A. and Bremner, S. S. (1978). The binding of [³H]diazepam to rat brain homogenates. *J. Pharmacol. Exp. Ther.*, **206**, 405

94 Toffano, G., Guidotti, A. and Costa, E. (1978). Purification of endogenous protein inhibitor of high affinity binding of gamma-amino-butyric acid to synaptic membranes of rat brain. *Proc. Natl. Acad. Sci. USA*, **75**, 4024

95 Guidotti, A., Toffano, G. and Costa, E. (1978). An endogenous protein modulates the affinity of GABA and benzodiazepine receptors in rat brain. *Nature (London)*, **275**, 553

96 Mitchell, P. R. and Martin, I. L. (1978). The effects of benzodiazepines on K^+-stimulated release of GABA. *Neuropharmacol.*, **17**, 317

97 Chung Hwang, E. and van Woert, M. H. (1980). Antimyoclonic action of clonazepam: the role of serotonin. *Eur. J. Pharmacol.*, **60**, 31

98 Corne, J. J., Pickering, R. W. and Warner, B. T. (1963). A method for assessing the effects of drugs on the central actions of 5-hydroxytryptamine, *Br. J. Pharmacol. Chemother.*, **20**, 106

99 Chadwick, D., Gorrod, J. W., Jenner, P., Marsden, C. D. and Reynolds, E. H. (1978). Functional changes in cerebral 5-hydroxytryptamine metabolism in the mouse induced by anticonvulsant drugs. *Br. J. Pharmacol.*, **62**, 115

100 Nakamura, M. and Fukushima, H. (1976). Head twitches induced by benzodiazepines and the role of biogenic amines. *Psychopharmacology*, **49**, 259

101 Nakamura, M. and Fukushima, H. (1977). Effect of benzodiazepines on central serotonergic neuron systems. *Psychopharmacology*, **53**, 121

102 Nakamura, M. and Fukushima, H. (1978). Effects of reserpine, parachlorophenylalanine, 5,6-dihydroxytryptamine and fludiazepam on the head twitches induced by 5-hydroxytryptamine or 5-methoxytryptamine in mice, *J. Pharm. Pharmacol.*, **30**, 254

103 Pinder, R. M., Brogden, R. N., Speight, T. M. and Avery, G. S. (1977). Sodium valproate: a review of its pharmacological properties and therapeutic efficacy in epilepsy. *Drugs*, **13**, 81

104 Tomlinson, E. B. (1974). Progressive myoclonus epilepsy. The response to sodium di-n-propylacetate. *Proc. Aust, Assoc. Neurol.*, **11**, 203

105 Fahn, S. (1978). Post-anoxic action myoclonus: improvement with valproic acid. *N. Eng. J. Med.*, **299**, 313

106 Ferrandes, B. and Eymard, P. (1973). Méthode rapide d'analyse quantitative du dipropyl-acétate de sodium dans le sérum ou le plasma. *Ann. Pharmac. Français*, **31**, 279

107 Loiseau, P., Brachet, A. and Henry, P. (1975). Concentration of dipropylacetate in plasma. *Epilepsia*, **16**, 609

108 Godin, Y., Heiner, I., Mark, J. and Mandel, P. (1969). Effects of di-n-propylacetate, an anticonvulsant compound, on GABA metabolism. *J. Neurochem.*, **16**, 869

109 Harvey, P. Y. P. (1976). Some aspects of the neurochemistry of Epilim. In Legg, N. J. (ed.) *Clinical and Pharmacological Aspects of Sodium Valproate (Epilim) in the Treatment of Epilepsy*, pp. 130–134 (Tunbridge Wells: MCS Consultants)

110 Chung Hwang, E. and van Woert, M. H. (1980). Effect of valproic acid on serotonin metabolism. *Neuropharmacology*, **18**, 391

111 Wurtman, R. J. and Fernstrom, J. D. (1972). L-tryptophan, L-tyrosine and the control of brain monoamine synthesis. In Snyder, S. H. (ed.) *Perspectives in Neuropharmacology*, pp. 143–193. (Oxford: Oxford University Press)

112 Curzon, G. and Marsden, C. A. (1975). Metabolism of a tryptophan load in the hypothalamus and other brain areas. *J. Neurochem.*, **25**, 251

113 Gal, E. M., Young, R. B. and Sherman, A. D. (1978). Tryptophan loading: consequent effects on the synthesis of kynurenine and 5-hydroxyindoles in rat brain. *J. Neurochem.*, **31**, 237

114 Magnussen, I. and Engbaek, F. (1978). The efects of aromatic amino acid decarboxylase inhibitors on plasma concentrations of 5-hydroxytryptophan in man. *Acta Pharmacol. Toxicol.*, **43**, 36

115 Sorel, L. and Dusaucy-Bouloye, A. A. (1958). A propos de 21 cas d'hypsarhythmie de Gibbs: Son traitment spectaculaire par l'ACTH. *Acta Neurol. Belg.*, **58**, 130

116 Jeavons, P. M. and Bower, B. D. (1964). Infantile spasms. A review of the literature and a study of 112 cases. In *Clinics in Developmental Medicine*. No. 15, pp. 1–79. (London: W. Heinemann Medical Books with the Spastics Society)

117 Kinsbourne, M. (1962). Myoclonic encephalopathy of infants. *J. Neurol. Neurosurg. Psychiatry*, **25**, 271

118 Christoff, N. (1969). Myoclonic encephalopathy of infants. A report of two cases and observations on related disorders. *Arch. Neurol.*, **21**, 229

119 Korten, J. J., Notermans, S. L. H., Frenken, C. W. G. M., Gabreels, F. J. M. and Joosten, E. M. G. (1974). Familial essential myoclonus. *Brain*, **97**, 131

120 Phillips, J. R. and Eldridge, F. L. (1973). Respiratory myoclonus (Leeuwenhoek's disease). *N. Engl. J. Med.*, **289**, 1390

5

Treatment of torsion dystonia

C. D. Marsden

INTRODUCTION

Torsion dystonia is distressing and difficult to treat. Few of the diseases known to cause torsion dystonia (symptomatic dystonia) can be cured. Most patients with idiopathic torsion dystonia (dystonia musculorum deformans) do not respond dramatically either to drugs or surgery, the unwanted side-effects or complications of which may be worse than the illness itself. The purpose of this chapter is to review briefly what can be done to help such patients.

First, it is necessary to define the condition under discussion. Dystonia merely refers to abnormal muscle tone. Torsion dystonia refers to a syndrome of abnormal movements and postures. Some prefer to use the term athetosis to describe such abnormal movements. Hammond introduced athetosis as a description of distal slow writhing movements of the digits following stroke. Subsequently, athetosis was employed to cover more proximal movements of similar type, although many retained the term torsion dystonia to characterize such movements when they affected axial structures such as the neck and trunk, or the muscles of the shoulder and pelvic girdles. Indeed, confusion reached the stage that athetosis might be termed distal dystonia, while torsion dystonia could be described as proximal athetosis. Further difficulty arose from the customary description of certain forms of cerebral palsy distinguished by dystonic movements as athetoid cerebral palsy. Indeed, this, and many other types of symptomatic dystonia are often referred to as athetosis. In the face of the division of opinion I will continue to use torsion dystonia to describe both the typical proximal movements and those of distal athetosis.

Torsion dystonia is not a diagnosis in itself, but merely a description of a distinctive motor syndrome characterized by the presence of abnormal movements and postures produced by prolonged spasms of muscle contraction that distort the body into typical dystonic postures. The spasms may be repetitive (even rhythmic) or sustained, so producing either repeated abnormal movements or continuous abnormal postures. Any part of the body may be affected (except the external occular muscles and sphincters). The neck may be rotated (torticollis), extended (retrocollis), or flexed (anticollis); the trunk likewise may bend forward, sideways, or backwards; the arms usually are extended at the elbow and hyperpronated with flexed wrists and extended fingers. The legs usually are extended at the knees with the feet plantar-flexed and turned in. The abnormal movements of dystonia are distinguished from those of chorea and myoclonus by their prolonged duration, those of the latter conditions being brief muscle jerks.

There are many causes of the syndrome of torsion dystonia such as perinatal birth injury, Wilson's disease, Hallervorden–Spatz disease etc. Such causes of symptomatic dystonia[1,2] usually also cause more extensive brain damage to produce clinical features such as fits, dementia or pyramidal deficit in addition to the syndrome of torsion dystonia. In other patients there is no additional neurological deficit, birth history is unremarkable, and investigations including copper studies, are quite normal. Such patients are said to have idiopathic torsion dystonia, which can be inherited, either as an autosomal recessive or as an autosomal dominant trait[3,4].

Idiopathic torsion dystonia may take a number of forms[5]. In childhood the disease usually is progressive, particularly if it starts in the legs, and spreads to involve all four limbs (generalized dystonia). When the illness starts in adult life usually it does not affect the legs and often it remains confined to its site of onset (focal dystonia)[6-8]. Examples of focal dystonia include blepharospasm and oro-mandibular dystonia, spasmodic torticollis or retrocollis, truncal dystonia and dystonic writer's cramp[7,9]. Not infrequently in adults, the illness may start in the neck and spread to one or both arms, or vice versa (segmental dystonia).

The details of treatment of the various causes of symptomatic dystonia are beyond the compass of this review, and the treatment of athetosis is considered in Chapter 3. I will concentrate on the management of idiopathic torsion dystonia.

Unfortunately, next to nothing is known about the pathophysiology, biochemical pathology, or even the basic neuropathology of idiopathic torsion dystonia and its focal variants. No convincing histological changes in the brain have been detected by conventional light microscopy[10] and far too few brains have been examined biochemically to identify any specific neurotransmitter abnormality. In the face of this ignorance, treatment necessarily is empirical.

The different forms of torsion dystonia demand different management, but the drugs used to treat generalized dystonia are also those employed in focal and segmental dystonia. In addition to drugs, many patients seek and find various forms of physical treatment for their illness, such as acupuncture or biofeedback. Likewise, the principle of the stereotaxic surgical approach to the treatment of generalized dystonia also has been applied to some forms of focal and segmental dystonia. Finally, the management of any case of dystonia requires much more than drugs, surgery and physical treatment. In most patients the illness is lifelong, its consequences disfiguring, and its overall effects distressing. Secondary psychiatric disability is common and requires appropriate care and consideration.

I propose to discuss each of these various approaches to treatment in relation to the management of generalized and segmental idiopathic torsion dystonia, and then to consider the special problems involved in the treatment of the various forms of focal dystonia.

GENERALIZED AND SEGMENTAL DYSTONIA

Drug therapy

No drugs are known to cure idiopathic torsion dystonia, so all therapy is symptomatic. Since the illness is nearly always lifelong, drug treatment must be taken continuously. Transient remissions occur in about 5% of cases early in the course of the illness, but permanent recovery is very rare[11].

Most drugs used in neurology have been tried in dystonia. Few have any useful effect and those that do rarely produce more than limited improvement. Side-effects often outweight benefit. The extent to which the physician presses drugs on the patient is dictated by their disability. Severely affected patients will tolerate unpleasant side-effects for small improvements, while the mildly disabled individual often prefers no treatment.

The groups of drugs listed in Table 1 have been reported to be of benefit in some patients with generalized idiopathic torsion dystonia. In my experience of over 200 patients with the disease, I have found that most patients continue to take only a limited number of agents, namely anticholinergics, benzodiazepines, carbamazepine, and dopamine antagonists (either postsynaptic dopamine receptor blockers or presynaptic antagonists which dis- rupt dopamine storage or synthesis). Levodopa or other dopamine agonists such as bromocryptine require seperate consideration. which disrupt dopamine storage or synthesis). Levodopa or other dopamine agonists such as bromocriptine require separate consideration.

Anticholinergics such as benzhexol or orphenadrine are employed widely and are tolerated reasonably well. They produce no more than modest benefit, but this may be sufficient to restore adequate function in patients with early mild dystonia. There is some suggestion that the benefits of anticholinergics are dose-dependent and this is currently a subject of collaborative clinical trial in Great Britain and the United States. Side-effects are not too severe—dry mouth, constipation, blurring of vision—and often can be reduced to a minimum by introduction of low dosage and subsequent very gradual build-up to maximum tolerance. There is no evidence that one anticholinergic is better than another. Anticholinergics can be used safely with the other drugs to be considered.

Table 1   Drugs used to treat idiopathic torsion dystonia

Produce benefit in more than a few patients[17]	Produce benefit in the odd patient	Of no benefit
Diazapam and other benzodiazepines	Apomorphine[31]	Penicillamine
Anticholinergics	Baclofen[15]	Anticonvulsants (other
Carbamazepine	Quinine	than carbamazipine)
Levodopa	Alcohol	ACTH
Phenothiazines	Marihuana	Vitamin B_6
Haloperidol		Vitamin B_{12}
Pimozide		Parachlorophenylalanine[21]
Reserpine		5-Hydroxytryptophan[17]
Tetrabenazine		α-Methyl-p-tyrosine[21]
		Naloxone[17]
		Morphine[17]
		Amantadine[17]
		Propranolol[17]
		Other β-blockers

Benzodiazepines such as diazepam also are useful. Again there is suggestive evidence that their benefits are dose-dependent. Initial drowsiness can be avoided with the introduction in low dosage and very gradual increase. Patients with dystonia often can tolerate very large doses of diazepam without side-effects. None of the other benzodiazepines appears to offer any advantage over diazepam. Longer acting drugs such as clonazepam often cause persistent and unacceptable sleepiness.

Carbamazepine has been reported to have a remarkable effect in a few children with dystonia, apparently producing complete or near complete suppression of symptoms and signs in those who have responded[12-17].(Table 2). However, this is not a common experience and I have encountered only a single example of such a response to the drug. This 11-year-old girl had a focal dystonia of one leg for some 5 years prior to starting on carbamazepine, following which her disability gradually disappeared over a matter of 3 months. By far the majority of patients with torsion dystonia do not respond to carbamazepine. I have treated some 32 patients for periods of 2 to 6 months, in doses of between 100 and 1600 mg/day, but have seen useful benefit in only that one patient. It should be noted that other anticonvulsants do not appear to have produced such benefit as has been described for carbamazepine.

Table 2 Treatment of idiopathic torsion dystonia with carbamazepine

Author	Number of patients	Age at onset	Dose (mg/day)	Good response	Some response	No response
Geller et al.[12,13]	10	13–46	450–1600	6	3	1
Isgreen et al.[14]	16	4–29	200–1600	1	2	13
Langdon[15]	7	?	?	1	0	6
Coleman[16]	5	?	?	0	0	5
Marsden[17]	32	4–61	100–1600	1	3	28
Total				9 (13%)	8 (11%)	53 (76%)

Table 3 Treatment of idiopathic torsion dystonia with levodopa

Author	Number of patients	Age at onset (years)	Dose* (per day)	Good response	Some response	No response	Worse
Coleman[20]	8	5–15	50–150 mg/kg	4	3	1	0
Chase[21]	4	6–11	3–10 g	1	1	2	0
Mandell[22]	21	4–12	2–8 g	0	7	6	8
Barrett et al.[23]	7	4–10	4–7 g	0	0	7	0
Barbeau et al.[24]	14	?	?	4	0	10	0
Rajput[25]	1	6	1.5 g	1	0	0	0
Hongladarom[26]	1	1	1 g	1	0	0	0
Marsden[17]	38	4–56	$\frac{3}{4}$–8	0	3	30	5
Total				11 (12%)	14 (15%)	56 (59%)	13 (14%)

*Where Sinemet (275) was used, the dose has been multiplied by five to give figures roughly comparable to those of plain levodopa.

The patients who have responded to carbamazepine have been young (1–12 years of age) with mild early dystonia. Recovery usually has occurred on a moderate dosage and it has been suggested that high doses may not be beneficial (Fahn, personal communication).

The question arises as to whether the benefits obtained in those few patients who have responded to the drug are a real pharmacological effect or coincidental. About one in 20 patients with generalized dystonia with onset in childhood will describe an early, spontaneous remission of their illness, lasting months to years, and very rarely the disease apparently may disappear[11]. Whether the few examples of considerable response to carbamazepine are true therapeutic effects of the drug, or coincidental spontaneous remissions cannot be decided with confidence at this time. But the fact that drug-withdrawal may provoke clinical deterioration is in favour of a real pharmacological action, albeit in a small number of cases.

Levodopa also has been of dramatic benefit in some patients (Table 3). Soon after its introduction for the treatment of Parkinson's disease, levodopa was tried in a number of patients with idiopathic torsion dystonia. One rationale for this use of levodopa was the observation that levodopa could correct some of the dystonic features of chronic manganese poisoning in Chilean miners[18].

Coleman and Barnet[19] initially described therapeutic success in an unusual patient with hereditary dystonia (also a sib. was affected) who also exhibited insomnia and vomiting. At the meeting where this was reported both Cotzias and Barbeau also described benefit from levodopa in patients with idiopathic torsion dystonia. However, Barbeau commented that 'we have improved the rigidity and the akinesia that is sometimes seen with the dystonia, but the movements were not changed'.

Subsequently at a conference held at the National Institutes of Health on torsion dystonia, Coleman[20] reported benefit from levodopa in no less than seven of eight patients with the idiopathic form of the disease. These studies were open, but she also undertook a double-blind cross-over study on a pair of identical twins with torsion dystonia, with impressive results in favour of levodopa at least in one twin. Chase[21] also reported benefit in some patients at the same meeting, but Mandell[22] and Barrett *et al.*[23] reported less favourable or negative results with levodopa in torsion dystonia.

Subsequently others have reported benefit[24–26] (although the diagnosis of idiopathic torsion dystonia is open to question in some of these patients). However, the overwhelming (and usually unreported) experience of most neurologists has been that levodopa has little or no effect on the disease[17]. In 1973 Eldridge and his colleagues[27] questioned neurologists in the United States as to the value of levodopa in torsion dystonia. Of 425 who responded, 90 had treated 203 patients; 21% were said to have improved, 70% were unchanged, and 9% were worse. These authors also questioned 39 patients who had received levodopa; 5% said they were better, 61% said they were unchanged, and 34% said they were worse. Also while 39% of patients expressed the view that initially they were better on levodopa, only two (5%) indicated long-term improvement. This accords with my personal experience of the use of levodopa (or Sinemet/Madopar) in 38 patients with torsion dystonia[17]. Regrettably, despite administration of maximum tolerated doses for periods of at least 3 months and usually 6 or more, I have not encountered a single useful response, and none of my patients have continued on the drug. Dystonic spasms were made worse in a few patients.

The overall conclusion from these data is that levodopa has little or no effect on torsion dystonia. In 1972 Cooper[28] raised the possibilty that prior levodopa treatment actually might compromise the success of subsequent stereotaxic surgical treatment. No further evidence has been forthcoming to support this latter contention, but the general use of levodopa in idiopathic torsion dystonia has not really proved very beneficial. Yet a few patients undoubtedly have responded to levodopa and sometimes dramatically. The questions arises as to whether these individuals have a different disease.

Segawa and his colleagues[29, 30] have described a familial form of dystonia which does respond dramatically to levodopa, but which clearly differs from the usual case of idiopathic torsion dystonia. These patients develop increasing dystonia in the course of the day, but are greatly improved by sleep— hence the description as hereditary progressive dystonia with marked diurnal fluctuation. Similar patients have now been discovered not only in Japan, but also in Australia, the United States and Great Britain amongst different ethnic groups. Perusal of the case histories of those patients with dystonia who have responded dramatically to levodopa suggests that some, but not all, exibited marked diurnal fluctuations and may have been examples of the disease described by Segawa and his colleagues.

The overall conclusion must be that most forms of idiopathic torsion dystonic are not responsive to levodopa, but the drug may be effective in the rare examples of other distinctive diseases included in the general syndrome of torsion dystonia.

There have been few published reports of the use of *other dopamine agonists* in idiopathic torsion dystonia. Braham and Serova-Pinhas[31] reported dramatic relief of torsion dystonia by subcutaneous apomorphine (0.5–1 mg) in a child aged 12 and a man aged 47 years. However, subsequent oral use of the dopamine agonist, bromocriptine, has not met with such success, at least in my hands. I have treated eight children and five adults with idiopathic torsion dystonia with bromocriptine in doses of 10–60 mg daily with no benefit or deterioration[17].

Many *dopamine antagonists* have been used in the disease, with very variable results, few of which have been published. There is no doubt that the occasional patient is helped considerably by a phenothiazine, such as clor-promazine, or prochlorperazine, but usually at the expense of a degree of drug-induced parkinsonism. However, the response to such phenothiazines and other neuroleptics, such as haloperidol or pimozide, is variable and unpredictable[22,17]. Only a minority of patients have gained sufficient relief from such drugs to continue them. Some patients actually are made worse by phenothiazines or haloperidol. Another complication of such drug treat-ment is the emergence of what appears to be a tardive dyskinesia with orofacial movements typical of those seen in schizophrenic patients on long-term neuroleptic medication.

Reserpine and tetrabenazine[32], both of which deplete presynaptic dop-amine stores, also have been employed. Again some patients gain benefit, but also at the expense of parkinsonism and depression, which is even more distressing and usually results in discontinuation of therapy.

Many other drugs have been tried in this disease, as illustrated in Table 1, but none have found favour. Marihuana has been mentioned by a few patients to have effects comparable to those of diazepam, and alcohol also is used. In this context, the postural tremor so reminiscent of benign essential tremor that is seen in a significant proportion of patients with idiopathic torsion dystonia[5] is helped by alcohol and sometimes by propranolol, but these agents do not alter the dystonia.

There are hopes that GABA agonists such as muscimol may be of benefit, but baclofen has not produced useful improvement[15]. Likewise, the new synthetic enkephalins now available may have no effect since opiates and naloxone do not alter the condition.

Table 4 illustrates what patients finally decide helps most from a series collected by Eldridge and his colleagues[27] and from the early series of Marsden and Harrison[11]. My subsequent experience would confirm these general trends.

Table 4   Drugs chosen as most helpful by patients with idiopathic torsion dystonia

	Eldridge et al.[27]	Marsden and Harrison[11,17]
Number of patients	39	42
Diazepam	26%	24%
Phenothiazines/butyrophenones	7%	19%
Tetrabenazine	—	9%
Benzhexol	5%	9%
Levodopa	5%	0%

Surgery

This is not the place to discuss details of surgical results or techniques, which in any case, are dealt with in Chapter 10. I shall briefly review the principles involved so as to provide guidance on the choice of patient, timing of operation, and likely outcome based on personal experience.

The introduction of stereotaxic surgery for the treatment of Parkinson's disease was soon followed by its application in torsion dystonia. Since 1955, Cooper has amassed the greatest experience in this field, having operated on no less than 226 patients by 1976[33–35]. Few other surgeons have great experience with torsion dystonia, and many have not pursued the principles enunciated by Cooper as rigorously as their advocate, so it is difficult to assess the significance of the less favourable results obtained by others[40].

Sterotaxic thalamotomy is the surgical treatment of choice but the lesion should, according to Cooper, be aimed at the posterior half of the ventro-lateral (VL) nucleus of the thalamus and should extent 1–2 mm into the posterior ventrolateral (VPL) and posterior ventromedial (PVM) nuclei as well as the centrum medianum (CM). This is a bigger lesion than that employed in Parkinson's disease, and may require multiple lesion placement at one or more operations (as is the case in about 60% of his cases). The aim should be to destroy all the thalamic inputs from the medial globus pallidus and cerebellum (via brachium conjunctivum) which terminate in this area. In Cooper's words 'persistence in the pursuit of surgical relief of dystonia is essential', and 'many of the patients in whom abolition of dystonic symptoms has been achieved would not have been relieved of their symptoms if a single operation had been performed, or if we had become discouraged by lack of success or return of symptoms following the initial surgical procedure'[35].

Cooper's results are shown in Table 5, along with those recorded in other smaller series containing more than 10 patients collected by Eldridge in his review in 1970[3]. Eldridge concluded from the literature that about 70% of patients were said to have had some long-term benefit from surgery, while the rest had no sustained improvement or were worse. Cooper[34] also notes that 'following surgical relief of symptoms, one-third of the cases demonstrated sufficient return to symptoms of warrant re-operation'.

Against this background of the apparent success of surgery must be set the risks. There is a substantial failure rate approaching 30% in the best of hands and nearer 50% in many centres. Each operation carries a small risk of producing hemiplegia, a risk that may approach 1% although deficit usually recovers with time. A unilateral lesion usually does not impair speech, but generalized torsion dystonia requires bilateral lesions, which carry the risk of producing a striatal pseudobulbar palsy with soft voice and poor articulation. Speech disturbance after bilateral thalamotomy occurs in up to 15% of patients and although recovery often occurs gradually in the months following surgery, severe residual disability may occur. The risks of speech impairment are particularly great among the third of patients with generalized torsion dystonia who exhibit speech involvement prior to surgery. Finally, one has to consider the impact of neurosurgical procedures on

Table 5 Results of surgical treatment of idiopathic torsion dystonia

Author	Number of patients	Number of bilateral lesions	Percentage				
			Worse	No change	Moderate improvement	Marked improvement	
Cooper[34,35]	208	122	12	18	45	25	
Marsden and Harrison[11]	18	9	—	39	28	33	
Markham and Rand[36]	11	—	—	22	33	44	
Samotokin and Bulgakov[37]	18	—	—	44	– 56 –		
Voitnya and Kandel[38]	20	—	—	16	20	64	
Laponogov[39]	14	—	—	—	50	50	

Cases of symptomatic dystonia cannot be separated clearly from those with idiopathic dystonia in all the series quoted. Nor is the degree of improvement and its duration always obvious. The figures given as results should be taken as a general guide.

children, particularly as the operation is best undertaken without general anaesthesia so as to be able to monitor the effect of incremental lesions. All these problems must be taken into account in deciding who to consider for surgical treatment.

A unilateral thalamotomy is of little or no value in generalized dystonia. Such patients require bilateral lesions with the increased risks to speech. Thalamotomy is most effective in relieving contralateral limb dystonia, and least effective in relieving axial or truncal dystonia. These principles underlie the common experience that surgery is most effective (and safest) when a unilateral lesion is employed to relieve an isolated contralateral focal limb dystonia.

In general, surgery is not contemplated until all avenues of medical therapy have been exhausted. Even then, it is usually only justified where disability is severe. In children, surgery is best delayed until around the age of 10–12 years by which time co-operation during the operation can be obtained. Delay until this age also has the advantage of allowing time for spontaneous remission to occur which, although a rare event, does happen in 5% or less of cases[11].

Table 6   Other treatments that have been used in torsion dystonia

Limited benefit	No benefit[3,17]
Psychotherapy[41]	Hypnosis
Sex therapy[17]	Abreaction
Biofeedback[42,43]	Psychoanalysis
	Dream interpretation
	Group therapy
	Aversion therapy
	Massed practice
	Systemic desensitisation
	Behaviour therapy
	Acupuncture
	Electroconvulsive therapy
	Leucotomy

Other treatments

Many other forms of treatment have been tried in torsion dystonia (Table 6). Most are ineffective and need not be considered further. Their use reflects the all too frequent initial referral of patients with this disease to psychiatrists and the latter's failure to recognize its organic origin. However, mention must be made of the use of psychotherapy[41] and sex counselling in the management of patients with torsion dystonia. Those disabled by disfiguring generalized dystonia face considerable problems of emotional and sexual development during adolesence and puberty. Indeed, these difficulties not infrequently over-ride the physical incapacity produced by the disease. Supportive psychotherapy is undoubtedly of the utmost importance in the management of such patients and is an essential part of the relationship between the neurologist and patient. Formal psychiatric referral may be required for the handling of severe depressive illness and expert sex counselling may be invaluable.

Bio-feedback[42,43] has little to play in the management of generalized torsion dystonia, for it is impossible for the patient to apply himself to the number of muscles involved in producing the widespread spasms. However, it has been used in focal dystonias, such as spasmodic torticollis (see below).

Treatment of the individual case

At the outset it is important to explain to the patients and their relatives that treatment does not cure the illness but is aimed to suppress the muscle spasms as far as is possible. It is also necessary to explain that control is often incomplete and that many drugs may have to be tried in order to establish which is going to be of most use and what dose is going to be most effective. It must admitted that in many patients no satisfactory treatment is established. These pessimistic but honest views may be tempered with a full explanation of the disease including the observation of a small but definite chance of spontaneous remission.

In the very mildest case drug treatment may not be indicated at all, particularly in children where side-effects may interfere with schooling. Where therapy is required I start with benzhexol 2.5 mg twice daily increasing gradually over a matter of many weeks to 5 mg four times daily or higher if tolerated. If relief is inadequate I then add carbamazepine starting in a dose of 100 mg at night and increasing again over a matter of many weeks to as much as 1.2–1.6 g daily as dictated by side-effects and blood carbamazepine levels. Throughout this period many patients also take a benzodiazepine, usually diazepam, for relief of anxiety and muscle tension. If neither benzhexol nor carbamazepine produce any benefit they are stopped. I then turn to tetrabenazine starting in a dose of 12.5 mg three times daily and increasing to as much as 50 mg three times daily as dictated by side-effects. If tetrabenazine fails, I then switch to haloperidol 1 mg twice daily increasing daily gradually up to as much as 8 mg twice daily as dictated by side-effects. If haloperidol is of no value I would then start on a course of levodopa in the form of Sinemet (levodopa combined with carbidopa) or Madopar (levodopa combined with benserazide) again introduced in small dosage gradually increased to the maximum tolerated.

The general principles followed with all these drugs is to introduce them in small dosage initially and then gradually increase over a matter of weeks or months to the maximum the patient can tolerate, which is then continued for a period of 2–4 months to complete a full trial of each medication. If adequate relief is obtained with simple drugs such as benzhexol and diazepam there is no need to pursue further clinical trials. Therapeutic aims should not be set too high. There is often no question of the patient being returned to normal and it is better to settle for a moderate degree of relief of discomfort and disability with simple drugs with little side-effects rather than instituting further clinical trials with the more powerful compounds such as the neuroleptics or levodopa.

During the slow process of working through the trials of the individual drugs mentioned the question of surgery will sooner or later be raised. My practice is to postpone a decision as to surgery for as long as possible, firstly to make quite certain all medical avenues have been adequately explored, secondly to allow the patients and relatives to grasp fully the implications of surgery, and thirdly to allow the passage of time to define the extent and rate of progression of the illness. In the case of children such delay often allows surgery to be contemplated at the optimum age after the age of 10 years or so. If all drug treatment fails and the patient is grossly disabled by their dystonia then surgery would be advised but my own practice is to try and persuade patients with less disabling degrees of dystonia to accept and live within the limits of their disability. Obviously such decisions are a matter of fine judgement and the time spent during initial drug trials during which the patient gets to know and trust his doctor does much to help form balanced judgements.

FOCAL DYSTONIAS

Spasmodic torticollis

Spasmodic torticollis is the commonest focal dystonia and its treatment is exceedingly difficult. The same drugs that are used to treat generalized dystonia are employed to treat spasmodic torticollis but often with a conspicuous lack of success (Table 7). The experience described by Shaw and his colleagues[45] is typical of that of most of us who treat large numbers of such patients. Of 18 cases of spasmodic torticollis treated with maximum tolerated doses of levodopa, amantadine, tetrabenazine or haloperidol, only two showed any useful response, one to levodopa and another to haloperidol.

Although there have been no formal trials of benzodiazepines such as diazepam or anticholinergics such as benzhexol, there is no doubt that these drugs are widely prescribed and frequently continued by many patients.

Previous reports of the use of levodopa in spasmodic torticollis have not been encouraging. None of the remaining 16 patients treated by Shaw et al. had any lasting benefit, and earlier authors also obtained negative results. There have been few reports of the use of other dopamine agonists in spasmodic torticollis. Tolosa described very modest benefit following injection of apomorphine[50]. Lees et al.[51] found that bromocriptine in doses of up to 80 mg daily was ineffective in nine of ten patients but did appear to help a single patient (the one who had previously responded to levodopa in an earlier trial carried out by these authors). Lithium has been reported to be of benefit in a single patient whose torticollis followed exposure to carbon monoxide 6 years earlier[52].

Table 7   Drug treatment of spasmodic torticollis

	Number of cases	Excellent	Moderate	Nil
Levodopa				
Barrett et al.[23]	3	0	0	3
Ansari et al.[44]	6	0	0	6
Shaw et al.[45]	17	1	3	13
Total	26	1	3	22
Haloperidol				
Gilbert[46, 47]	6	3	1	2
Shaw et al.[45]	6	1	0	5
West[48]	3	0	0	3
Couch[49]	17	8	6	2
Total	31	12	7	12
Amantadine				
Gilbert[46]	4	3	1	0
Shaw et al.[45]	9	0	0	9
West[48]	10	0	0	10
Total	23	3	1	19
Tetrabenazine				
Shaw et al.[45]	9	0	1	8
Swash et al.[32]	3	0	1	2
Total	12	0	2	10

The results obtained with haloperidol also have been conflicting. Few authors have been able to confirm the earlier excellent results claimed by Gilbert[46], but Couch[49] reported a careful double-blind cross-over study of haloperidol (in doses of up to 7 mg daily) in a group of 16 patients, 14 of whom improved on active drug, a statistically significant difference. Nor have amantadine and tetrabenazine been of much use. Indeed, Matthews *et al.* in a recent review concluded that, 'we found no indication of any form of curative treatment and the outcome appears to have changed little since Gowers (1893) stated that, "prognosis must be grave in every developed case"'[53]. Even in those few patients who do seem to respond to therapy there must be doubt, for significant spontaneous remissions occur (usually in the first 5 years) in a proportion of patients, perhaps some 5–10%[54].

In the face of such therapeutic difficulty it has been natural to turn to surgery, and both stereotaxic thalamotomy[55] and local denervation[56] have been widely used in spasmodic torticollis. Initial enthusiasm for thalamotomy has dwindled both because the operation turned out to be unreliable and because the bilateral lesions required often caused severe and prolonged speech disturbance, a risk unacceptable in what is essentially a benign condition. Following his earlier report on beneficial effects of thalamotomy on torticollis, Cooper described less favourable experience with a series of 120 such patients and concluded that although the operation may work on occasion, 'I personally never operate on torticollis any more because of the fact that one-third failed. The operation has to be bilateral which means there is a 12–14% risk of dysphonic speech. Therefore, unless a patient is virtually incapacitated or in great pain, we don't operate on them'[57]. Few surgeons now employ thalamotomy for torticollis and most have returned to cervical rhizotomy.

The standard operation has been that devised by Dandy[56] in which the upper three cervical motor roots are sectioned bilaterally at laminectomy and one or both spinal accessory nerves also are divided. The results reported with cervical rhizotomy have been conflicting. Sorensen and Hamby[58] reported success in the majority of 71 patients operated upon but this has not been the experience of others. Meares[54], for instance, concluded that those receiving rhizotomies may fare worse than unoperated cases. Recurrence of residual torticollis after surgery is common and other disadvantages such as head lolling and the late appearance of painful spondylosis also pose problems. Indeed a flabby neck with persistent abnormal movements is often the end result of rhizotomy. This may be partly due inadequate denervation, and some surgeons cut, intrathecally, the upper four cervical motor roots on one side (that to which the head moves) and the upper three roots on the other side, as well as cutting the spinal accessory intrathecally on both sides at the level of the first root, and the spinal accessory in the neck on the side that sternomastoid is contracting as well. Walsh reported results in 33 such patients, 26 of whom were improved and were said to be satisfactory[59]. Bertrand and his colleagues advocate combined unilateral stereotaxic thalamotomy with rhizotomy[60], but this has not gained widespread favour. (See also Chapter 10).

The general conclusion drawn from these various surgical approaches to treatment of torticollis is that all involve risk and discomfort and none achieves cure in a disease whose main disability is usually social. Accordingly, my own practice is to postpone surgery for as long as possible in the hope that the patient may be one of the lucky few who undergo a spontaneous remission or that they may come to terms with their illness. Only in those with persisting torticollis which renders work impossible or social life intolerable do I consider surgery, and in those circumstances I would favour rhizotomy.

In view of the relative lack of efficacy of both medication and surgery, a number of behavioural techniques have been employed to try and modify spasmodic torticollis. In particular, biofeedback methods have been used widely. Cleeland[61] in an early study described the successful use of EMG feedback from the contracting sternomastoid muscles as an audio-signal, combined with an electric shock delivered to the fingers triggered when muscle activity exceeded a threshold. Eight of ten patients with torticollis were able to reduce the intensity and frequency of their muscle spasms using this technique, and six of the ten patients maintained improvement after stopping therapy for periods of between 1–40 months. Korein and his colleagues[42,43] reported more extensive investigation of the use of sensory feedback therapy in 48 patients with spasmodic torticollis. EMG activity recorded from surface electrodes over the actively contracting neck muscles was fed back to the patient both as a tone and as a visual display. Therapeutic sessions lasting approximately 45 min were undertaken three to five times a week over a period of 8–12 weeks. If treatment progressed satisfactorily, visual feedback was withdrawn and the patient used auditory feedback and a mirror. Finally the patient was advised to continue using a mirror only. Twenty-six of the 48 patients with torticollis obtained a response to feedback which carried over to periods between treatment sessions. Improvement persisted for 3 months after stopping all therapy in 20 of these patients. Those who gained benefit tended to be younger and to have had the illness for a short period of time. In a subsequent report, the same authors found that 37 of 69 patients obtained benefit which persisted between treatments, and 30 of these reported improvement persisting after the end of treatment for periods of months to years.

These studies show that the majority of patients with torticollis can control their muscle spasms while receiving sensory feedback therapy. A proportion, perhaps about 40%, carry over benefit between treatments during a course of therapy. While some of these patients consequently relapse, a large number are reported to continue to benefit for months or even years after the course of treatment has finished. Further studies are required to confirm these findings and to establish whether such techniques will be of general use in the treatment of spasmodic torticollis.

Writer's cramp

There is debate as to the nature of writer's cramp, but it is this author's opinion that virtually all types are fragments of focal dystonia[5,7]. There can be no doubt that this is the case when manual acts other than writing are involved and patients develop typical dystonic postures on wielding a knife or fork, tool, pen, or other implement. Indeed, some such patients with *dystonic writer's cramp* clearly have dystonia elsewhere, such as torticollis. When the condition is confined solely to the act of writing (*simple writer's cramp*), the matter is less clear-cut. However, I have now seen a sufficient number of such patients who have subsequently gone on to develop typical dystonic writer's cramp to convince me that even the simple form is a manifestation of focal dystonia. Writing is, for most of us, our most skilled manual act, so writer's cramp is commonest. But others who use their hands for different skilled acts may develop craft or occupational palsies peculiar to their trade. Typist's cramp is now common while telegraphist's cramp used to be[62]. Every conceivable form of cramp is seen amongst musicians— pianist's cramp, violinist's or cellist's cramp, and even flutist's cramp.

The treatment of writer's cramp is unsatisfactory. Few drugs have any useful effect. Benhexol may give some relief; diazepam may help anxiety, but neither usually cure the condition. I have not been impressed with the value of any other drugs.

A variety of re-education programmes have been employed. Initial attempts at avoidance conditioning using electrical shocks delivered to the hand whenever it gripped the pen excessively or deviated from a prescribed training course claimed success[63], but have not gained wide use. Crisp and Moldofsky[64] described benefit in seven patients from general relaxation, correction of abnormal writing posture and re-education of hand-writing accompanied by formal psychotherapy, a regime based on a psychosomatic rationale[65]. My experience of such an approach has not been so rewarding and I have not known it help those patients whom I have referred for such treatment. Bindman and Tibbetts[66] obtained no success with psychotherapy and re-education (or hypnosis) in four patients. They also examined the potential of sensory feedback therapy using EMG activity recorded by surface electrodes over the flexor tendons to the index and thumb fed back as a sound. This produced a rapid relaxation during writing in four of six patients, one of whom relapsed during the follow-up. As in the case of torticollis, there has been insufficient assessment of the value of sensory feedback therapy in writer's cramp, particularly in regard to long-term benefits of such treatment.

There are reasons to suppose that unilateral thalamotomy might well be of benefit in isolated writer's cramp, but the risks of operation for such a limited focal dystonia in an otherwise normal person have prevented me from referring a patient for such surgical treatment.

Blepharospasm – oromandibular dystonia (Brueghel's syndrome; also called Meige syndrome)

Spasms of eye closure (blepharospasm) and spasms of mouth opening or mouth closure (oromandibular dystonia) may occur separately or together[9]. Like spasmodic torticollis and writer's cramp, this curious illness occurs as an isolated focal dystonia in adults and is equally difficult to treat. Spontaneous remissions are rare. The full range of drugs that have been used to treat generalized dystonia have been tried, mostly with no success. Anticholinergics and benzodiazepines give a little relief and the occasional patient will obtain benefit from tetrabenazine or a dopamine receptor antagonist, but most do not[9].

A variety of surgical techniques have been used in an attempt to relieve blepharospasm. Alcohol injection into the peripheral branches of the facial nerve innervating orbicularis oculi[67] are painful and produce only temporary relief, recurrence occurring within a few months, so have been discarded. Similarly, myomectomy of orbicularis oculi[68] has not proved satisfactory. The technique most widely employed is to section the upper branches of the facial nerve as they emerge from the parotid gland[69,70]. Great care is necessary to identify each branch by electrical stimulation so that all supplying orbicularis oculi are cut. In addition, buccal branches must also be divided as these may have anastomosing fibres to the eye muscles and also are a source of re-innervation, which leads to recurrence within the first 6–12 months and may require re-operation. Bilateral surgery should always be done to preserve facial symmetry. Successful surgery stops blepharospasm but leaves the patient with a paralysed expressionless, blank upper half to the face. This may be disguised by wearing dark spectacles. Other complications are uncommon but include exposure keratitis and parotid fistulae.

Surgery for blepharospasm is indicated in those cases in which the frequency of eye spasm is such as to render the patient functionally blind, or when the disorder leads to such psychological trauma as to leave the individual a social recluse. It is wise to undertake a preliminary anaesthetic block to show the patient the effects and appearance of the bilateral facial nerve paralysis that will replace the blepharospasm after surgery.

There is no surgical treatment for oromandibular dystonia, but the occasional patient may require surgical division of crico-pharyngeus to relieve severe dysphagia.

Spasmodic dysphonia (laryngeal dystonia)

It is only recently that this condition has been recognized in the neurological literature[5,71]. Most affected patients are referred to otolaryngologists who term the disorder 'spastic dysphonia' and frequently but erroneously consider it to be hysterical in origin. The characteristic strained tight soft voice is due to dystonic spasm of the phonatory muscles.

No drugs are known to help the condition but unilateral section of one recurrent laryngeal nerve has improved speech[72]. The rationale for this operation is that excessive adduction of the vocal cords occurs during speech in patients with spasmodic dysphonia and is held to be responsible for the strained voice. Certainly after recurrent laryngeal nerve section many patients exhibit improved clarity of voice, return of pitch control, and loss of straining. Again it is sensible to undertake an initial local anaesthetic block or crush of the nerve to show the patient what will happen after surgery.

OTHER DYSTONIAS

Paroxysmal dystonia

The characteristic abnormal postures and movements of idiopathic torsion dystonia initially occur only on specific motor acts (action dystonia). At other times, as when sitting still or lying on the bed, there is nothing abnormal to find. As the disease progresses dystonic movements and postures occur more frequently and spontaneously.

There are other diseases in which paroxysms of explosive dystonic movements and postures occur, lasting for short periods of time, with complete recovery between attacks. In some such patients consciousness is lost and the event is clearly a fit often accompanied by EEG changes in the opposite hemisphere to the limbs involved. The most obvious example of such an event would be the tonic adversive seizure due to frontal lobe discharge.

There are other patients with paroxysms of dystonia who retain clarity of consciousness throughout the attacks and who never develop overt epilepsy. two types of this condition have been recognized[72]. The commonest is paroxysmal kinesigenic choreoathetosis. This condition is often familial, commences in childhood, is characterized by episodes of usually unilateral dystonic or choreoathetoid movements lasting for 5 minutes or less, and always is precipitated by movement (or by startle which provokes movement). Consciousness is not lost and the EEG usually is normal during the attack, but treatment with anticonvulsants is very successful in preventing episodes. Non-familial paroxysmal tonic spasms of the limbs may also occur in multiple sclerosis and other structural brain lesions.

The second form of paroxysmal dystonia, familial paroxysmal dystonic choreoathetosis, always is inherited as an autosomal dominant trait, begins in early childhood, is characterized by attacks lasting for over 10 minutes to a few hours in which the limbs of one side or both suddenly adopt bizarre dystonic postures. Such attacks occur infrequently, perhaps two or three times a month, appear spontaneously and are not precipitated by movement are unaccompanied by alteration of consciousness or the EEG, and are not prevented by ordinary anticonvulsants but may be helped by clonazepam.

Drug-induced acute dystonia

Some 2–5% of patients prescribed a neuroleptic drug such as a phenothiazine or butyrophenone develop, usually within the first 48 hours of intake, a bizarre acute dystonic reaction. Such events are distressing and often are painful, but usually can be abolished by intravenous injection of an anticholinergic drug or benzodiazepine.

CONCLUSIONS

The treatment of the various dystonias described here obviously is unsatisfactory. This reflects gross ignorance as to the cause and pathophysiology of most of these conditions. It is remarkable that even in severe generalized idiopathic torsion dystonia, no pathological abnormality has been detected in the brain at *post mortem* by conventional methods. Nor has any physiological abnormality been detected during life by any of the techniques currently available. Even the clinical pharmacology of dystonia is uncertain. Drugs affect another category of abnormal movements, chorea, sufficiently reproducibly and sufficiently obviously to allow a fairly concrete statement as to the pharmacological sensitivity of the condition. Dopamine antagonists improve chorea, while dopamine agonists make it worse (provided they are not administered in doses small enough to selectively stimulate presynaptic dopamine receptors thereby producing a paradoxical decrease in dopaminergic neurotransmission). Likewise cholinergic drugs improve chorea, while anticholinergics make it worse. From this data it is possible to conclude that chorea is associated with dopaminergic over-activity and cholinergic under-activity.

No such clear picture emerges from the clinical pharmacology of torsion dystonia. There is a suggestion that activation of dopaminergic mechanisms may cause dystonia from the observation that levodopa may provoke dystonic abnormal movements in some patients with Parkinson's disease, but these are far less common than chorea and oro-facial dyskinesia. Likewise, dopamine antagonists sometimes improve dystonia but often do not. The inconsistency of the clinical pharmacology of dystonia with regard to dopamine agonists and antagonists may reflect the possibility that dystonia arises from activation of only one set of dopamine systems. It is now recognized that more than one type of dopamine receptor exists in the brain and the development of more specific and selective dopamine agonists and antagonists may provide new tools for treating dystonia.

The availability of valid animal models of dystonia certainly would aid the development of new drugs. Unfortunately, few such animal models exist. It is possible to produce torticollis experimentally in primates either with a unilaterally electrolytic lesion or with 6-hydroxydopamine injected in the ventral tegmental area of the mid-brain[74,75]. Such head turning produced by either method can be manipulated pharmacologically. In general, dopamine agonists intensify such experimental torticollis, and dopamine antagonists inhibit it.

The mutant mouse described as dystonic by Duchen and his colleagues[76] is widely quoted as a possible animal model of the disease, for the curious writhings of such animals do have a superficial resemblance to human dystonia. However, neuropathology shows that these animals have extensive damage to peripheral and central sensory pathways, changes that are not found in human idiopathic torsion dystonia. The dystonic mouse is more a model of human pseudo-athetosis which occurs as a result of peripheral sensory damage or posterior column sensory loss.

One of the few clues to the cause of dystonia comes from observations on manganese poisoning. The neurological sequelae of chronic manganese exposure in Chilean miners includes an extrapyramidal syndrome many of whose features are those of dystonia. Barbeau and his colleagues[77] have followed this lead with extensive studies on experimental manganese poisoning in animals and examination of manganese metabolism in patients with dystonia, but so far there is no hard evidence to suggest that this or other heavy metal poisoning can be held responsible for other cases of idiopathic torsion dystonia.

Perhaps the most promising avenue towards understanding human dystonia may come from elucidating the pathophysiological mechanisms involved in the production of acute dystonic reactions to neuroleptic drugs. Some progress has been made in this direction because identical events can be provoked in a proportion of primates[78,79]. Pharmacological study of such animals suggests that acute dystonic reactions are due to the compensatory increased turnover and release of dopamine produced on acute administration of a neuroleptic acting upon dopamine receptors rendered supersensitive by the first administration of a neuroleptic. It is to be hoped that the pursuit of clues such as this may eventually lead to greater understanding of the mechanisms responsible for dystonia and those improvements in treatment which are so urgently needed.

References

1 Zeman, W. and Whitlock, C. C. (1968). Symptomatic dystonias. In Vinken, P. J. and Bruyn, G. W. (eds.) *Handbook of Clinical Neurology, Diseases of the Basal Ganglia*. Vol. 6. pp. 544–566 (Amsterdam: North-Holland)

2 Fahn, S. and Eldridge, R. (1976). Definition of dystonia and classification of the dystonic states. In Eldridge, R. and Fahn, S. (eds.) *Dystonia, Advances in Neurology*. Vol. 14, pp. 1–5. (New York: Raven Press)

3 Eldridge, R. (1970). The torsion dystonias: literature review and genetic and clinical studies. *Neurology (Minneap.)*, 20, 1

4 Eldridge, R. and Gottlieb, R. (1976). The primary hereditary dystonias: genetic classification of 768 families and revised estimate of gene frequency, autosomal recessive form, and selected bibliography. In Eldridge, R. and Fahn, S. (eds.) *Dystonia, Advances in Neurology*. Vol. 14, pp. 457–474 (New York: Raven Press)

5 Marsden, C. D. (1976a). Dystonia: the spectrum of the disease. In Yahr, M. D. (ed.) *The Basal Ganglia*, pp. 351–367. (New York: Raven Press)

6 Marsden, C. D., Harrison, M. J. G. and Bundey, S. (1976). Natural history of idiopathic torsion dystonia. In Eldridge, R. and Fahn, S. (eds.) *Dystonia, Advances in Neurology*. Vol. 14, pp. 177–186 (New York: Raven Press)

7 Marsden, C. D. (1976b). The problem of adult-onset idiopathic torsion dystonia and other isolated dyskinesias in adult life (including blepharospasm, oromandibular dystonia,

dystonic writer's cramp and torticollis or axial dystonia). In Eldridge, R. and Fahn, S. (eds.) *Dystonia, Advances in Neurology*. Vol. 14, pp. 259–276 (New York: Raven Press)

8 Cooper, I. S., Cullinan, T. and Riklan, M. (1976). The natural history of dystonia. In Eldridge, R. and Fahn, S. (eds.) *Dystonia, Advances in Neurology*. Vol. 14, pp. 157–169 (New York: Raven Press)

9 Marsden, C. D. (1976c). Blepharospasm-oromandibular dystonia syndrome (Brueghel's syndrome). *J. Neurol. Neurosurg. Psychiatry*, **39**, 1204

10 Zeman, W. (1970). Pathology of the torsion dystonias (dystonia musculorum deformans). *Neurology (Minneap.)*, **20**, 79

11 Marsden, C. D. and Harrison, M. J. G. (1974). Idiopathic torsion dystonia (dystonia musculorum deformans); a review of forty-two patients. *Brain*, **97**, 793

12 Geller, M., Kaplan, B. and Christoff, N. (1974). Dystonic symptoms in children. *J. Am. Med. Assoc.*, **229**, 1755

13 Geller, M., Kaplan, B. and Christoff, N. (1976). Treatment of dystonic symptoms with carbamazepine. In Eldridge, R. and Fahn, S. (eds.) *Dystonia, Advances in Neurology*. Vol. 14, pp. 403–410 (New York: Raven press)

14 Isgreen, W. P., Fahn, S., Barrett, R. E., Snyder, S. R. and Chutorian, A. M. (1976). Carbamazepine in torsion dystonia. In Eldridge, R. and Fahn, S. (eds.) *Dystonia, Advances in Neurology*. Vol. 14, pp. 411–416 (New York: Raven Press)

15 Langdon, R. (1976). In Eldridge, R. and Fahn, S. (eds.) *Dystonia, Advances in Neurology*. Vol. 14, pp. 418–419 (New York: Raven Press)

16 Coleman, M. (1976). In Eldridge, R. and Fahn, S. (eds.) *Dystonia, Advances in Neurology*. Vol. 14, pp. 417 (New York: Raven Press)

17 Marsden, C. D. (1979). Treatment of torsion dystonia. A review based upon the experience of management of 259 cases. (In preparation)

18 Mena, I., Court, J., Fuenzaldia, S., Papavasiliou, P. S. and Cotzias, G. C. (1970). Modification of chronic manganese poisoning—treatment with L-DOPA or 5-OH tryptophan. *N. Engl. J. Med.*, **282**, 5

19 Coleman, M. P. and Barnet, A. (1969). L-dopa reversal of muscular spasm, vomiting and insomnia in a patient with an atypical form of familial dystonia. *Trans. Am. Neurol. Assoc.*, **94**, 91

20 Coleman, M. (1970). Preliminary remarks on the L-dopa therapy of dystonia. *Neurology (Minneap.)*, **20**, 114

21 Chase, T. N. (1970). Biochemical and pharmalogic studies of dystonia. *Neurology (Minneap.)*, **20**, 122

22 Mandell, S. (1970). Treatment of dystonia with L-dopa and haloperidol. *Neurology (Minneap.)*, **20**, 103

23 Barrett, R. E., Yahr, M. D. and Duvoisin, R. C. (1970). Torsion dystonia and spasmodic torticollis—results of treatment with L-dopa. *Neurology (Minneap.)*, **20**, 107

24 Barbeau, A. (1976). In Eldridge, R. and Fahn, S. (eds.) *Dystonia, Advances in Neurology*. Vol. 14, pp. 421 (New York: Raven Press)

25 Rajput, A. H. (1973). Levodopa in dystonia musculorum deformans. *Lancet*, **1**, 432

26 Hongladarom, T. (1973). Levodopa in dystonia musculorum deformans. *Lancet*, **1**, 1114

27 Eldridge, R., Kanter, W. and Koerber, T. (1973). Levodopa in dystonia. *Lancet*, **2**, 1027

28 Cooper, I. S. (1972), Levodopa-induced dystonia. *Lancet*, **2**, 1317

29 Segawa, M., Ohmi, K. and Itoh, S. (1971). Childhood basal ganglia disease with remarkable response to L-DOPA, 'hereditary basal ganglia disease with marked diurnal fluctuation'. *Therapy*, **24**, 667

30 Segawa, M., Hosaka, A., Miyagawa, F., Nomura, Y. and Imai, H. (1976). Hereditary progressive dystonia with marked diurnal fluctuation. In Eldridge, R. and Fahn, S. (eds.) *Dystonia, Advances in Neurology*. Vol. 14, pp. 215–233 (New York: Raven Press)

31 Braham, J. and Sarova-Pinhas, I. (1973). Apomorphine in dystonia musculorum deformans. *Lancet*, **2**, 432

32 Swash, M., Roberts, A. H., Zakko, H. and Heathfield, K. W. G. (1972). Treatment of involuntary movement disorders with tetrabenazine. *J. Neurol. Neurosurg. Psychiatry*, **35**, 186

33 Cooper, I. S. (1970). Neurosurgical treatment of dystonia. *Neurology (Minneap.)*, **20**, 133

34 Cooper, I. S. (1976a). Dystonia: surgical approaches to treatment and physiologic implications. In Yahr, M. D. (ed.) *The Basal Ganglia*, pp. 369–383 (New York: Raven Press)

35 Cooper, I. S. (1976b). 20-year follow up study of the neurosurgical treatment of dystonia musculorum deformans. In Eldridge, R. and Fahn, S. (eds.) *Dystonia, Advances in Neurology*. Vol. 14, pp. 423–447 (New York: Raven Press)

36 Markham, C. H. and Rand, R. W. (1961). Physiological and anatomical influences on dystonia. *Trans. Am. Neurol. Assoc.*, **86**, 135

37 Samotokin, B. A. and Bulgakov, N. B. (1964). Stereotaxic operations in the treatment of Parkinson's disease and someother extrapyramidal hyperkinesia. *Vesten. Khir.*, **95**, 59

38 Voityna, S. V. and Kandel, E. I. (1966). Clinical picture and surgical treatment of dystonia musculorum deformans (torsional). *Vop. Nierokhir.*, **30**, 23

39 Laponogov, O. A. (1969). Immediate results of stereotaxic operations in the treatment of extrapyramidal hyperkinesias. *Vop. Nierokhir.*, **33**, 12

40 Hankinson, J. (1969). Stereotaxic surgery. In Brain, R. and Wilkinson, M. (eds.) *Recent Advances in Neurology and Neuropsychiatry*. Vol. 8, pp. 147–174 (London: J. & A. Churchill)

41 Eldridge, R., Riklan, M. and Cooper, I. S. (1969). The limited role of psychotherapy in torsion dystonia. *J. Am. Med. Assoc.*, **210**, 705

42 Korein, J. and Brudny, J. (1976). Integrated EMG feedback in the management of spasmodic torticollis and focal dystonia: a prospective study of 80 patients. In Yahr, M. D. (ed.) *The Basal Ganglia*, pp. 385–424 (New York: Raven Press)

43 Korein, J., Brudny, J., Grynbaum, B., Sachs-Frankel, G., Weisinger, M. and Levidow, L. (1976). Sensory feedback therapy of spasmodic torticollis and dystonia; results in treatment of 55 patients. In Eldridge, R. and Fahn, S. (eds.) *Dystonia, Advances in Neurology*. Vol. 14, pp. 375–402 (New York: Raven Press)

44 Ansari, K. A., Webster, D. and Manning, N. (1972). Spasmodic torticollis and L-dopa. *Neurology (Minneap.)*, **22**, 670

45 Shaw, K. M., Hunter, K. R. and Stern, G. M. (1972). Medical treatment of spasmodic torticollis. *Lancet*, **1**, 1399

46 Gilbert, G. J. (1972). Medical treatment of spasmodic torticollis. *Arch. Neurol.*, **27**, 503

47 Gilbert, G. J. (1972). Haloperidol in spasmodic torticollis. *Lancet*, **2**, 234

48 West, H. H. (1977). Treatment of spasmodic torticollis with amantadine: a double-blind study. *Neurology (Minneap.)*, **27**, 198

49 Couch, J. R. (1976). In Eldridge, R. and Fahn, S. (eds.) *Dystonia, Advances in Neurology*. Vol. 14, p. 419. (New York: Raven Press)

50 Tolosa, E. S. (1978). Modification of tardive dyskinesia and spasmodic torticollis by apomorphine. *Arch. Neurol.*, **35**, 459

51 Lees, A., Shaw, K. M. and Stern, G. M. (1976). Bromocryptine and spasmodic torticollis. *Br. Med. J.*, **1**, 1343

52 Couper-Smartt, J. (1973). Lithium in spasmodic torticollis. *Lancet*, **2**, 741

53 Matthews, W. B., Beasley, P., Parry-Jones, W. and Garland, G. (1978). Spasmodic torticollis: a combined clinical study. *J. Neurol. Neurosurg. Psychiatry*, **41**, 485

54 Meares, R. (1971). Natural history of spasmodic torticollis, and effect of surgery. *Lancet*, **2**, 149

55 Cooper, I. S. (1964). Effect of thalamic lesions on torticollis. *N. Engl. J. Med.*, **70**, 967

56 Dandy, W. E. (1930). Operation for treatment of spasmodic torticollis. *Arch. Surg.*, **20**, 1021

57 Cooper, I. S. (1976c). In Eldridge, R. and Fahn, S. (eds.) *Dystonia, Advances in Neurology.* Vol. 14, p. 449. (New York: Raven Press)

58 Sorensen, B. F. and Hamby, W. B. (1966). Spasmodic torticollis: results in 71 surgically treated patients. *Neurology (Minneap.)*, **16**, 867

59 Walsh, L. (1976). Surgical treatment of spasmodic torticollis. *Proc. Inst. Neurol. Madras*, **6**, 36

60 Bertrand, C., Molina-Negro, P. and Martinez, S. N. (1978). Combined stereotactic and peripheral surgical approach for spasmodic torticollis. *Proceedings of 7th Symposium of the World Society for Stereotaxic and Functional Neurosurgery*, Sao Paulo.

61 Cleeland, C. S. (1973). Behavioral technics in the modification of spasmodic torticollis. *Neurology (Minneap.)*, **23**, 1241

62 Ferguson, D. (1971). An Australian study of telegraphist's cramp. *Br. J. Ind. Med.*, **28**, 280

63 Sylvester, J. D. and Liversedge, L. A. (1960). Treatment of writer's cramp. In Eysenck, H. J. (ed.) *Behaviour Therapy and Neuroses*, p. 334, (Oxford: Pergamon Press)

64 Crisp, A. H. and Moldofsky, H. (1965). A psychosomatic study of writer's cramp. *Br. J. Psychiatry*, **111**, 841

65 Moldofsky, H. (1971). Occupational cramp. *J. Psychosom. Res.*, **15**, 439

66 Bindman, E. and Tibbetts, R. W. (1977). Writer's cramp: a rational approach to treatment. *Br. J. Psychiatry*, **131**, 143

67 Gurdjian, E. S. and Williams, H. W. (1928). Surgical treatment of intractable cases of blepharospasm. *J. Am. Med. Assoc.*, **91**, 2053

68 Fox, S. A. (1951). Relief of intractable blepharospasm. *Am. J. Ophthalmol.*, **34**, 1351

69 Reynolds, D. H., Smith, J. L. and Walsh, T. J. (1967). Differential section of the facial nerve for blepharospasm. *Trans. Am. Acad. Ophthalmol. Otolaryngol.*, **71**, 656

70 Coles, W. H. (1973). Essential blepharospasm. *South. Med. J.*, **66**, 1407

71 Aminoff, M. J., Dedo, H. H. and Izdebski, K. (1978). Clinical aspects of spasmodic dysphonia. *J. Neurol. Neurosurg. Psychiatry*, **41**, 361

72 Dedo, H. H. (1976). Recurrent laryngeal nerve section for spastic dysphonia. *Ann. Otol. Rhinol. Laryngol.*, **85**, 451

73 Lance, J. W. (1977). Familial paroxysmal dystonic choreoathetosis and its differentiation from related syndromes. *Ann. Neurol.*, **2**, 285

74 Battista, A. F., Goldstein, M., Miyomoto, T. and Matsumoto, Y. (1976). Effect of centrally acting drugs on experimental torticollis in monkeys. In Eldridge, R. and Fahn, S. (eds.) *Dystonia, Advances in Neurology.* Vol. 14, pp. 329–337 (New York: Raven Press)

75 Crossman, A. R. and Sambrook, M. A. (1978). Experimental torticollis in the monkey produced by unilateral 6-hydroxydopamine brain lesions. *Brain Res.*, **149**, 498

76 Duchen, L. W. (1976). Dystonia musculorum: an inherited disease of the nervous system in the mouse. In Eldridge, R. and Fahn, S. (eds.) *Dystonia, Advances in Neurology.* Vol. 14, pp. 353–365 (New York: Raven Press)

77 Barbeau, A., Inoue, N. and Cloutier, T. (1976). Role of manganese in dystonia. In Eldridge, R. and Fahn, S. (eds.) *Dystonia, Advances in Neurology.* Vol. 14, pp. 339–351. (New York: Raven Press)

78 Meldrum, B. S., Anlezark, G. M. and Marsden, C. D. (1977). Acute dystonia as an idiosyncratic response to neuroleptics in baboons. *Brain*, **100**, 313

79 Marsden, C. D. and Jenner, P. (1980). Pathophysiological mechanisms of extrapyramidal side-effects of neuroleptic drugs. *Psychol. Med.*, **10**, 55

6

Treatment of tics and Tourette syndrome

A. K. Shapiro, E. Shapiro and R. D. Sweet

DEFINITION OF TIC

Tics are defined as involuntary contractions of functionally related groups of skeletal muscles in one or more parts of the body, involuntary noises or involuntary words. These symptoms are brief, rapid, sudden, unexpected, repetitive, inappropriate, stereotypic, irresistible, and of variable intensity; occur at irregular intervals; and usually involve a number of muscles in their normal synergistic relationships. Symptoms may be stable for periods but usually change spontaneously over time, decrease during non-anxious distraction or concentration, disappear during sleep, and increase with tension. Tics can be voluntarily suppressed for a variable period of time, but the effort causes an increase in tension and the symptoms eventually must be discharged.

Tic disorders may be transient or chronic. There are at least three tic conditions which should be differentiated. It is probable that tic disorders represent a continuum from the mild transient tic of childhood to the most complex, severe multiple tics of Gilles de la Tourette syndrome.

CLASSIFICATION OF TIC DISORDERS

Transient tic disorders

'Transient tic disorder of childhood' is the most common tic condition. The symptoms are usually called 'habit tics' by paediatricians, and parents are advised to ignore them as they will go away in time. The onset of the symptoms is in childhood or early adolescence and the duration is at least 1 month but usually not more than 1 year. The most common movement is an eye blink or a facial tic. However, the whole head, torso or limbs may be involved. One or more tics may occur simultaneously, sequentially or at different times. Vocal tics occur infrequently. The symptoms can be voluntarily suppressed for minutes to hours and the intensity can vary over weeks or months.

Chronic motor tic

The age of onset is in childhood or after 40. When the onset is in adult life the tic tends to be limited to a single muscle group. The major symptoms are usually motor. Vocal tics occur infrequently, are not loud or intense and are often caused by thoracic, abdominal or diaphragmatic contractions.

The intensity and type of symptoms tend to be constant during the course of the illness and the symptoms can be voluntarily suppressed for minutes to hours. The course of the illness is life-long.

Chronic multiple tic or Tourette syndrome

Chronic multiple tic or Tourette syndrome has its onset between 2 and 15 years, similar to the age of onset for transient tic disorder. The tics usually involve the head and frequently other parts of the body, torso, and limbs. Multiple vocal tics are always present. They include various complicated sounds, words, or coprolalia (involuntary utterance of obscene words), which occur in 60% of patients. Other features of this disorder may include echolalia (repetition of another's last words or phrases), palilalia (repetition of one's own last words or phrases), echokinesis (imitation of the movements of others), and mental coprolalia (involuntary obscene thoughts). The movements can be voluntarily suppressed for minutes to hours. The number, type and intensity of symptoms varies over weeks or months and the illness is characterized by a fluctuating, waxing and waning, clinical course.

Typically the first symptom is a single tic, most frequently an eye blink. Initial symptoms also include tongue protrusion, squatting, sniffing, hopping, skipping, throat clearing, stuttering, sounds, words, or coprolalia. In many patients the initial symptoms are multiple and include combinations of motor and vocal tics. New symptoms are added to or replace old symptoms over months or years. Tourette syndrome is usually chronic and life-long.

AETIOLOGICAL CONCEPTS ABOUT TOURETTE SYNDROME

History of aetiological concepts

In the past, neurologists did not differentiate among tics, dystonias, writer's cramp, nail biting, chorea, enuresis, compulsions and so on. Trousseau[1] described complex multiple tics with vocalizations and echolalia but referred to them as a sub-order of chorea.

The first recorded history of a patient with Tourette syndrome was Itard's[2] description of the Marquis de Dampierre. She was subsequently seen by Charcot and discussed by his pupil Gilles de la Tourette[3] in a paper describing nine patients in 1885. Tourette characterized the illness as consisting of generalized motor tics and noises, always accompanied by echolalia and often by coprolalia. Tourette emphasized echolalia because he did not differentiate this syndrome from the jumping Frenchmen, Latah and Myriachit, in which echolalia was a prominent symptom. Echolalia occurs in only 35% of patients[4]. Tourette was rewarded by Charcot for his classic description of Tourette syndrome by having the syndrome named after him.

In this early period between 1825 and 1900, tics were thought to be the result of degenerative hereditary antecedents and family backgrounds were frequently characterized as alcoholic, epileptic, and so on.

The aetiological emphasis shifted from hereditary antecedents to the mental or psychic state of the patient in an important treatise on tics by Meige and Feindel in 1902[5] which was translated into English in 1907. Ticqueurs were described as infantile and emotionally unstable. Tourette syndrome was differentiated from tics as a separate illness of a more morbid nature and could result in insanity.

The emphasis on a psychological aetiology for tics and Tourette syndrome then dominated the literature for 70 years. Ferenczi[6] labelled the illness a narcissistic disorder. Abraham[7] diagnosed and emphasized an anal-sadistic conflict. Beginning in 1943, Mahler and her colleagues[8] published a series of papers, which described tics as the expression of an emotional conflict between gratification of and defense against instinctual impulses attributed to parental restrictions of motor restlessness in constitutionally predisposed children.

Psychopathology was believed to exist not only in the patient but in the family as well. Kanner[9] felt that tics were caused by rigid and overdemanding parents. Bruch and Thurm[10] and Dunlap[11] blamed family tensions. Zausmer[12] believed that the crucial psychological factor was the disturbed and anxiety-producing mother–child relationship.

In the 1950s there was an upsurge of interest in tics and Tourette syndrome characterized by the collection and study of a large number of patients[12-17]. Although some authors were still concerned with psycho-pathological causes others became interested in organic factors. Pasamanick[13] attributed the aetiology of tics to cerebral injury since tics are frequently associated with hyperactivity and epidemic encephalitis and that more males than females have tics.

Current concepts and study of aetiology

In 1968[18] we postulated that tics and Tourette syndrome are caused by a primary organic disease of the central nervous system and were unrelated to unconscious psychological, familial or other psychological conflicts. The evidence for this conclusion is supported by studies described in detail in our book on Tourette syndrome[19].

We found higher male to female ratio similar to other organic conditions such as infant mortality, minimal brain dysfunction (MBD), dystonia musculorum deformans, childhood autism, and other organic illnesses. A higher than expected frequency of organic stigmata was found in patients suggesting an organic aetiology: factors such as 42% of patients with organic signs on the Bender-Gestalt test, 68% with overall ratings of organicity on psychological testing, 22.8% with left-handedness or ambi-dexterity, 57.1% with soft signs of neurological abnormality, 46.8% (about 25% of adults and 71% of children) with EEG abnormalities, and 57.9% with symptoms of MBD. Many of these CNS abnormalities are found in children with signs and symptoms of MBD. In addition, the low prevalence of Tourette syndrome in the population suggests a specific physiological factor since most people do not respond to psychological, social or cultural stress with Tourette syndrome.

We conducted a controlled study of the popular psychodynamic formu-lation that tics and other symptoms of Tourette syndrome were the symbolic expression of a massive, unconscious conflict about the expression of hos-tility and aggression which resulted in reaction formation, obsessions, compulsions, symptom substitution and ultimately revealed an underlying psychotic process. Our expectations were confirmed by our results that psychopathological states such as hysteria, inhibition of aggression, obsess-ive–compulsive traits, schizophrenia or other psychoses did not characterize patients with Tourette syndrome more than a matched outpatient psychi-atric sample.

The introduction of psychopharmacological drugs in the 1950s led to the successful use of haloperidol in the treatment of Tourette syndrome. The effectiveness of haloperidol, a known dopamine blocker, without symptom substitution, contributes additional support for an organic aetiology for Tourette syndrome and gave new direction to the treatment and study of the neurophysiology of Tourette syndrome.

TREATMENT

History of treatment

Almost every medicinal, surgical and other therapeutic modality was used at one time or another to treat tics and Tourette syndrome without any success. These included: conium, bromides, chloral hydrate, opium, morphine, laudanum, the basic extract, atropine, curare, chloroform, ether, zinc, valerianate, valerian, gelsemium, quinine, cannibus indica, arsenic, strong mustard plasters, cocaine, kola, coca, antipyrine, sulfanol, lecithin, cautery to the vertebral column, cold, hot and tepid douches, body packs and warm fomentations.

Surgical treatment included elongation, section or ligature of the spinal accessory nerve, resection of the trigeminal nerve, spinofacial anastamoses and tonsillectomy. Other treatment included: rhythmic traction of the tongue, thoracic compression, phrenic electrization, static sparks, diet, nutrition, general hygiene, hydrotherapy, morning and evening bath followed by energetic friction of the skin, massage, electricity, and waking and hypnotic suggestion.

In addition, techniques similar to present day behavioural manipulations included: systematized mental discipline, forced immobility, motor discipline, training antagonists, respiratory drill or gymnastics, systematized exercises, mirror drill, systematic discipline, isolation with bed rest and encouragement.

Table 1 Recasting of the data summarizing the results of treatment collected by Abuzzahab and Anderson (1973)

Treatment modality	No. of treatment trials[a]	Reported improvement					
		For less than 6 months or of unknown duration		For more than 6 months		Total improvement	
		n	%	n	%	n	%
Psychological[b]	228	60	26.3	21	9.2	81	35.3
Somatic[c]	41	6	15.0	3	7.3	9	22.0
Chemotherapy[d]	155	24	15.0	7	4.5	31	20.0
Antipsychotic drugs[e]	81	21	26.0	18	22.2	39	48.1
Haloperidol	63	14	22.0	42	66.7	56	88.9
Total	568	125	22.0	91	16.0	21.6	38.0

[a] Because many patients were treated with several treatment modalities, the total number of patients = 430 and the total treatment trials = 568.

[b] Psychotherapy, hypnotherapy, hydrotherapy, isolation, sleep therapy, bed rest, behaviour therapy, physiotherapy.

[c] Lobotomy, leukotomy, thalamotomy, CO_2 inhalation therapy, shock therapy.

[d] Sedatives: Chloral hydrate, ethchlorynol, bromides, barbiturates, meprobamate, ethanol, chlordiazepoxide, diazepam, oxazepam, hydroxyzine, methaqualone, arsenic, paraldehyde. Antidepressants: imipramine, amitriptyline, nortriptyline, doxepin, protriptyline, isocarboxazid, phenelzine, iproniazid. Stimulants: amphetamine, d-amphetamine, methamphetamine, methylphenidate. Anticonvulsants: diphenylhydantoin, primidone, trimethadione, ethosuximide, paramethadione. Antiparkinsonians: belladonna, trihexyphenidyl, benztropine mesylate, orphenadrine, diphenhydramamine, amantadine, levodopa.

[e] Antipsychotics: chlorpromazine, promazine, triflupromazine, thioridazine, prochlorperazine, trifluoperazine, chlorprothixene, fluphenazine, perphenazine, thiothixene, piperacetazine, promethazine, reserpine, rauwolfia alkaloids.

During the early twentieth century, neurologists increasingly began to attribute disorders of unknown origin to psychological conflicts. This trend snowballed and culminated in a massive over-psychologizing in medicine, and has resulted in over 160 different systems of psychotherapy[20], and the use of treatment for tics and Tourette syndrome which vary from psychoanalysis to EST[19].

It was inevitable that psychopharmaceuticals would be tried in Tourette syndrome after their introduction in 1954. In 1961, haloperidol, a buty-rophenone antipsychotic drug, was used successfully in Europe in single patients with Tourette syndrome by Seignot[21] and Caprini and Melotti[22]. In 1963, Challas and Brauer[23] reported successful use of haloperidol in two patients; Shapiro and Shapiro[18] described similar results for three patients in 1968 and 34 in 1973[24]. Since that time, haloperidol has been used successfully in hundreds of patients[19].

The literature on treatment was comprehensively reviewed by Abuzzahab and Anderson[25] who described 430 patients who had received 568 treatments of various types. The data was recast by us[19] in Table 1.

The last column summarizes the percentage of improvement for various treatments after 6 months. Six month follow-up is necessary for reliable and valid evaluation, because of the spontaneous waxing, waning and fluctuation of symptoms in Tourette syndrome. This is illustrated by comparing improvement reported at less than 6 months with more than 6 months follow-up. The percentage improvement is the same or decreases at 6 months for all treatment modalities except haloperidol. The percentage improvement after 6 months is 66.7% for haloperidol compared to 9.2% for all psychological treatments and 12% for psychotherapy alone. The data indicates that haloperidol is strongly, but antipsychotic drugs are moderately, associated with clinical improvement for the symptoms of Tourette syndrome.

CHEMOTHERAPY OF TOURETTE SYNDROME

The pharmacologic action of haloperidol in blocking dopamine receptor sites, and its success in decreasing tics in Tourette syndrome, stimulated us to study classes of drugs known to have their major pharmacologic action on specific neurotransmitters. This strategy may help elucidate the neuropharmacology of Tourette syndrome and contribute to the development of new chemotherapy for the illness.

Dopamine antagonists

Haloperidol (Haldol)

Studies of treatment with haloperidol. The efficacy of haloperidol in the treatment of Tourette syndrome was supported by several retrospective clinical studies[18,19,24,26].

We reviewed the treatment of the first 80 patients treated by us. Their ages ranged from 6 to 67 years and they were evaluated an average of 2.9 years (range 7 months to 8.5 years) after initial evaluation[19]. Sixty-two patients were on medication, 11 had discontinued medication, one had mild symptoms not requiring treatment, 4 had complete remission of symptoms for more than 1 year and two were deceased—both suicides.

Of the sixty-two patients on medication, 59 were on haloperidol alone or combined with another medication. Eighty per cent of these patients had an average decrease in symptoms of 80% whereas patients who were not on medication ($n = 12$) had an average decrease of only 24.3%. This difference was significant at the $p < 0.001$ level.

The study also confirmed an earlier finding that patients continued to improve over time with treatment[24]. The median improvement was 80% for patients treated less than 2 years, 85.8% for patients treated 2–4 years and 94% for patients treated more than 4 years. The variability for improvement also decreases over time so that improvement after 4 years for 12 patients was never lower than 70%.

We have treated over 600 patients with haloperidol, some for as long as 14 years. Many individual patients were given placebos, in single-blind clinical studies, and many more were clinically evaluated with and without medication as part of clinical management. Although long-term double-blind studies have not been done, we believe that haloperidol is the drug of choice for the treatment of Tourette syndrome.

Current treatment regime. Our initial treatment regimen employed high dosages of haloperidol (up to 500 mg daily) to control 100% of the symptoms followed by stepwise lowering of the dosage to a maintenance level to achieve maximum benefit with minimum side-effects. Our current treatment is to titrate the dosage upward in very small increments to the same end-point, and is described in detail elsewhere[19].

Symptomatic control can be achieved within 1 day if necessary by rapid hourly oral or parenteral increases of haloperidol. Rapid treatment, which usually requires hospitalization, is rarely necessary, however, and most patients are treated intially with 0.25 mg of haloperidol and 0.5 mg of benztropine mesylate (Cogentin) – both medications taken at bedtime. Haloperidol is increased 0.25 mg every fifth day and reaches a steady blood level state in about 4 days. Benztropine mesylate is used initially at a daily night-time dosage of 0.5 mg to control acute dystonia which occurs in 9% of patients and akinesia which occurs in about 25% of patients during the first 2 weeks of treatment. It may be increased later on in therapy to control extrapyramidal effects and usually can be discontinued when these adverse side-effects disappear. Haloperidol induces enzyme inhibition early in treatment and enzyme stimulation later in treatment. Because of these pharmacodynamic effects, genetic differences in the metabolism of the drug and the spontaneous variation of symptomatology, treatment is empirical and requires constant management. Haloperidol does not cure tics or Tourette syndrome, it merely suppresses symptoms. It works as well in patients with mild or severe symptoms and acute or chronic illness.

Tolerance to haloperidol does not develop and exacerbation or decrease of symptoms is due to spontaneous waxing, waning and fluctuation of symptoms which are characteristic of the syndrome.

The main indication for treatment is cosmetic reduction of symptoms to prevent gross muscular dysregulation, vocal outbursts and to minimize adverse psychosocial effects on the patient from the environment.

Patients are taught to slowly vary the dosage of medication according to the severity of their symptoms and are usually evaluated every 6 months, during subsequent chronic treatment.

Based on extensive experience, we recommend that the treating physician should be thoroughly familiar with the use of psychopharmaceuticals and knowledgeable about and experienced with, the treatment of tics and Tourette syndrome.

Adverse effects of treatment. The pattern of side-effects differs among patients. Early side-effects may include acute dystonia, akinesia, akathesia, xerostoma and mild gastrointestinal upset. Other side-effects which may occur with increased dosage include mydriasis, loss of accommodation for near vision, constipation, increased appetite, weight gain and extrapyramidal side-effects.

Cognitive impairment, as well as the loss of motivation or drug-induced feelings of depression, are major limitations to the use of high dosages of haloperidol. Antiparkinson and stimulant drugs help reduce their intensity.

Tardive dyskinesia, an unfortunate complication of treatment with all antipsychotic drugs, appears to be related to chronic and high dosages of these drugs. Only one patient treated with haloperidol for Tourette syndrome has been reported in the literature: a 15-year-old psychotic boy with Tourette syndrome was treated for 2 years with 50 mg of haloperidol, 100 mg of amitriptyline and 2 mg of trihexyphenidyl[27]. In the dosages used by us (mean 5.0 mg, range 1.5 to 15 mg) none of our patients have developed tardive dyskinesia. Although we have observed that many patients develop minor fibrillation of the muscles of the tongue and slight mannerism of the hands, none of these symptoms progress to tardive dyskinesia. The tendency in the literature to designate these symptoms as incipient or overt tardive dyskinesia is a grievous error in our opinion.

We have observed only two patients with withdrawal dyskinesia, both treated elsewhere. A 22-year-old male who had been treated with 60 mg of haloperidol for about a year, and a 13-year-old male who had been treated with 30 mg of haloperidol for several months, both developed tardive dyskinesia, as well as severe extrapyramidal effects and cognitive impairment. The dosages for both patients were reduced to 6 mg of haloperidol; all traces of dyskinesia and other adverse effects disappeared in 1 month and tic symptoms were controlled 80–90%.

Blood levels. To monitor treatment more effectively, 23 haloperidol blood levels, using a specific radioimmunoassay[28,29], were obtained for 12 male and four female patients who ranged in age from 9 to 28 years and had been treated with haloperidol for up to 4 years at dosages ranging from 0.5 to

71 mg/day (median 3.0 mg/day). Nine patients were excluded from the analysis for the following reasons: five patients ingested haloperidol 2–7 h before blood was drawn, two patients were not taking haloperidol, two determinations were done for one patient who was on 30 and 71 mg of haloperidol. For the remaining 14 patients, blood was drawn an average of 14.4 h after ingesting haloperidol (SD = 2.1, range 11–18), the average age was 15.8 (SD = 5.1, range 10–28), average weight was 28.4 kg (SD = 28.9, range 31.8–86.4), average daily dosage of haloperidol was 2.96 mg (SD = 2.04, range 0.5–7.0), average mg/kg was 0.06 (SD = 0.05, range 0.001–0.192); the average blood level was 3.8 ng/ml haloperidol (SD = 2.85, range 1.0–10.5). The correlation coefficient between mg/kg haloperidol and blood level was 0.81 ($p < 0.001$) for the 14 patients and 0.98 ($p < 0.001$) for the total sample of 23 patients. However, for the 14 patients treated with therapeutic dosages of haloperidol, the amount of ingested haloperidol or blood level was unrelated to therapeutic response, or adverse side-effects, sex, age, weight, chronicity of illness and length of treatment. The minimum effective blood level of haloperidol is about 2.0 ng/ml.

Although these results indicate that blood levels are not useful currently for monitoring treatment with haloperidol, further refinement and study of this technique is highly desirable.

Pimozide (Orap)

Pimozide, or diphenylbutyliperidine, is reported to be a specific dopamine blocker.

Three reports have been found in the literature about the effect of pimozide on tics. Pimozide was reported successful in the treatment of 186 children aged 5–15 with various behaviour problems including tics, the mean effective dosage reported as 1–2 mg per day[30]. In a clinical report of 33 children with various types of tics, 22 (67%) were described as cured, four (12%) improved and seven (21%) failures[31].

Pimozide was compared with haloperidol and placebo in an acute double-blind cross-over study of five patients by Ross and Moldofsky[32]. The dosage of pimozide or haloperidol was increased 2 mg every other day to a total dosage of 12 mg over a period of 12 days. Both medications significantly decreased tic symptoms but pimozide was reported to result in significantly fewer complaints of tiredness. Similar results are described for about 25 patients who were treated clinically with pimozide for more than a year[33].

These results stimulated us to clinically evaluate pimozide in patients with inadequate responses to or adverse effects from haloperidol. We treated 16 patients with dosages varying from 4 to 60 mg/day. The average dosage was 8 mg/day—about two to three times higher than equivalent clinical dosages of haloperidol. Six patients had a better response (higher therapeutic to toxic ratio) with haloperidol, five with pimozide and there was no difference between the two medications in five patients. Therapeutic and adverse effects, including lethargy, sedation, akinesia and cognitive impairment, were similar in general for both drugs. Our clinical results suggest that some patients have a better response to pimozide than haloperidol and that pimozide should be tried in patients with inadequate response to haloperidol and other drugs. Pimozide has not been approved for use in the United States, although it is approved in Canada and many other countries, and therefore requires an IND from the Food and Drug Administration (FDA) for use in the United States.

Penfluridol (Semap)

Penfluridol, a diphenylbutylpiperidine derivative, is a long lasting medication with a duration of 5–7 days and is thought to be a more specific dopamine blocker without norepinephrine or serotonin blocking effects. It has been reported to have fewer side-effects in general than similar drugs[34], particularly less akinesia[35], and its extrapyramidal effects are readily controlled with anticholinergic agents. Potential advantages of penfluridol include oral administration, ease of administration, especially in children, and reported infrequent adverse side-effects compared with other antipsychotic drugs.

We clinically treated a 10-year-old male Tourette patient, previously treated with haloperidol and pimozide, at a dosage of 60 mg of penfluridol twice weekly. Although symptoms improved 85% and side-effects were minimal, it is difficult to compare the results with the other dopamine antagonists because of frequent spontaneous variations in this patient's clinical course. Further evaluation of penfluridol is warranted, especially in patients with inadequate responses to haloperidol. These clinical evaluations are currently in progress. Penfluridol, a non-approved drug in the United States and Canada, requires an IND from the FDA for use in the United States. Mammary and pancreatic tumours have been reported with chronic high dosages in 2-year-old rats.

Phenothiazines

Chlorpromazine. Chlorpromazine has been reported as both effective and ineffective for the treatment of Tourette syndrome[36–40]. We recently saw a patient successfully treated for a prolonged period by another physician with chlorpromazine. However, because of ocular opacities, chlorpromazine was discontinued and the patient has been successfully switched to haloperidol. Another patient developed 'fog states' on haloperidol and was successfully treated with an initial dosage of 900 mg and subsequent maintenance dosage of 300 mg of chlorpromazine.

Mesoridazine. Mesoridazine has been tried in seven Tourette patients for as long as 6 months, without marked or sustained improvement.

Other Phenothiazines. Many other phenothiazines have been used, including fluphenazine. Clinical reports indicate they are less useful than haloperidol, although controlled, comparative studies have not been done[19,25].

Miscellaneous dopamine antagonists

Tetrabenazine (Nitoman). Tetrabenazine, a benzoquinolizine derivative, impairs catecholamine storage selectively in the CNS. We gave tetrabenazine up to 300 mg/day to 14 Tourette patients. Initial improvement occurred in 12 patients, in association with sedation and akinesia, but the improvement was not sustained after 2 months. Five patients discontinued medication because of incapacitating side-effects. Only one patient, previously treated with 40 mg/day of haloperidol, has been successfully treated with tetrabenazine at a dosage of 75–100 mg/day for over 5 years. Recent substitution of 0.1 mg/day of reserpine is reported by the patient to work as well as tetrabenazine. However, we have not been able to observe a clinically meaningful difference in tic frequency on the above medications or when the patient is not on any medication.

Our impression is that improvement on tetrabenazine is secondary to the sedation and akinesia that occurs with initial treatment and that improvement is not sustained after the disappearance of these adverse side-effects.

Clozapine. Clozapine, an antipsychotic, which blocks dopamine receptors and has few extrapyramidal effects and no reports of tardive dyskinesia, was evaluated in a double-blind cross-over study over 4 to 7 weeks in seven patients at a dosage varying between 8 and 10 mg/kg per day[41]. There were no significant therapeutic effects. These negative results are inconsistent with the dopamine hypothesis for Tourette syndrome, and it is significant that six of the seven patients had a previous good response to haloperidol. Adverse side-effects included drowsiness, marked somnolence, salivation and leukopenia.

α-Methylparatyrosine. Alpha methylparatyrosine, which inhibits tyrosine hydroxylase, the rate limiting enzyme in catecholamine synthesis, was administered to six Tourette patients at a maximum dosage of 3000 mg/day[42]. Improvement of tic symptoms was obtained in three patients, especially the dystonic neck and trunk movements of two. There was no improvement in three patients. The major limitation of this medication is its adverse side-effects. Microscopic, needle-like crystals were observed in the urine of four patients, and the creatine clearance of two patients fell to 50–60 ml/min when crystalluria appeared. In addition, akinesia, akathesia, lethargy and enuresis were sufficiently pronounced to cause improved patients to discontinue medication.

Disulfiram (Antabuse). Disulfiram is an inhibitor of the enzyme dopamine–β–hydroxylase (DBH) which catalyses the conversation of dopamine to norepinephrine. Based on the theory that inhibiting DBH should decrease the concentration of norepinepherine and enhance the accumulation of dopamine, two Tourette patients were given 1.5 mg/day of disulfiram. Both patients reported an increase in tic frequency while on the medication. The increase in symptoms persisted and was not reversed when one patient stopped the medication. The second patient remained on the medication for only 4 days and increase in tics were not observed. Further studies of the effect of disulfiram is warranted by these results.

Dopamine agonists

Dihydroxyphenylalanine (Levodopa)

Levodopa, a precursor of dopamine and norepinephrine which increases brain dopamine concentration, should result in increased tic activity.

We gave three Tourette patients levodopa in increasing doses to a maximum of 3000 mg/day. At the maximum dosage of 3000 mg/day, tics in a 26-year-old man increased forcefully up to twice their original frequency. The movements, however, were choreoathetoid and dystonic and clearly different from tics. Tics in a second patient on 1000 to 1500 mg/day did not increase. A third patient on 1500 mg/day discontinued the medicine because of irritability and nausea and the effect on his tics could not be evaluated. Levodopa was also given to a 38-year-old man in doses up to 6 mg/day without increase in tics[43], although the effect of levodopa might have been mitigated by the concomitant use of 900 mg/day of chlorpromazine. Other investigators have informally described an increase of tics with the administration of levodopa, although this effect has not been documented in a well-controlled study.

The evidence of an imbalance in transmitter functions for Tourette syndrome has to be interpreted cautiously.

Apomorphine

Apomorphine, a strong dopamine agonist, was given subcutaneously by us to two Tourette patients in 0.5, 1.0 and 1.5 mg doses. Nausea was reported by both patients at the higher dose. There was a slight reduction in tic frequency. It is difficult to know if the decrease in symptoms resulted from the medication or the adverse side-effects.

Feinberg and Carroll[44] gave apomorphine subcutaneously to two Tourette patients and reported that apomorphine reduced their tics even in the presence of *d*-amphetamine. They noted a dose–response relationship since the beneficial effect occurred at a dosage low enough to avoid nausea or significant sedation.

These results suggest the possibility of an inhibitory effect on presynaptic dopamine neurons.

Piribedil

Piribedil is a putative stimulator of dopamine receptors. We gave 3 mg of piribedil intravenously to two patients. This dosage resulted in drowsiness and a slight decrease in tics. In one patient, an oral dosage of up to 160 mg/day resulted in nausea but no effect on tics.

Feinberg and Carroll[44] used piribedil in doses from 40 to 240 mg/day in two patients without effect.

Stimulants

Meyerhoff and Snyder[45] noted increased tics with *d*- compared with *l*-amphetamine in an 8-year-old girl with hyperactivity and tics. However, Feinberg and Carroll[44] reported an increase of tic frequency with both amphetamine isomers in two patients.

Although Golden[46,47] reported the onset of tics in 17 of 32 children treated with methylphenidate in a retrospective study of a selected sample, Denckla[48] reported that only 1.3% of 1520 children treated with stimulants developed tics, and that the tics disappeared in all but one patient when the drug was discontinued. We have not found a relationship between stimulants, including methylphenidate, and tics in patients given the drug before being treated with haloperidol, and we have not observed any increase in tics when it was given to decrease akinesia while on haloperidol. An occasional patient on a very high dosage of 80 to 100 mg/day began 'twitching', similar to many patients on high dosages of stimulants. Stimulants may increase tics, not because of any specific effect on catecholamine mechanisms, but merely as a non-specific stressor. Based on our experience, we do not believe that the use of stimulants can cause Tourette syndrome or will be a major problem when appropriately used in the management of side-effects caused by haloperidol. We do not see any strong contraindication for its use in children with MBD. However, further observation is warranted.

Serotonin agonists

L-5-Hydroxytryptophan (5HTP)

The serotonin agonist, L-5-hydroxytryptophan (5HTP), in combination with carbidopa, was reported to be effective in amelioration of tics and self-mutilation (tongue and lip biting) in one patient by van Woert *et al.*[49].

However, van Woert (in a personal communication) reported this medication to be ineffective in nine other patients[50] and it elicits hypomanic excitement.

L–tryptophan (LTP)

We treated two patients with L–tryptophan, an amino acid precursor of serotonin. Nausea was reported by a 46-year-old patient on 6.5 g/day but disappeared when the dosage was decreased to 5.5 g/day. The second patient, an 18-year-old boy, was evaluated in a double-blind procedure alternating placebo and LTP. He was also given MK 486 and 100 mg/day of pyridoxine. The medication had no significant effect on the tics.

Tricyclic antidepressants

Tricyclic antidepressants, which block the reuptake of serotonin in presynaptic neurons, are discussed in the section on 'Antidepressants' (see below).

Serotonin antagonists

Methysergide

Methysergide, a serotonin antagonist, in doses to 10 mg/day for 2 weeks, was given to two of our patients with Tourette syndrome. They reported an initial but unsustained reduction in tics.

Cholinergic agonists

Physostigmine

Physostigmine is an agonist of acetylcholine by inhibiting acetylcholinesterase. Physostigmine (1 mg) together with methyl scopolamine (1 mg) were given subcutaneously to five of our Tourette patients. Three patients showed no change after physostigmine and two others were mildly improved. Side-effects included abdominal cramps, lightheadedness and euphoria.

Deanol (Deaner)

Deanol, a possible generator of acetylcholine in the CNS, was given to two Tourette patients at a maximum dosage of 2 g/day without altering the frequency of tics from baseline levels. Side-effects included lightheadedness and nervousness. The addition of deanol (1200 mg/day) to perphenazine (36 mg/day) did not result in improvement of tic symptoms in another patient with Tourette syndrome[51].

Choline

Three patients were treated with choline by us. A 20-year-old male was given 40 g/day of choline as an outpatient. Tic frequency was decreased approximately 40% without side-effects but the patient discontinued using choline because of the offensive fish odour that invariably occurs. A 16-year-old male was given 1.2 g/day of choline as an in-patient but the medication induced nausea and emesis and was discontinued before an adequate clinical trial could be conducted. Choline at a dosage of 20 g/day was also ineffective in a 26-year-old patient.

Lecithin, which does not cause a fish-like odour, may be better tolerated and warrants a trial in patients with Tourette syndrome.

Cholinergic antagonists

Benztropine

Benztropine (2 mg), an antagonist of acetylcholine, was given to five of our Tourette patients subcutaneously. The tic symptoms increased briefly in three patients and markedly in one of them. One patient reported no tics for an hour after the injection and another reported no change in frequency of tics.

Antidepressants

The effects of antidepressants on tics and Tourette syndrome is unclear and contradictory. In a literature review up to 1973, antidepressants were reported as causing deterioration in 13 of 17 patients[25]. However, the antidepressants included various types of tricyclic and monoamine inhibitor drugs which have very different neuropharmacological effects. Tricyclic antidepressants differentially block presynaptic reuptake of norepinephrine (NE) or 5–hydroxytryptamine (5HT) and have little effect on dopamine (DA), and MAO inhibitors interfere with the metabolism of catecholamines and indolamines. Because it is difficult to generalize the results for different antidepressants, each drug and drug category will be discussed separately.

Tricyclic antidepressants

Imipramine (Tofranil). Imipramine is a tricyclic antidepressant with both NE and 5HT reuptake blocking properties. Two recent clinical reports describe exacerbation of Tourette syndrome by imipramine[52,53].

An 11.5-year-old male began treatment with haloperidol which successfully controlled his symptoms until the age of 13 when his symptoms exacerbated. Haloperidol (dosage not given) was withdrawn for 2 weeks and 25 mg/day imipramine was reported to exacerbate the symptoms within 2–3 days. Since symptoms usually return after discontinuing haloperidol within about 4 days to 2 weeks and occasionally 1 month[19,54], the return of symptoms could have been due to stopping haloperidol or spontaneous change in symptoms and not due to the use of imipramine.

The second patient was a 21-year-old male[53] who was treated with 8 mg/day of haloperidol with slight improvement. Imipramine, 75 mg/day, was added and both medications were continued for 1 month. The symptomatic improvement disappeared and the patient returned to his prehaloperidol symptom level. Imipramine was discontinued and the patient gradually returned to the level of improvement achieved with haloperidol. Because of inadequate clinical response, haloperidol was increased to 60 mg/day. The clinical history does not exclude the possibility that tics could have increased spontaneously or after adaptation to (akinesic or other sedative effects of) haloperidol and were only coincidentally associated with the use of imipramine.

In contrast to these reports, a 44-year-old male[55], who participated in extensive metabolic studies, was treated with varying dosages of haloperidol (1–30 mg/day), together and alternating with imipramine and placebo. The authors report that 75 mg/day of imipramine suppressed the tics although the length of the follow-up period was not reported.

Amitriptyline (Elavil). Amitriptyline is a tricyclic antidepressant with predominant 5HT reuptake blocking properties. A negative effect of amitriptyline was described for a 31-year-old male with Tourette syndrome who was being treated with 4 mg/day of haloperidol[53]. The patient became depressed and was treated with amitriptyline. His mood improved on 40–60 mg/day without effect on his tics but at a dosage of 75 mg/day, profuse hyperhidrosis developed and the tics worsened. Discontinuation of amitriptyline resulted in return to pretreatment tic levels after 2–3 days. However, the patient became depressed and was eventually hospitalized because of severe depression. The deteriorating clinical course for the patient makes it difficult to ascribe the exacerbation of tics to amitriptyline.

Chlorimipramine (Anafranil). Chlorimipramine is a non-FDA approved tricyclic antidepressant with predominant 5HT reuptake blocking effects. It was reported in a double-blind study[56] to improve 80–90% of symptoms when clinically evaluated by therapists, although there was no significant difference between active and inactive drug when evaluated by patients and symptoms did not increase when placebo was substituted for active medication.

A careful double-blind cross-over study compared chlorimipramine and desimipramine (both at a maximum dosage of 150 mg) with placebo in six patients[57]. There were no signifcant differences between active and inactive agents. Four of the six patients had previously had a good response to haloperidol.

We have used chlorimipramine (up to 300 mg, with and without halo-peridol) in eight patients without significant beneficial or deleterious clinical effects on tics.

Desimipramine (Norpramin, Pertofrane). Desimipramine is a tricyclic with predominant NE reuptake blocking properties. In a double-blind cross-over study[57], at a dosage of 150 mg/day for 4 weeks there were no significant beneficial or adverse effects. Four of the six patients had a previously good response to haloperidol.

Monoamine oxidase inhibitors. MAO inhibitors increase brain levels of NE, DA and 5HT. They have been tried by us (and others), alone or with haloperidol, without beneficial therapeutic effect or increase in tics at dosages below the toxic level.

Conclusion. We have used many antidepressants in our early clinical attempts to treat Tourette syndrome, without beneficial or deleterious effects on Tourette symptoms, except in a range which causes toxic effects. Antidepressants have also been used by us to counteract the sedative and depressant side-effects of haloperidol without beneficial effect or deleterious effects on tics when used in appropriate therapeutic dosages. However, if the dosage of the antidepressant or haloperidol or their combined use exceeds the therapeutic dosage and reaches toxic levels, the clinical condition of the patient may deteriorate. Some of the reported adverse effects may be due to the toxic dosages caused by combining haloperidol and an antidepressant, since both drugs inhibit each other's metabolism, and result in potentiating the dosage levels for both drugs. The absence of beneficial or deleterious effects of chlorimipramine described previously tend to support these conclusions.

The results of the controlled studies of chlorimipramine and desimi-pramine and the accumulated clinical experience with imipramine and the MAO inhibitors supply little evidence for either beneficial or adverse effects for antidepressants and supply no evidence for the DA, NE or 5HT hypo-thesis for Tourette syndrome. Some of the disparate clinical findings might be due to spontaneous or other irrelevant factors that occurred during the clinical observations. Controlled studies are necessary to resolve these contradictory findings, especially because of the implication for various catecholamine hyptheses for tics and Tourette syndrome.

Lithium

Lithium, at blood levels between 0.8 and 1.0 mmol/l, has been reported as effective in two Tourette patients, maximal benefit occurring after 3 weeks of treatment[58]. Improvement of these patients was reported to have been maintained for 3.5 months[59].

We have used lithium, at blood levels between 0.8 and 1.5 mmol/l, in combination with haloperidol, in six patients. Lithium had no significant therapeutic effect on Tourette symptoms, although it improved the mood of one severely agitated patient.

The effectiveness of lithium for tics or Tourette syndrome is highly questionable and requires further study before it can be recommended.

Barbiturates

All of the barbiturates have been used to suppress tic symptoms but are effective only at dosages that cause sedation and impaired cognitive functioning. Their use is further limited by the development of tolerance, addiction and withdrawal effects.

Benzodiazepines

Drugs in this category include chlordiazepoxide (Librium), diazepam (Valium), flurazepam (Dalmane), clorazepate (Tranxene), clonazepam (Clonopin) and others. They are pharmacologically similar to barbiturates and other sedatives, except for a greater and safer toxic-to-therapeutic ratio. As with other sedatives, increasing dosages of benzodiazepines result in: antianxiety effects, sedation, hypnosis, anaesthesia, coma and death, and can cause addiction and withdrawal effects[60].

The results for a clinical trial of clonazepam (Clonepin) in seven patients with Tourette syndrome[61] suggest potential benefit for the vocalizations of three patients and some reduction of tics in two others. However, it is difficult to evaluate the enduring effect because of the naturally fluctuating course of the illness and the preliminary nature of the observations.

The results are offset, however, by the observation that more than 60% of our patients had been treated with benzodiazepines by other physicians without significant and enduring therapeutic effects.

Other antianxiety–sedative–hypnotic drugs

Many other drugs in this category have been used unsuccessfully in the past. These include glycol derivatives such as meprobamate (Miltown, Equanil), piperidinediones, such as methyprylon (Noludar) and glutethimide (Doriden), tertiary alcohols such as ethchlorvynol (Placidyl), carbamatles, chloral derivatives, paraldehyde, bromides, antihistamines such as hydroxyzine (Atarax, Vistaril), methaqualone (Quaalude) and many others.

Potentially serious adverse effects of these drugs further limit their usefulness.

Anticonvulsants

Phenytoin (Dilantin)

Sixty of our patients had been treated previously with adequate dosages of phenytoin without therapeutic benefit. We have used phenytoin with and without haloperidol and in combination with other drugs and have not observed beneficial effects on tics or Tourette syndrome.

However, there is no contraindication to the use of phenytoin, or other anticonvulsants in patients with both Tourette syndrome and epilepsy. Two of our patients with grand mal and one with petit mal epilepsy were successfully treated with the combination of both medications.

Carbamazepine (Tegretol)

Carbamazepine at dosages of 600–800 mg/day had been reported as very effective in five male, Polish patients between 12 and 14 years of age who previously had been treated unsuccessfully with haloperidol[62].

We used carbamazepine initially in combination with α-methyl-para-tyrosine in one patient who had developed fog states on haloperidol[19]. The medication did not control the fog states nor did it help the tic symptoms.

Two patients with a history of psychomotor seizures and Tourette syndrome were treated with carbamazepine and other anticonvulsants without benefit. Subsequently, we used carbamazepine in a range of 1000–1800 mg/day in 11 Tourette patients who had had adverse side-effects to haloperidol. The medication had no beneficial effect on symptoms. Adverse effects included: nausea, ataxia, vertigo, sedation, diplopia, dysarthria, numbness and incoordination.

We concluded that carbamazepine was ineffective in controlling the tics and vocalizations of Tourette syndrome and that the adverse side-effects were a further limitation of treatment with this medication.

Other anticonvulsants

Other patients have been referred to us who previously had been treated unsuccessfully with ethoxucimide (Zarontin) and primidone (Mysoline). We have not used and know of only one patient who had been treated unsuccessfully with valproic acid (Depakene).

Miscellaneous chemotherapy

Baclofen (Lioresal)

This drug, an analogue of the putative neurotransmitter inhibitor γ-amino-butyric acid (GABA), has been used by other physicians and has been reported to be ineffective by seven of our patients.

Corticosteroids

An English abstract of a Polish paper[63], which has not been translated in its entirety, described the successful treatment of four patients with prednisone and three patients with haloperidol and thioridazine. A recent clinical report[64] described the treatment of an 11-year-old boy who developed symptoms of Tourette syndrome after an acute infection. Some of the subsequent laboratory findings were abnormal. He was treated with 30 mg/day of prednisone for 2 weeks and 15 mg/day for 3 months. Symptoms disappeared after 3 days and did not recur after prednisone was discontinued after 3 months. The patient has been asymptomatic for 4 years.

The brief description of symptomatology is characteristic of Gilles de la Tourette syndrome except for trembling of the body, body tensing and dystonic-like flexion and arching. The history of an acute infection followed by elevated antistreptolysin-O titres, C-reactive protein and rheumatoid arthritis suggests a residual encephalitis which provoked the tic symptoms. Interpretation of the aetiology and effects of treatment are difficult. The tic symptom could have been the result of a short-lived idiopathic Tourette syndrome, provoked by the residual encephalitis or caused by the streptococcal infection which resulted in rheumatic fever and the symptoms of Sydenham's chorea. Careful differential diagnosis of Tourette syndrome and Sydenham's chorea would be important for subsequent treatment. Improvement in the symptoms could have been spontaneous or from the corticosteroid therapy. Because of long-term side-effects of corticosteroids, chronic use for Tourette syndrome is impractical.

Psychotomimetics

Lysergic acid diethylamide (LSD). LSD has been reported as effective in controlling muscular but not vocal tics in a single patient[65]. Several of our patients had used LSD with variable effect, some reporting no effect, others an increase or decrease of symptoms.

Tetrahydrocannabinol (Marijuana). This drug has been used by many of our patients with variable effect, some reporting a decrease, others an increase or no effect on tics.

Propranolol (Inderal)

Propranolol, a β–adrenergic blocking agent, extensively used in cardiology, was used empirically in seven patients because of its reported effectiveness in the treatment of somatic anxiety. All of the patients had previously responded to haloperidol but adverse side-effects limited its usefulness. The first patient, an 18-year-old boy diagnosed as having 'chronic tic' (see earlier section on diagnosis), achieved 25% reduction of his symptoms on 6 mg/day of haloperidol and a slow onset of cognitive impairment. At a dosage of 400 mg/day of propranolol, tics decreased by 60–80% and improvement has persisted for 8 months. There were no side-effects. The second patient, a 20-year-old boy, had a 60% decrease on 6–8 mg/day of haloperidol. Because of concomitant lethargy, he was slowly titrated to 100 mg/day of propranolol with 40% decrease in tic symptoms and no side-effects. A third patient reported no therapeutic benefit on tics or side-effects on 1000 mg/day of propranolol. A 17-year-old boy prematurely discontinued the medication at a dosage of 200 mg/day. Two patients discontinued their medication at dosages of 320 and 150 mg/day because of adverse side-effects which appeared to be placebo-induced. A 13-year-old boy had about 40% improvement at a dosage of 250 mg/day but the medication had to be stopped because of bradycardia (which varied between 40 and 60 beats per minute).

Our clinical impression is that propranolol is not useful for Tourette syndrome, but may deserve further clinical trials in patients with chronic tic.

Clonidine (Catapres)

Clonidine, a centrally active imidazoline antihypertensive medication, reduces brain turnover of norepinephrine at low dosages. Seven of eight patients with Tourette syndrome and severe behavioural problems treated with clonidine at dosages which varied between 0.05 and 0.6 mg daily had significant improvement in symptoms[66]. We treated 25 patients with clonidine in dosages of 0.05 to 2.0 mg daily. Three other physicians, in a personal communication, reported treating approximately 20 patients with clonidine. The percent improvement of symptomatology reported for these 45 patients varies between 10 and 20%. Clonidine may be effective in a subgroup of patients with Tourette syndrome. Further studies comparing clonidine, haloperidol and placebo are necessary to confirm this clinical report.

Antihistamines

Many different antihistamines have been used, alone or in combination with other drugs, in over 60 of our patients. Antihistamines, like other sedative drugs, have slight beneficial effects only at dosages causing sedation, and are without enduring therapeutic benefit.

Megavitamins

Forty patients have tried megavitamins, alone or together with different trace elements, and often with concomitant haloperidol. This treatment has been therapeutically unsuccessful except for the beneficial effect of haloperidol.

Feingold Diet

The Feingold Diet has been used with various degrees of stringency or completeness in 20 patients without therapeutic benefit.

Psychotherapy

As noted earlier, the average improvement after 6 months for various types of psychological treatments is 9.2% and 12% for psychotherapy alone[19,25]. A majority of the 800 patients evaluated and treated by us since 1971 have had some form of psychological treatment for their tics which included psychoanalysis, individual psychotherapy, group therapy, family therapy and so on. All patients reported that psychotherapy had no effect on their tics, although some described improved functioning after psychotherapy for non-tic psychological problems. Therefore, we do not recommend psychotherapy as a treatment for tics or Tourette syndrome. However, if there are indications of an emotional disturbance concomitant with or subsequent to having Tourette syndrome, psychotherapy may be indicated. Our belief is that the aetiology of the disorder is organic and that psychological procedures are ineffective in controlling neurological symptoms.

Hypnosis

About 20% of our total sample have been unsuccessfully treated with hypnosis. Schneck[67] reported an unsuccessful case. Erickson[68] reports successful use of hypnosis in two patients, who, according to our diagnostic criteria, did not have Tourette syndrome.

Behaviour therapy

In 1958, the use of modern behavioural approaches to the treatment of tics was initiated. We were stimulated to critically evaluate the use of behavioural techniques for tics and Tourette syndrome after a favourable positive report about its effectiveness was published by an American Psychiatric Association Task Force on Behaviour Therapy[70,71]. We concluded after review of 31 case studies[19] that behaviour therapy yields about 20–25% success, which is similar to the percentage reported for a variety of psychological treatment used less than 6 months or non-specific spontaneous change. Our interpretation is similar to the observation made by Yates[72] that Tourette syndrome 'may best be treated by the drug (haloperidol) rather than the tedious procedure of massed practice and tend to confirm the presumed organic basis of the syndrome'.

Approximately 40 of our patients have been unsuccessfully treated with some form of behaviour therapy. A dramatic example was a 14¼-year-old male patient who had Tourette syndrome since the age of five, although the diagnosis was not made until the age of 11. The patient was then treated serially with intensive psychotherapy, family therapy, hypnosis, transcendental meditation, chemotherapy and finally, during a 9 month hospitalization at a university centre, with behaviour therapy. The patient's condition deteriorated and the parents were advised to seek indefinite residential treatment. The family chose instead to bring him to us for treatment with haloperidol. After 2 months of outpatient treatment, at a dosage of 6.75 mg/day of haloperidol and 1 mg of benztropine mesylate, 90–98% of symptoms were suppressed with minimal side-effects.

At follow-up evaluation, 3.5 years later, the patient has maintained his improvement of over 90% suppression of tics without side-effects at a dosage of 5.5 mg/day of haloperidol. He is now 18 years old and about to enter college.

At the present time, without better studies and more definitive data, we have concluded that the behaviour therapies are ineffective for Tourette syndrome.

Surgery

Several surgical procedures have been used to treat Tourette patients[73]. One of the procedures includes surgical ablation, usually cryotherapy, of localized areas of the extrapyramidal system. Stereotypic radiographic guidance is used to place a lesion in the lateral thalamus. This procedure was done in one of our patients who had surgery bilaterally with 60% reduction of symptoms. Symptoms were further reduced to 80% with haloperidol which became available after the surgery. A mild dysarthria was the only adverse side-effect of the surgery. Another female patient had a left cryothalamectomy at the age of 41. Movements on the right side and barking almost disappeared but movements continued on the left side and in the trunk. The movements returned in 1 month, however, and she had a second procedure which was reported as successful. Improvement unfortunately did not endure.

Another surgical approach involves coagulation of the rostral intralaminar and medial nuclei of the thalamus bilaterally in patients with obsessive–compulsive neurosis and Tourette syndrome. The authors report 70, 90 and 100% suppression of tics in three patients[74].

Similar stereotactic surgery was tried on three patients with Tourette syndrome[75]. The authors used a modified Leskill apparatus, the ventricular structures were outlined by air, and the DM and iLa nuclei were destroyed by radiofrequency coagulation. Two patients had complete remissions for over a year. Unfortunately, symptoms returned in both patients, and followed a prolonged period of mental confusion in one patient. The third patient had a small reduction in compulsive symptomatology, but the symptoms returned after 9 months. A second intervention was unsuccessful. The authors conclude that stereotactic surgery is not useful for the treatment of Tourette syndrome.

Remission of tics has been reported following bilateral surgical lesions in one Tourette patient[76].

Neurosurgical procedures, as now used, are not recommended because of the equivocal, limited and unsustained therapeutic benefit and the possibility of irremediable central nervous system damage. Precisely identifying the causitive lesion in Tourette syndrome might lead to the development of more specific and useful surgical procedures.

CONCLUSION

The data reviewed in this paper lead to several conclusions.

The most important task is to identify the cause for tics and Tourette syndrome. The evidence suggests a central nervous system organic aetiology. The clinical symptomatology and course, as well as the differential response to haloperidol and other drugs, suggests that there may be more than one illness or aetiology for tics and Tourette syndrome.

The evidence for various aetiological theories is inconclusive. Although the most likely aetiological hypothesis for tics and Tourette syndrome is malfunction of the basal ganglia, there is no support for this hypothesis.

Abnormal levels of metabolism have not been consistently demonstrated for various neurotransmitters such as homovanillic acid, vanylmandelic acid and 5-hydroxyindolacetic acid in the cerebral spinal fluid; dopamine-β-hydroxylase, norepinephrine and amino-oxidase activity in plasma MAO activity in platelets, and catechol-o-methyltransferase in erythrocytes.

The evidence derived from clinical use of various drugs does not suggest abnormalities for norepinephrine, serotonin and acetylcholine. The weight of the clinical evidence, particularly the effectiveness of haloperidol, suggests abnormal dopamine effects, either presynaptic levels or postsynaptic sensitivity. However, the ineffectiveness of clozapine, a known postsynaptic dopamine blocker, is inconsistent with the dopamine hypothesis. Clozapine has few extrapyramidal effects, including akinesia and cognitive impairment, both of which occur with haloperidol and most other antipsychotic drugs. The effectiveness of haloperidol in the treatment of tics and Tourette syndrome, therefore, may be related in some way to factors causing, mediating, or associated with these adverse side-effects rather than a primary dopamine effect. Carefully controlled clinical studies with different antipsychotics, with specific dopamine blocking effects and adverse side-effects, together with reliable ratings of clinical effectiveness and side-effects, should permit evaluation of this hypothesis.

Although there are no long-term and well controlled studies that demonstrate the effectiveness of haloperidol in comparison with placebo, psychological treatment or other drugs; considerable clinical experience indicates that haloperidol is presently the drug of choice for the treatment of tics and Tourette syndrome. Other dopamine antagonists such as pimozide and penfluridol, are alternative drugs that should be tried in patients with inadequate response to haloperidol or who develop adverse side-effects. The comparative clinical efficacy of these medications should be further evaluated in long-term and well controlled clinical studies.

Although the therapeutic impact of haloperidol on the treatment of tics and Tourette syndrome has been dramatic, offering hope to patients and often permitting normal functioning, there is a need to develop more effective drugs with fewer side-effects that can be used effectively by all physicians. Complexities and subtleties of treatment with haloperidol now require management by expert psychopharmacologists.

A major difficulty hampering study of the aetiology and treatment of tics, Tourette syndrome and other movement disorders is the reluctance of private industry, governmental and private funding agencies to financially support the research necessary for further progress.

References

1 Trousseau, A. (1873). *Clinique médical de l'hôtel Dieu de Paris*, 2, 267
2 Itard, J. M. G. (1825). Memoire sur quelques fonctions involuntaires des appareils de la locomotion de la prehension et de la voix. *Arch. Gen. Med.*, 8, 385
3 Gilles de la Tourette, G. (1885). Étude sur une affection nerveuse caractérisée de l'incoordination motrice accompagnée d'écholalie et de coprolalie. *Arch Neurol.*, 9, 158
4 Shapiro, A. K., Shapiro, E. and Wayne, H. L. (1973). The symptomatology and diagnosis of Gilles de la Tourette's syndrome. *J. Am. Acad. Child Psychiatry*, 12, 702
5 Meige, H. and Feindel, E. (1907). *Tics and Their Treatment*. Translated and edited by S. A. K. Wilson, (New York: William Wood & Co.)
6 Ferenczi, S. (1921). Psycho-analytical observations on tic. *Int. J. Psychoanal.*, 2, 1
7 Abraham, K. (1927). Contributions to a discussion on tic. In *Selected Papers of Karl Abraham, M.D.*, Translated by B. D. Strachey (London: Hogarth Press)
8 Mahler, M. S. and Rangell, L. (1943). A psychosomatic study of maladie des tics. *Psychiatry Q.*, 17, 579
9 Kanner, L. (1957). *Child Psychiatry*. (Springfield: Charles C. Thomas)
10 Bruch, H. and Thum, L. C. (1968). Maladie des tics and maternal psychosis. *J. Nerv. Ment. Dis.*, 146, 446
11 Dunlap, J. R. (1960). A case of Gilles de la Tourette's disease (maladie des tics): A study of the intrafamily dynamics. *J. Nerv. Ment. Dis.*, 130, 340
12 Zausmer, D. M. (1954). The treatment of tics in childhood: A review and follow-up study. *Arch. Dis. Child.*, 29, 537
13 Pasamanick, B. and Kawi, A. (1956). A study of the association of prenatal and paranatal factors in the development of tics in children. *J. Pediatr.*, 48, 596
14 Torup, E. (1962). A follow-up study of children with tics. *Acta Pediatr.*, 51, 261
15 Kelman, D. H. (1965). Gilles de la Tourette's disease in children. A review of the literature. *J. Child Psychol., Psychiatry*, 6, 219

16 Fernando, S. J. M. (1967). Gilles de la Tourette's syndrome. *Br. J. Psychiatry*, **113**, 607

17 Corbett, J. A., Matthews, A. M., Connell, P. H. and Shapiro, D. A. (1969). Tics and Gilles de la Tourette's syndrome: A follow-up study and critical review. *Br. J. Psychiatry*, **115**, 1229

18 Shapiro, A. K. and Shapiro, E. (1968). Treatment of Gilles de la Tourette's syndrome with haloperidol. *Br. J. Psychiatry*, **114**, 345

19 Shapiro, A. K., Shapiro, E., Bruun, R. D. and Sweet, R. D. (1978). *Gilles de la Tourette Syndrome*. (New York: Raven Press)

20 Shapiro, A. K. (1977). The placebo effect. In Clark, W. G. and Guidice J. del (eds.) *Principles of Psychopharmacology*. (New York: Raven Press)

21 Seignot, M. J. N. (1961). Un cas de maladie des tics de Gilles de la Tourette guéri par de R-1625. *Ann. Med. Psychol.*, **119**, 578

22 Caprini, G. and Melotti, V. (1961). Un grave sindrome ticcosa guarita con haloperidol. *Riv. Sper. Freniat.*, **85**, 191

23 Challas, G. and Brauer, T. (1963). Tourette's disease: Relief of symptoms with R-1625. *Am. J. Psychiatry*, **120**, 283

24 Shapiro, A. K., Shapiro, E. and Wayne, H. L. (1973). Treatment of Gilles de la Tourette syndrome with haloperidol: Review of 34 cases. *Arch. Gen. Psychiatry*, **28**, 92

25 Abuzzahab, F. S. and Anderson, F. O. (1973). Gilles de la Tourette's syndrome: International registry. *Minn. Med.*, **56**, 492

26 Bruun, R. D., Shapiro, A. K., Shapiro, E., Sweet, R. D., Wayne, H. L. and Solomon, G. E. (1976). A follow-up of 78 patients with Gilles de la Tourette's syndrome. *Am. J. Psychiatry*, **133**, 944

27 Caine, E. D., Margolin, D. I., Brown, G. L. and Ebert, M. H. (1978). Gilles de la Tourette's syndrome, tardive dyskinesia and psychosis in an adolescent. *Am. J. Psychiatry*, **135**, 241

28 Perel, J. and Shostak, M. (1979). Personal communication

29 Shostak, M. and Perel, J. (1976). Radioimmunoassay for haloperidol. *Fed. Proc.*, **35**, 531

30 Messerschmitt, P. (1972). The use of pimozide in pediatric psychiatry. *Thesis for the Doctorate of Medicine,* presented to the Faculte de Medicine de Paris, (Abstracted by McNeil Laboratories)

31 Debray, P., Messerschmitt, P., Longchamp, D. and Herbault, M. (1972). The use of pimozide in child psychiatry. *Nouv. Presse Méd.*, **1**, 2917

32 Ross, M. S. and Moldofsky, H. (1977). Comparison of pimozide with haloperidol in Gilles de la Tourette's syndrome. *Lancet*, **1**, 103

33 Moldofsky, H. (1978). Personal communication

34 Ayd, F. (1972). Penfluridol: A long-acting oral neuroleptic. *Int. Drug Ther. Newsletter*, **7**, 13

35 Quitkin, F., Rifkin, A., Kane, J., Ramos-Lorenzi, J. R. and Klein, D. F. (1978). Long-acting oral vs injectable antipsychotic drugs in schizophrenics. *Arch. Gen. Psychiatry*, **35**, 889

36 Mesnikoff, A. (1959). Three cases of Gilles de la Tourette syndrome treated with psychotherapy and chlorpromazine. *Arch. Neurol. Psychiatry*, **81**, 710

37 Bochner, S. (1959). Gilles de la Tourette's disease. *J. Ment. Sci.*, **105**, 1078

38 Eisenberg, L., Ascher, E. and Kanner, L. (1959). A clinical study of Gilles de la Tourette's disease (maladie des tics) in children. *Am. J. Psychiatry*, **115**, 715

39 Walsh, P. J. F. (1962). Compulsive shouting and Gilles de la Tourette's disease. *J. Clin. Psychol.*, **20**, 52

40 Levy, B. S. and Ascher, E. (1968). Phenothiazines in the treatment of Gilles de la Tourette's disease. *J. Nerv. Ment. Dis.*, **146**, 36

41 Caine, E. D., Polinsky, R. J., Kartzinel, R. and Ebert, M. H. (1979). The trial use of Clozapine for abnormal involuntary movement disorders. *Am. J. Psychiatry*, **136**, 317

42 Sweet, R. D., Bruun, R. D., Shapiro, A. K. and Shapiro, E. (1976). The pharmacology of Gilles de la Tourette's syndrome (chronic multiple tic). In Klawans, H. L. (ed.). *Clinical Neuropharmacology*. Vol. 1, pp. 81–105. (New York: Raven Press)

43 DiGiacomo, J. N., Fahn, S., Glass, J. B. *et al* (1971). A case with Gilles de la Tourette's syndrome: Recurrent refractoriness to haloperidol and unsuccessful treatment with L-DOPA. *J. Nerv. Ment. Dis.*, **152**, 115

44 Feinberg, M. and Carroll, B. J. (1977). Effects of dopamine agonists and antagonists in Tourette's syndrome. Paper presented at the *VIth World Congress of Psychiatry*, August 28-September 3, Honolulu, Hawaii

45 Meyerhoff, J. L. and Snyder, S. H. (1973). Gilles de la Tourette's disease and minimal brain dysfunction: Amphetamine isomers reveal catecholamine correlates in an affected patient. *Psychopharmacologia*, **29**, 211

46 Golden, G. S. (1974). Gilles de la Tourette's syndrome following methylphenidate administration. *Dev. Med. Child Neurol.*, **16**, 76

47 Golden, G. S. (1977). The effect of central nervous system stimulants on Tourette syndrome. *Ann. Neurol.*, **2**, 69

48 Denckla, M. B., Bemporad, J. R. and McKay, M. C. (1976). Tics following methylphenidate administration. *J. Am. Med. Assoc.*, **235**, 1349

49 Van Woert, M. H., Yip, L. C. and Balis, M. E. (1977). Purine phosphoribosyltransferase in Gilles de la Tourette syndrome. *N. Engl. J. Med.*, **296**, 210

50 Van Woert, M. H. (1979). Personal communication

51 Pinta, E. R. (1977). Deanol in Gilles de la Tourette syndrome: A preliminary investigation. *Dis. Nerv. Syst.*, **38**, 214

52 Fras, I. and Karlavage, J. (1977). The use of methylphenidate and imipramine in Gilles de la Tourette disease in children. *Am. J. Psychiatry*, **134**, 195

53 Fras, I. (1978). Gilles de la Tourette's syndrome. Effects of tricyclic antidepressants. *N.Y. State J. Med.*, **78**, 1230

54 Shapiro, A. K. (1977). Treatment of Gilles de la Tourette syndrome. Letter to the editor, *J. Am. Med. Assoc.*, **238**, 29

55 Messiha, F. S. and Knopp, W. (1976). A study of endogenous dopamine metabolism in Gilles de la Tourette's disease. *Dis. Nerv. Syst.*, **37**, 470

56 Yaryura-Tobias, J. A. and Neziroglu, F. A. (1977). Gilles de la Tourette syndrome: A new clinico-therapeutic approach. *Prog. Neuropsychopharmacol.*, **1**, 335

57 Polansky, R. (1978). Paper presented at the *Tourette Syndrome Association Meeting*, October 7th, New York

58 Messiha, F. S., Erickson, H. M. and Goggin, J. E. (1976). Lithium carbonate in Gilles de la Tourette's disease. *Res. Commun. Chem. Pathol. Pharmacol.*, **15**, 609

59 Erickson, H. M. Jr., Goggin, J. E. and Messiha, F. S. (1976). Comparison of lithium and haloperidol therapy in Gilles de la Tourette syndrome. In Messiha F. S. and Kenny, A. D. (eds.). *Advances in Experimental Medicine and Biology*. Vol. 90, pp. 197–205. (New York: Fienum Press)

60 Shapiro, A. K. (1976). Psychopharmacology. In Grenell, R. G. and Gabay, S. (eds.) *Biological Foundations of Psychiatry*, pp. 793–836. (New York: Raven Press)

61 Gonce, M. and Barbeau, A. (1977). Seven cases of Gilles de la Tourette's syndrome: Partial relief with clozapan: A pilot study. *Can. J. Neurol. Sci.*, **4**, 279

62 Zawadski, A. (1972). Treatment of maladie des tics with carbamazepine. *Pediatr. Pol.*, **47**, 1105

63 Popielarska, A., Kuliqowska, M. and Mazur, M. (1972). Ozeapole Gilles de la Tourette 1 próbach jego leczenia na podstawie Wtasnych obserwacji. *Pediatr. Pol.*, **47**, 1097

64 Kondo, K. and Kabasawa, T. (1979). Improvement in Gilles de la Tourette syndrome after corticosteroid therapy. *Ann. Neurol.*, **4**, 387

65 Smith, C. G. (1969). Gilles de la Tourette syndrome treated with LSD. *Irish J. Med. Sci.*, **2**, 269

66 Cohen, D. J., Young, J. G., Nathanson, J. A. *et al.* (1979). Clonidine in Tourette's syndrome. *Lancet*, **2**, 551

67 Schneck, J. M. (1960). Gilles de la Tourette's disease. *Am. J. Psychiatry*, **117**, 78

68 Erickson, M. H. (1964). Experimental hypnotherapy in Tourette's disease. *Am. J. Clin. Hypnosis*, **7**, 325

69 Yates, A. (1958). The application of learning theory to the treatment of tics. *J. Abnorm. Soc. Psychol.*, **56**, 175

70 Task Force Report 5: Behavior Therapy in Psychiatry. Washington, D.C., American Psychiatric Association, 1973

71 Shapiro, A. K. (1976). The behavior therapies: Therapeutic breakthrough or latest fad? *Am. J. Psychiatry*, **133**, 154

72 Yates, A. (1970). Tics. In Costello, C. (ed.) *Symptoms of Psychopathology.* (New York: John Wiley & Sons)

73 Cooper, I. S. (1969). *Involuntary Movement Disorders.* (New York: Hoeber Medical Division, Harper and Row)

74 Hassler, R. and Dieckmann, G. (1970). Traitment stereotaxique des tics et cris inarticulés ou coprolalalique considérés comme phénoomène d'obsession motrice au cours de la maladie Gilles de la Tourette. *Rev. Neurol, (Paris)*, **123**, 89

75 deDivitiis, E., D'Errico, A. and Cerillo, A. (1977). Stereotactic surgery in Gilles de la Tourette syndrome. *Acta Neurochirurgica*, **73** (Suppl.), 24

76 Baker, E. F. W. (1962). Gilles de la Tourette syndrome treated by bimedial frontal leucotomy. *Can. Med. Assoc. J.*, **86**, 746

7

Treatment of tardive dyskinesia

G. W. Paulson

INTRODUCTION

Tardive dyskinesia (TD) is not now considered rare or controversial and may be the most frequently diagnosed iatrogenic disease of the nervous system. Diagnosis of TD in individual cases can occasionally be difficult, but in contrast to a decade ago the existence of TD is unquestioned. There is no serious effort at this time to attribute tardive dyskinesia to tics or to habits, nor to the 'stereotypies' of schizophrenia nor even to voluntary mannerisms in edentulous or senile patients. Although diagnosis and aetiology is no longer controversial, uncertainty characterizes concepts of treatment. Dozens of therapeutic approaches have been suggested, none are completely accepted and none are invariably effective. This article reviews treatment, but does not confirm one ideal treatment among the many suggested categories of medication or supplementary nonmedical therapies of TD.

DIAGNOSIS OF TD

The diagnosis of TD is an observational skill and no laboratory test suggests or establishes the label. The characteristic patterns have been described in most of the references used for this review. Any patient who receives psychotropic medications may develop TD, although older patients and those with brain damage are particularly vulnerable[1,2]. Use of phenothiazines in teenagers or in the young can also lead to persistent movements, since high potency antipsychotics are particularly likely to be used in adolescents[3-5]. After the first case reports, many articles on TD have listed percentage of population groups which manifested the phenomena with results varying from 2–50% of certain groups of mental patients[6-9]. Nonpsychotic patients can be affected[10].

No definitive biochemical or electrophysiological abnormalities are seen in TD, although with special leads an artifact produced by the glossolingual electrical potential can be detected in the EEG. 'Mitten' patterns in the EEG of patients with TD have also been reported, but are also not diagnostic[11].

There is no reliable quantitative measure of TD and also no reliable estimation of the effect of therapy, although Crane and others have offered several scales as research tools[12]. Subjective observations fill the literature. TV or movies may be the best monitors currently available for research purposes. Gardos *et al.*[13] have reviewed techniques of assessment of TD and noted the usefulness of:

(1) Global rating which can employ specific clinical features such as drawing an Archimedes screw or check of handwriting;

(2) Multi-item rating scales first employed in a series of articles by the major North American evangelist against TD, Doctor George Crane. From personal experiences with earlier ratings in parkinsonism most neurologists consider rating scales to be deceptive, since actual disability may not lessen even while the scales improve;

(3) Videotaping also has defects as a sole measurement system, particularly since the tape itself requires a rating scale. The rating clinician may be uninformed of technical change in the production of the videotape, or may be unaware of the phenomenon of spontaneous oral facial dyskinesias.

A conscientious clinician can be biased by a history of phenothiazine ingestion in his patients and may over diagnose TD. Organic disorders that mimic TD can be overlooked as with a recent 20-year-old patient diagnosed as TD for 3 months when in fact he had Wilson's disease. Tarsy[14] describes a similar case. The clinician must remember that millions of psychotic and non-psychotic patients have used phenothiazines without developing TD and phenomena similar to TD can follow exposure to therapeutic agents other than phenothiazines. The limb and mouth movements in TD are as variable as were the extrapyramidal features described after the epidemic of encephalitis lethargica 60 years ago[15]. Individuals with TD have a unique nervous system and develop unique combinations of unilateral phenomena: truncal sway, postural distortions, respiratory distress, buccolingual movements, or fleeting finger movements. In some reports, intended to evaluate therapy of TD, the criteria for the original diagnosis can be questioned. Even when diagnosis is secure, measurements of improvement are rarely well defined and despite contrary expressions[16,17] tardive dyskinesia is *not* usually permanent. Researchers or clinicians may claim credit for spontaneous improvements.

Movies were often suggested and sometimes actually utilized for confirmation, and in several studies two or more clinicians have independently measured and graded the movements. Many neurologists and psychiatrists interested in TD have seen patients with AIMS (Abnormal Involuntary

Movements), which were only partially due to tardive dyskinesia or AIMS totally confusing in distribution and character. In individual cases: facial synkinesia, combinations of chorea or athetosis, dystonia, and/or similar disorders will require distinction from TD. Variations in TD from moment to moment are remarkable, although there is little evidence regarding the effect of time of day, diet, and similar physiological processes on TD. Some observations in the literature have been affected by these or other unknown variables. The level of activation can influence the severity of TD and should be the same whenever patients or treatments are compared[18]. As a rule the movements are better observed with subtlety and indirection rather than by an overt or penetrating observation that alerts the patient[19]. Rapidity in diagnosis does not always enhance precision since such speed can be an inducement to quick and superficial assessment, even if ease of diagnosis in most cases with TD is a delight for the slipshod clinician.

In addition to informal observation and movies, numerical quantitative measures of TD have been attempted. After identification of body parts such as mouth, tongue, fingers, legs, or trunk; a gradation system from 1–4 + is employed and reproducibility is possible with such measurements. One movement, the buccolingual dyskinesia, is so distinctive to TD and is so infrequent in other disorders that the presence of lingual AIMS may be recorded as just presence or absence, a plus or minus measurement.

PREVENTION OF TD

Prevention is clearly the primary goal in TD and one preventive measure suggested is 'drug vacation'. Some patients with serious psychiatric illnesses may do as well with an intermittent use of psychotropic medication, as with prolonged steady use and certainly brief periods of absence from medications are rarely hazardous. Whenever an informal effort is made to reduce medications in a State institution, up to 50% of the patients adjust without phenothiazines for as long as a month. Over a period of a year, at least two-thirds of chronic patients will be placed back on medicines because of psychiatric or behavioural disturbances. In addition to the use of drug vacations as protection for the patient, brief trials 'off medicine' may also signal the onset of TD[20], since TD frequently first appears when medicine is reduced. Extensive, longlasting and very severe TD is harder to manage than the milder forms of the disorder and may even increase mortality by affecting respiratory function[21–23]. Phenothiazines may affect cardiac function[24], but there is no known linkage between TD and cardiac problems. Abdominal distress can occur with TD[25].

There have been suggestions in the recent literature that patients should sign a specific release which mentions the dangers of TD whenever phenothiazines are initiated[26]. Certainly patients who have developed tardive dyskinesia and who are in need of continual medication should be apprised of the risk and their families should also be informed. Furthermore, those at particular risk such as women, the aged, or those with organic disease, should be specifically informed of the possibility of TD and drug vacations are particularly relevant for this group. There is no data suggesting that adjunctive medication, including anticholinergics, will prevent TD.

DRUG TREATMENT OF TARDIVE DYSKINESIA

As Klawans[27] has emphasized, the pathology, pathophysiology, and natural history of TD are all incompletely understood, and therefore it is not surprising that treatment remains unsatisfactory. Table 1 lists some of the medications that have been suggested as treatment for TD. The early literature suggested reserpine and related drugs for TD[28–31] and these agents continue to be used, based on the concept of dopaminergic factors in TD and a known decreased activity of dopamine in the presence of reserpine. Reserpine can produce a depletion of dopamine by effects on uptake or on storage. Fahn[32] has recently suggested that reserpine when combined with α–methyltyrosine, may give a dramatic improvement in TD. Other chemicals which have also been reported to deplete or suppress neurohumours such as dopamine include the monoamine oxidase inhibitors[33], methyldopa[34] and tetrabenazine. Some observers have suggested that tetrabenazine, not readily available in the USA, is the best medication to control the movement disorders of Huntington's chorea[35] and tetrabenazine has been suggested for TD[36–39]. It is possible that the effect of tetrabenazine on TD will be transient but this drug remains a useful agent in therapy of TD.

Efforts to replace choline have been reported based on the classical but presumed seesaw balance between choline and dopamine in extrapyramidal disease. If there is dopaminergic hypersensitivity and cholinergic hypofunction in TD[40] then it seems as logical to increase choline stores as to block dopamine receptors. Choline has been administered directly, with reportedly beneficial results[41,42], but is poorly tolerated by many patients because of the 'fishy odour'. Lecithin is a more convenient way to administer choline,

Table 1   Partial list of medications that have been reported to help with TD

Amantadine	Clonazepam	Papaverine
α–Methyldopa	D–Amphetamine	Phenothiazines
α–Methyltyrosine	Deanol	(particularly CPZ)
Antihistamines	Diazepam	Pimozide
Apomorphine	Dimethyl aminoethanol	Pyridoxine
Baclofen (Lioresal)	Imipramine	Reserpine
Barbiturates	Lecithin	Tetrabenazine
Butyrophenones	Levodopa	Serotonin
(haloperidol)	Lithium	Valproate
Choline	Manganese	

according to the studies of Barbeau[43] in ataxia and has also been postulated as potentially beneficial for tardive dyskinesia[44]. As part of the systematic assay of many agents by the US National Institute of Health other cholinergic compounds such as arecholine[45] remain under active study at present, but so far none have been dramatically helpful. Administration of dimethylaminoethenol (deanol) has been of particular interest since this agent may work by mechanisms similar to choline. Reports regarding this agent display the usual history of all agents reported to 'cure' TD. At first there were several dozen brief papers regarding deanol, most of which were very encouraging, but later papers raised serious questions as to the effectiveness of the agent[46-54]. After there was less certainty[55,56] as to the effect, higher doses were used and then a few observers suggested that only certain types of TD will respond to deanol. It indeed may be true that subtypes of TD exist[57]. Nervertheless, the first flash of cheerful reports has gradually paled. Negative reports are probably less likely to be published than any initial encouraging observation, and certainly deanol is still utilized in many neurological centres for the treatment of TD. Nevertheless, there is no firm evidence at this time that this particular agent is any more helpful than many similar agents which do at times benefit certain patients.

Anticholinergics have not been helpful in tardive dyskinesia, although, of course, they can block some of the acute extrapyramidal symptomatology of phenothiazines. The acute dystonic reaction of recent phenothiazine use and the pseudoparkinsonism of prolonged drug use are usually independent of TD, although in a few cases features of parkinsonism and TD may overlap. In fact, if TD fluctuates a great deal then when the movements of TD are less obvious parkinsonian features may coexist to a limited degree; reminding one of the complex mixture of beneficial effects and troublesome side-effects of levodopa. The use of anticholinergics jointly with phenothiazines, in order to suppress parkinsonian symptoms, has been condemned on the basis of a theoretical tendency of these agents to increase chances of TD as well as of lack of proof that anticholinergics offer significant benefit.

Dopaminergic agents such as levodopa and Sinemet have not been used frequently since both theoretical and clinical studies indicate they are not helpful in TD, in fact may worsen the disorder. Several informal reports have suggested that small doses of levodopa can be useful in TD and this might well be the case in patients with a dystonic response or rigidity associated with TD. Nevertheless, on theoretical grounds levodopa is not likely to be helpful and has been generally avoided[58]. Informal trials of pyridoxine, which is needed for decarboxylation, or of decarboxylase inhibitor alone have not showed major benefit[59,60] from these agents, although the effect of large doses of pyridoxine must be checked. One of the reasons pyridoxine was tried was its apparent ability to reduce the effectiveness of levodopa and thus lessen dyskinesia secondary to an overdose of levodopa.

Several agents that affect the GABA (γ-aminobutyric acid) system have been reported beneficial in TD, but informal reports suggest that these also have limited value. Baclofen (Lioresal) has been studied in several movement disorders, since this antispasm agent is a compound somewhat analagous to GABA. It was reported to be useful initially, in one encouraging report[61]; but later studies by Simpson[62] have refuted the initial optimism. Three patients seen in our office for TD were not dramatically benefitted by baclofen. There may be a need to test agents such as isoniazid, which can affect GABA aminotransferase, but clear-cut effects on TD are not yet reported for this drug. Perry[63] has suggested that occasional patients are dramatically improved by isoniazid when chorea is due to the hereditary disorder of Huntington's disease. Others are less sure of the effect of isoniazid, and at this time isoniazid is not considered a 'miracle cure' for either Huntington's disease or for TD. Sodium valproate[64-65] has been used in levodopa-induced chorea and for TD because of the suggestion that valproate can produce changes in brain GABA. Details of the use of valproate are not yet clear, but it does seem that valproate offers modest prospects, if any, for utilization in tardive dyskinesia. In addition to valproate, other anticonvulsants including newer ones such as clonazepam[66] are rarely useful. In fact chorea can result from an excess of anticonvulsants such as phenytoin[67-69].

Papaverine, which is used frequently as a presumed vasodilator in the aged, has also been suggested in TD and for the dyskinesia due to levodopa, but appears only modestly effective[70,71].

The antihistamines have been evaluated in TD, usually informally and without written reports. There is little evidence that this group of agents is helpful in TD, although since Benadryl (diphenhydramine hydrochloride) is an established drug for parkinsonism it, in particular, has been used in TD. Benadryl is helpful for parkinsonism not only as a mild sedative, but as an anticholinergic compound. TD is worsened, or is more apparent, in patients who are at rest than when active and TD is different in other ways than parkinsonism, and it is not to be expected that antihistamines would help TD. One of these drugs of interest in neurology, Periactin (cyproheptadine hydrochloride) is also not helpful[72]. Other antihistamines[73,74] can *produce* a dyskinesia similar to TD. Of particular note are the amphetamine group of drugs used therapeutically for narcolepsy and for the hyperactive child. Even normal individuals may note bruxism, chewing movements and twitching when receiving significant doses of these agents and at least one child has been seen in our office who developed what appeared to be mild Tourette's syndrome while on these agents; with relief from tics when the agents were withdrawn. There are numerous case reports confirming the ability of some antihistamines and of dextroamphetamine compounds to induce or increase dyskinesia[75-79].

The effect of alcohol on benign tremor is one of the most striking and inexplicable therapeutic phenomena in neurology, but there has been no systematic study of the effect of alcohol on TD or in other extrapyramidal disorders, either as therapy or as a predictor of the tendency to develop a movement disorder. Some patients with Huntington's disease (HD) seem unusually vulnerable to alcohol, but no one has reported an attempt to elicit subclinical dyskinesias in either TD or HD by use of alcohol. There are suggestions that the acute dystonia secondary to phenothiazines can be worsened by alcohol[80] and I have had one patient with Tourette's syndrome who developed severe transient dystonia while on haloperidol when beer was added.

Amantadine is used frequently at present to ameliorate some of the parkinsonian side-effects of phenothiazines; but there is no evidence that this agent will be any more useful than the anticholinergics.

Lithium is an agent which has a complex impact upon receptor sites and especially upon catecholamine receptor sites. In addition lithium manifests complex effects on sodium, cell membranes etc. The major neurological side-effect of lithium is a tremor which resembles benign essential tremor. The mechanism of the production of this tremor is as elusive as that of benign or of withdrawal tremor; but certainly lithium itself does produce tremor, and with excessive doses myoclonus and coarse dyskinetic movements may appear. Despite this, when used in therapeutic ranges some authors have demonstrated a useful effect of lithium on TD[81-83]. Lithium in larger doses can produce an exacerbation of TD[84,85].

Barbiturates have been rarely mentioned as treatment for TD, but Lipsius,[86] in a letter in the *American Journal of Psychiatry*, reviews a 55-year-old patient with probable TD who developed slow mouth movements which were increased in a setting of fear or anxiety. On phenobarbital 30 four times daily, she was calmer, slept well and no longer had abnormal mouth and tongue movements. Whether barbiturates function as a general sedative or in a more direct therapeutic fashion in patients with TD is uncertain[87].

Lastly, the use of the phenothiazines themselves[88,89], or of related compounds such as the butyrophenones, can certainly dampen the movements in patients with TD. In fact these agents are more commonly mentioned as therapy for TD than any single group of agents. The literature in this area is immense, but as is usual in TD consists particularly of case reports. The justification for such case reports may lie less in their scientific validity than in the remarkable impact TD has had upon different clinicians who rediscover this iatrogenic disease.

TREATMENT OF RELATED DISORDERS

Therapeutic efforts in other conditions and in animal models are surveyed in other chapters in this book. The repeated suggestion that dopamine receptor supersensitivity is present in TD has been studied by several techniques, in both humans and animals, although results remain inconclusive. One technique, that of Tamminga *et al.*[90], sought biochemical evidence of changes in growth hormone and prolactin secretion in patients with TD. If there was a meaningful change it was a decreased response to dopa stimulation following therapy with phenothiazines. Chronic therapy with phenothiazines has been reported, however, to increase binding of dopamine at receptor sites[91].

Animal studies and animal models are often disappointing as indicating a direct analogy to human disease. There has been difficulty in eliciting a movement similar to TD in primates, though extensive studies in rodents have been reported by the Klawans group and others. Gnawing or restlessness in rodents is not equivalent to TD in humans, however; and even the primate model is different. The effect of chlorpromazine in primates is dosage related and appears soon after the drug is administered. Initial articles[92] suggested that haloperidol was unlikely to lead to a movement disorder in primates, but later reports confirm the presence of 'TD' after haloperidol was administered to monkeys[93]. At this time there has been no systematic study of the effect of treatment on these disorders of movement in the primate. It is also known that haloperidol can produce TD in humans, in contrast to earlier opinions[94].

Although it is unwise to assume direct comparison between animal models and human disease, and also spurious to link TD with other movement disorders; there is theoretical overlap with TD and other extrapyramidal disorders.

Huntington's disease has been reviewed in this monograph and most of the therapy suggested for HD has been tried in TD. Some agents reported to be useful in HD have apparently not been tried in TD, such as the dipropylacetic acid used by Bachman *et al.*[95]. Tourette's syndrome has been successfully treated with phenothiazines, catecholamine antagonists, as well as with antidopaminergic medications. Haloperidol[96] is probably the most commonly used medication but pimozide (a piperidine) was reported in one double-blind[97] study to be at least as efficacious as haloperidol. Sweet and others[98] have suggested that antagonists to presynaptic catecholamines are as useful as are compounds with an antidopaminergic effect. An occasional overlap between TD and Tourette's has been reported by Caine *et al.*[99] and others[100].

OTHER MEASURES FOR THE MANAGEMENT OF TARDIVE DYSKINESIA

Prevention can hardly be over emphasized. It is unnecessary and unwise to use psychotropic agents to control minor neurotic conditions and mild anxiety. The occurrence of TD in non-psychotic individuals seems an unnecessary tragedy, as well as a classic iatrogenic error and a 'succulent legal plum'. TD is more common in patients with brain damage and may occur more frequently when phenothiazines are combined with electro-shock, lobotomy, and similar major therapeutic measures[101]. Females, especially older females, may be at particular risk although depressed patients and schizophrenics and neurotic patients are all vulnerable[102]. The use of anticholinergics can potentiate the development of TD, and pre-existent parkinsonism can increase chances of TD[103]. It is also possible that other disorders, even spontaneous oral facial movements[104] can increase the vulnerability to phenothiazines.

In addition to limiting phenothiazines to those patients who really need them, and to an insistence on particular caution in vulnerable individuals, it must be emphasized that there is little evidence that doses of phenothiazines higher than the equivalence of 400 mg of chlorpromazine add to the anti-psychotic benefit from these agents. There is, of course, not universal agreement regarding this limiting level[105]. In addition to limiting the dosage of antipsychotic medication the duration of therapy should be as brief as feasible. Drug holidays have been suggested and these combined with an awareness of TD by the clinician may lead to a minimal number of cases which generate concern.

NON-MEDICAL MEASURES

Since the patient's movements are usually most apparent when relaxed, heightened alertness and increased general activity might be of value for some patients. Some manage to reduce the cosmetic impact of the move-ments by chewing gum. A few can, and do, exert a temporary voluntary control over the movements. As of this time, no specific exercises or activity measures have been suggested, nor has the influence of exercise upon this and upon similar neurological disorders been studied in detail. Since the edentulous state can lead to restless mouth movements, ill fitting dentures may be assumed to augment the movements and therefore adequate dental care should be suggested to these patients.

Biofeedback has been used as therapy for disorders of the basal ganglia for several years[106,107]. Most reports have concerned the effect of biofeedback measures on dystonia, and though reports are enthusiastic the level of genuine or sustained improvement is uncertain. As with cutaneous stimu-lation for pain, initial benefit will often fade with time, although for enthusi-astic, devoted, or gullible patients physical measures may be helpful.

Korein and Brudny[108] have reviewed the philosophical basis of negative feedback and discuss the value of feedback measures in disorders of the basal ganglia. Clinical observation in dystonic patients, who often use touch or rubbing of fingers or nose or neck in geste antagonistique, suggested that electrical feedback might be even more effective. Eighty patients with dystonic syndromes were presented with a quantitative auditory and/or visual feedback. Electrical signals did serve to help the patient gain control over the defective muscle activity; 56% of the patients noted improvement. Some patients were unable to form a pattern of reciprocal innervation. Dementia, psychiatric trouble, or the combined influence of medications may all lessen the effectiveness of this treatment mode. No one has utilized educational measures such as sensory feedback in order to control the movements of tardive dyskinesia. Farrar[109] has reported the use of biofeedback as a help with spontaneous orofacial dyskinesia, but controlled studies in TD are not reported.

The treatment of the acute dyskinetic reaction secondary to phenothiazines offers little insight into the overall management of TD. Acute dystonia or dyskinesia can occur after only a few doses of medication and may be manifested by retrocollis and torticollis, trismus, or even opisthotonus. The symptoms can be relieved by benztropine, caffeine, diphenhydramine, or even diazepam. In fact, as in any movement disorder, if the movement is severe enough to endanger the patient, induction of sleep will stop the movement. Early reports suggested the use of barbiturates, and such hypnotics or sedatives could be employed in the severe cases of dystonia that interfere temporarily with respiration. Nevertheless, in general the management of the acute phenothiazine-induced dystonia is less troublesome than that of TD, if only because the acute reaction is so transient.

Surgery has been done in a few cases[110] but is not an accepted approach in TD.

Among all the medications that have been suggested can be seen lack of proof of the varied major views regarding causation of TD[111, 112]. The denervation sensitivity hypothesis has been most enthusiastically suggested in numerous writings by Harold Klawans[113–116] with a concept that receptor endings have become inappropriately sensitive in TD and have been modified biochemically and pathologically. This might explain the calming effect of phenothiazines on TD; as well as the development of TD when phenothiazines are discontinued. The calming effect of the phenothiazines could be not only 'the hair of the dog that bit you', but specific replacement of the chemical agent most likely to block receptor sites. Neuroleptic drugs produce complex effects at several sites and depletion of stores, or blockade of receptors, may lead to increased synthesis and paradoxical effects[117, 118]. The large number of phenothiazines, butyrophenones, and related compounds that can treat TD makes it hard to pick any single best agent to illustrate this concept.

It seems possible that several concepts in neurological management are illustrated by TD:

(1) Iatrogenic disease is hard to recognize[119], and incidence will vary markedly depending on population groups studied and the doses used.

(2) A metabolic or biochemical insult to the nervous system may, if severe enough, become an anatomic one.

(3) Drug 'vacations' might be considered for many agents that affect the CNS.

(4) If drugs affect more than one system in the CNS, and they usually do, then the pathophysiology of side-effects will be hard to unravel.

(5) If subclinical damage occurs, or is present, many agents may appear to affect the changed area. Whenever a deterioration occurs it may reflect the action of an agent on the damaged regions and when malfunction occurs the damaged area appears to be involved. Thus numerous agents appear to work by a similar mechanism when in fact the initial insult changed patterns of vulnerability to all agents.

WHAT MAJOR QUESTIONS REMAIN?

(1) Is the mechanism one of dopamine blockage followed by super sensitivity of receptors, excess dopamine, inadequate cholinergic, catecholamine imbalance, or a combination of all of these? Do anticholinergics fail to help or increase the risk[120]?

(2) Is there a difference in patients with buccolingual-masticatory form and the other varieties of TD?

(3) Does 'natural' ageing of the CNS increase tendency for TD in the elderly and if so, how? For example, is the oral form related to age?

(4) For medicolegal, or moral reasons, is informed consent required before using phenothiazines?

(5) Why are so few patients troubled by the movements, even when AIMS are grossly apparent?

(6) Are there other 'tardive' effects of drugs on the CNS to which we remain blind. Should vacation periods be considered for other medications used for the CNS (i.e. anticonvulsants)?

(7) How, and where, does the biochemical effect of phenothiazines lead to the apparent anatomic disorder of TD, and what are the mechanisms leading to such persistent biochemical lesions?

MANAGEMENT OF THE INDIVIDUAL CASE

In view of lack of a certain single mechanism, and lack of a certain single cure[121-127], how can one manage a patient with TD? First the history of that single patient must be ascertained, with particular attention to precipitating factors and to the true need for antipsychotic medicine. Secondly, other organic diseases must be considered, with appraisal of the severity of the movement disorder. The possibility of cortical atrophy may require evaluation[128,129]. The role of mechanical measures, particularly dentition and need for adequate physical activity should be considered. If the patient has only mild TD and is off medications little therapy may be needed. For moderate cases one can try barbiturates or diazepam, agents which may tranquilize by another biochemical mechanism than is true for phenothiazines. In the more severe cases use of haloperidol or tetrabenazine may be considered; but such use should be at the lowest level that allows reasonable comfort, and used with the goal of an eventual reduction or elimination of medication. Withdrawal from phenothiazines should be done slowly in patients on chronic medication.

Other psychotropic medication, such as lithium or librium (chlordiazepoxide hydrochloride) may be required and the tricyclic medications and anticholinergics should be used with caution. In rare life threatening situations, such as respiratory distress from TD, induction of sleep will offer a temporary respite. A combination of agents or use of agents under current experimentation, such as α–methyltyrosine, may eventually be considered the best drug therapy. Surgery will rarely be useful; critical individualized care is the goal.

The issue of informed consent regarding TD should be considered by the physician, particularly for those at risk. Each time phenothiazines are prescribed the concepts of prevention (low dosage, brief therapy, drug vacations, no anticholinergics) should be considered.

GENERAL CONCLUSIONS

The first important principle of therapy is prevention and for all patients, and especially for those at risk, phenothiazines should be administered cautiously. The second principle, one that cannot be presented with as much certainty as the first principle, is that there is no single optimal treatment for TD. In patients who are in distress with TD after phenothiazines are terminated careful use of dopamine antagonists such as reserpine, or of choline agonists such as deanol can be justified. Severe cases may require replacement of lesser doses of phenothiazines and gradual staged reduction of dosage over a period of weeks.

Treatment, as reviewed, remains unsatisfactory but newer concepts offer great promise. New drugs, such as clozapine, may offer antipsychotic effects with less extrapyramidal toxicity[130]. There is increased interest and research in the role of choline and lecithin, not only in TD but in numerous other disorders[131]. Balance between several neurotransmitters, the effects of normal ageing in the CNS, and the uncertain nature of the insult resulting from phenothiazine use all complicate understanding of TD. Nevertheless, continued study of TD by researchers, and clinical awareness of such research, can be expected to enrich understanding of all extrapyramidal disorders.

References

1 Crane, G. E. (1973). Persistent dyskinesia. *Br. J. Psychiat.*, **122**, 395

2 Crane, G. E. (1974). Factors predisposing to drug-induced neurologic effects. *Adv. Biochem. Psychopharmacol.*, **9**, 269

3 Polizos, P. and Engelhardt, D. M. (1973). Neurological consequences of psychotropic drug withdrawal in schizophrenic children. *J. Autism. Child.*, **3**, 247

4 Paulson, G. W., Rizvi, C. A. and Crane, G. E. (1975). Tardive dyskinesia as a possible sequel of long-term therapy with phenothiazines. *Clin. Pediatr.*, **14**, 953

5 Chiles, J. A. (1978). Extrapyramidal reactions in adolescents treated with high-potency antipsychotics. *Am. J. Psychol.*, **135**, 239

6 Crane, G. E. (1968). Tardive dyskinesia in patients treated with major neuroleptics; a review of the literature. *Am. J. Psychiatry*, **124**, 40

7 Schiele, B. C., Gallant, D., Simpson, G., Gardner, E. A. and Cole, J. O. (1973). Tardive dyskinesia. A persistent neurological syndrome associated with antipsychotic drug use. *Ann. Intern. Med.*, **79**, 99

8 Crane, G. E. and Smeets, R. A. (1974). Tardive dyskinesia and drug therapy in geriatric patients. *Arch. Gen. Psychiatry*, **30**, 341

9 Jus, A., Pineau, R., Lachance, R., Pelchat, G., Jus, K., Pires, P. and Villeneuve, R. (1976). Epidemiology of tardive dyskinesia. *Dis. Nerv. Syst.*, **37**, 210

10 Klawans, H. L., Bergen, D., Bruyn, G. W. and Paulson, G. W. (1974). Neuroleptic induced tardive dyskinesia in nonpsychotic patients. *Arch. Neurol.*, **30**, 338

11 Kane, J., Wegner, J. and Struve, F. (1978). The mitten pattern as a potential EEG predictor of tardive dyskinesia. *Psychopharmacol. Bull.*, **14**, 35

12 Crane, G. E. and Naranjo, E. R. (1971). Motor disorders induced by neuroleptics. A proposed new classification. *Arch. Gen. Psychiatry*, **24**, 179

13 Gardos, G., Cole, J. O. and LaBrie, R. (1977). The assessment of tardive dyskinesia. *Arch. Gen. Psychol.*, **34**, 1206

14 Tarsy, D. (1978). Dr. Tarsy replies. *Am. J. Psychiatry*, **135**, 386

15 Jelliffe, S. E. (1929). Oculogyric crises as compulsive phenomena in postencephalitis. Their occurrence, phenomenology and meaning. *J. Nerv. Ment. Dis.*, **69**, 59

16 Paulson, G. W. (1968). 'Permanent' or complex dyskinesias in the aged. *Geriatrics*, **23**, 105

17 Carruthers, S. C. (1971). Persistent tardive dyskinesia. *Br. J. Med.*, **3**, 572

18 Paulson, G. W. (1975). Tardive dyskinesia. *Am. Rev. Med.*, **26**, 75

19 Symington, G. R., Leonard, D. P., Shannon, P. J. and Vajda, F. J. E. (1978). Sodium valproate in Huntington's disease. *Am. J. Psychiatry*, **135**, 352

20 Quitkin, F., Rifkin, A., Gochfeld, L. and Klein, D. F. (1977). Tardive dyskinesia: are first signs reversible? *Am. J. Psychiatry.*, **134**, 84

21 Casey, D. E. and Rabins, P. (1978). Tardive dyskinesia as a life threatening illness. *Am. J. Psychiatry*, **135**, 486

22 Mehta, D., Mallya, A. and Volavka, J. (1978). Mortality of patients with tardive dyskinesia. *Am. J. Psychol.*, **135**, 371

23 Weiner, W. J., Goetz, C. G., Nausieda, P. A. and Klawans, H. L. (1978). Respiratory dyskinesia: extrapyramidal dysfunction and dyspnea. *Ann. Intern. Med.*, **88**, 327

24 Chouinard, G. and Annable, L. (1977). Phenothiazine-induced EEG abnormality. *Arch. Gen. Psych.*, **34**, 951

25 Lemere, F. (1977). Tardive dyskinesia of the abdomen. *J. Am. Med. Assoc.*, **238**, 306

26 Sovner, R., DiMascio, A., Berkowitz, D. and Randolph, P. (1978). Tardive dyskinesia and informed consent. *Psychosomatics.*, **19**, 172

27 Klawans, Jr., H. L. (1973). The pharmacology of extrapyramidal movement disorders. In *Monographs in Neural Sciences*. Vol. II, p. 136 (New York: Karger)

28 Villeneuve, A. and Bozormenyi, Z. (1970). Treatment of drug-induced dyskinesia. *Lancet*, **1**, 353

29 Sato, S., Daly, R. and Peters, H. (1971). Reserpine therapy of phenothiazine induced dyskinesia. *Dis. Nerv. Syst.*, **32**, 680

30 Crane, G. E. (1973). Mediocre effects of reserpine on tardive dyskinesia. *N. Engl. J. Med.*, **288**, 104

31 Kobayaski, R. M. (1977). Drug therapy of tardive dyskinesia. *N. Engl. J. Med.*, **296**, 257

32 Fahn, S. (1978). Treatment of tardive dyskinesia with combined reserpine and α-methyl-tyrosine. *Ann. Neurol.*, **4**, 169

33 Bucci, L. (1971). The dyskinesia: a new therapeutic approach. *Dis. Nerv. Syst.*, **32**, 324

34 Kazamatsuri, H., Chien, C. and Cole. J. O. (1972). Treatment of tardive dyskinesia. *Arch. Gen. Psychiatry*, **27**, 824

35 Huang, C. Y., McLeod, J. G., Holland, R. T. and Elliot, C. (1976). Tetrabenazine in the therapy of Huntington's chorea. *Med. J. Aust.*, **1**, 583

36 MacCallum, W. A. (1970). Tetrabenazine for extrapyramidal motor disorders. *Br. J. Med.*, **1**, 760

37 Goodwin-Austin, R. B. and Clark, T. (1971). Persistent phenothiazine dyskinesia treated with tetrabenazine. *Br. J. Med.*, **4**, 25

38 Kazamatsuri, H., Chien, C. and Cole, J. O. (1972). Treatment of tardive dyskinesia, i: clinical efficacy of a dopamine-depleting agent, tetrabenazine. *Arch. Gen. Psychiatry*, **27**, 95

39 Kazamatsuri, H., Chien, C. and Cole, J. O. (1973). Long-term treatment of tardive dyskinesia with haloperidol and tetrabenazine. *Am. J. Psychiatry*, **130**, 479

40 Gerlach, J., Reisby, N. and Randrup, A. (1974). Dopaminergic hypersensitivity and cholinergic hypofunction in the pathophysiology of tardive dyskinesia. *Psychopharmacologia.*, **34**, 21

41 Klawans, H. L. and Rubovits, R. (1974). Effect of cholinergic and anticholinergic agents on tardive dyskinesia. *J. Neurol. Neurosurg. Psychiatry*, **37**, 941

42 Growdon, J. H., Hirsch, M. J., Wurtman, R. J. and Wiener, W. (1977). Oral choline administration to patients with tardive dyskinesia. *N. Engl. J. Med.*, **297**, 524

43 Barbeau, A. (1978). Phosphatidylcholine (Lecithin) in neurologic disorders. *Neurology*, **28**, 358

44 Growdon, J. H., Gelenberg, A. J. and Doller, J. (1978). Lecithin can suppress tardive dyskinesia. *N. Engl. J. Med.*, **298**, 1029

45 Nutt, J. G., Rosin, A. and Chase, T. N. (1978). Treatment of Huntington's disease with a cholinergic agonist. *Neurology*, **28**, 1061

46 Miller, E. M. (1974). Deanol: a solution for tardive dyskinesia? *N. Engl. J. Med.*, **291**, 796

47 Casey, D. E. and Denney, D. (1974). Dimethylaminoethanol in tardive dyskinesia. *N. Engl. J. Med.*, **291**, 797

48 Fann, W. E., Gerber, C. J. and McKenzie, G. M. (1974). Cholinergic suppression of tardive dyskinesia. *Psychopharmacologia.*, **37**, 101

49 Escobar, J. I. and Kemp, K. F. (1975). Dimethylaminoethanol for tardive dyskinesia. *N. Engl. J. Med.*, **292**, 317

50 Crane, G. E. (1975). Deanol for tardive dyskinesia. *N. Engl. J. Med.*, **292**, 926

51 Davis, K. L., Berger, P. A. and Hollister, L. E. (1975). Choline for tardive dyskinesia. *N. Engl. J. Med.*, **293**, 152

52 Hoy, R. (1975). Deanol for tardive dyskinesia. *N. Engl. J. Med.*, **292**, 926

53 Granacher, R. P. and Baldessarini, R. J. (1975). Deanol for tardive dyskinesia. *N. Engl. J. Med.*, **292**, 926

54 Widroe, H. J. and Heisler, S. (1976). Treatment of tardive dyskinesia. *Dis. Nerv. Syst.*, **37**, 162

55 Tarsy, D. and Bralower, M. (1977). Deanol acetamidobenzoate treatment in choreiform movement disorders. *Arch. Neurol.*, **34**, 756

56 Penovich, P., Morgan, J. P., Kerzner, B., Karch, F. and Goldblatt, D. (1978). Double blind evaluation of deanol in tardive dyskinesia. *J. Am. Med. Assoc.*, **239**, 1997

57 Casey, D. E. (1976). Tardive dyskinesia: are there subtypes? *N. Engl. J. Med.*, **295**, 1078

58 Klawans, H. L. and McKendal, R. (1971). Observations on the effects of L-dopa on tardive linguo-facial-buccal dyskinesia. *J. Neurol. Sci.*, **11**, 189

59 Paulson, G. W. (1971). Use of pyridoxine in chorea. *Am. J. Psychol.*, **127**, 1091

60 DeVeaugh-Geiss, J. and Manion, L. (1978). High-dose pyridoxine in tardive dyskinesia. *J. Clin. Psychiatry*, **39**, 573

61 Korsgaard, S. (1976). Baclofen (Lioresal) in the treatment of neuroleptic-induced tardive dyskinesia. *Acta Psychiatry Scand.*, **54**, 17

62 Simpson, G. M., Lee, J. H., Shrivastava, R. K. and Branchey, M. H. (1978). Baclofen in therapy of tardive dyskinesia and schizophrenia. *Psychopharmacol. Bull.*, **14**, 16

63 Perry, T. L., MacLeod, P. M. and Hansen, S. (1977). Treatment of Huntington's chorea with isoniazid. *N. Engl. J. Med.*, **297**, 840

64 Price, P. A., Parkes, J. D. and Marsden, C. D. (1978). Sodium Valproate in the treatment of levodopa-induced dyskinesia. *J. Neurol. Neurosurg. Psychiatry*, **41**, 702

65 Gibson, A. C. (1978). Sodium valproate and tardive dyskinesia. *Br. J. Psychol.*, **133**, 82

66 Peiris, J. B., Boralessa, H. and Lionel, N. D. W. (1976). Clonazepam in the treatment of choreiform activity. *Med. J. Aust.*, **1**, 225

67 Shuttleworth, E., Wise, G. and Paulson, G. (1974). Choreoathetosis and diphenyl-hydantoin intoxication. *J. Am. Med. Assoc.*, **230**, 1170

68 Chadwick, D., Reynolds, E. H. and Marsden, C. D. (1976). Anticonvulsant-induced dyskinesia: A comparison with dyskinesias induced by neuroleptics. *J. Neurol. Neurosurg. Psychiatry*, **39**, 1210

69 DeVeaugh-Geiss, J. (1977). Aggravation of tardive dyskinesia by phenytoin. *N. Engl. J. Med.*, **298**, 457

70 Duvoisin, R. O. (1975). Antagonism of levodopa by papaverine. *J. Am. Med. Assoc.*, **231**, 845

71 Gardos, G. and Cole, J. O. (1975). Papaverine for tardive dyskinesia? *N. Engl. J. Med.*, **292**, 1355

72 Gardos, G. and Cole, J. O. (1978). Pilot study of cyproheptadine (periactin) in tardive dyskinesia. *Psychopharmacol. Bull.*, **14**, 18

73 Brait, K. A. and Zagerman, A. J. (1977). Dyskinesias after antihistamine use. *N. Engl. J. Med.*, **296**, 111

74 Hale, C. and Heins, T. (1978). Tardive dyskinesia and antihistamines. *Med. J. Aust.*, **1**, 112

75 Mattson, R. H. and Calverley, J. R. (1968). Dextroamphetamine-sulfate-induced dys-kinesias. *J. Am. Med. Assoc.*, **204**, 400

76 Fann, W. E., Davis, J. M. and Wilson, I. C. (1973). Methylphenidate in tardive dyskinesia. *Am. J. Psychiatry*, **130**, 922

77 Thach, B. T., Chase, T. N. and Bosma, J. F. (1975). Oral facial dyskinesia associated with prolonged use of antihistaminic decongestants. *N. Engl. J. Med.*, **293**, 486

78 Davis, W. A. (1976). Dyskinesia associated with chronic antihistamine use. *N. Engl. J. Med.*, **294**, 113

79 Extein, I. (1978). Methylphenidate-induced choreoathetosis. *Am. J. Psychol.*, **135**, 252

80 Lutz, E. G. (1976). Neuroleptic-induced akathisia and dystonia triggered by alcohol. *J. Am. Med. Assoc.*, **236**, 2422

81 Dalén, P. (1973). Lithium therapy in Huntington's chorea and tardive dyskinesia. *Lancet*, **1**, 107

82 Reda, F. A., Escobar, J. I. and Scanlan, J. M. (1975). Lithium carbonate in the treatment of tardive dyskinesia. *Am. J. Psychiatry*, **132**, 560

83 Simpson, G. M., Branchey, M. H. and Lee, J. H. (1976). Lithium in tardive dyskinesia. *Pharmakopsychiatr. Neuropsychopharmakol.*, **9**, 76

84 Crews, E. L. and Carpenter, A. E. (1977). Lithium-induced aggravation of tardive dyskinesia. *Am. J. Psychol.*, **134**, 933

85 Rosenbaum, A. H. (1978). Tardive dyskinesia and pharmacotherapy. *Am. J. Psychol.*, **135**, 506

86 Lipsius, L. H. (1977). Barbiturates and tardive dyskinesia. *Am. J. Psychol.*, **134**, 1162

87 Sovner, R. and Loadman, A. (1978). More on barbiturate and tardive dyskinesia. *Am. J. Psychiatry*, **135**, 382

88 Kazamatsuri, H., Chien, C. and Cole, J. O. (1972). Treatment of tardive dyskinesia, II. Short-term efficacy of dopamine-blocking agents, haloperidol and thiopropazate. *Arch. Gen. Psychiatry*, **27**, 100

89 Curran, J. P. (1973). Management of tardive dyskinesia with thiopropazate. *Am. J. Psychiatry*, **130**, 925

90 Tamminga, C. A., Smith, R. C., Pandey, G., Frohman, L. A. and Davis, J. M. (1977). A neuroendocrine study of supersensitivity in tardive dyskinesia. *Arch. Gen. Psychol.*, **34**, 1199

91 Burt, D. R., Creese, I. and Snyder, S. H. (1977). Antischizophrenic drugs: chronic treatment elevates dopamine receptor binding in brain. *Science*, **196**, 326

92 Paulson, G. (1976). Effects of chronic administration of neuroleptics: dyskinesias in monkeys. *Pharmacol. Ther. B.*, **2**, 167

93 Gunne, L. M. and Barany, S. (1976). Haloperidol induced tardive dyskinesia in monkeys. *Psychopharmacology*, **50**, 237

94 Jacobson, G., Baldessarini, R. J. and Manschreck, T. (1974). Tardive dyskinesia associated with haloperidol. *Am. J. Psychiatry*, **131**, 910

95 Bachman, D. S., Butler, I. J. and McKhann, G. M. (1977). Long-term treatment of juvenile Huntington's chorea with dipropylacetic acid. *Neurology*, **27**, 193

96 Shapiro, A. K., Shapiro, E. and Wayne, H. (1973). Treatment of Tourettes' syndrome. *Arch. Gen. Psychol*, **28**, 92

97 Ross, M. S. and Moldofsky, H. (1978). A comparison of pimozide and haloperidol in the treatment of Gilles de la Tourette syndrome. *Am. J. Psychol.*, **135**, 585

98 Sweet, R. D., Bruun, R., Shapiro, E. and Shapiro, A. K. (1974). Presynaptic catecholamine antagonists as treatment for Tourette syndrome. *Arch. Gen. Psychol.*, **31**, 857

99 Caine, E. D., Margolin, D. I., Brown, G. L. and Ebert, M. H. (1978). Gilles de la Tourette's syndrome, tardive dyskinesia, and psychosis in an adolescent. *Am. J. Psychol.*, **135**, 241

100 Klawans, H. L., Falk, D. K., Nausieda, P. A. and Weiner, W. J. (1978). Gilles de la Tourette syndrome after long-term CPZ therapy. *Neurology*, **28**, 1064

101 Uhrbrand, L. and Faurbye, A. (1960). Reversible and irreversible dyskinesias after treatment with perphenazine, chlorpromazine, reserpine and electroconvulsive therapy. *Psychopharmacologia.*, **5**, 408

102 Rosenbaum, A. H., Niven, R. G., Hanson, N. P. and Swanson, D. W. (1977). Tardive dyskinesia: relationship with a primary affective disorder. *Dis. Nerv. Syst.*, **38**, 423

103 Crane, G. E. (1978). Parkinsonism and tardive dyskinesia. *Am. J. Psychol.*, **135**, 619

104 Altrocchi, P. H. (1972). Spontaneous oral-facial dyskinesia. *Arch. Neurol.*, **26**, 506

105 Shader, R. I., Elkins, R., Ciraulo, D. and Salzman, C. (1978). On guidelines for maximum dosages. *Am. J. Psychiatry*, **135**, 499

106 Brudney, J., Korein, J., Levidow, L., Grynbaum, B., Lieberman, A. and Friedmann, L. (1974). Sensory feedback therapy as a modality of treatment in CNS disorders of voluntary movement. *Neurology*, **24**, 925

107 Albanese, H. and Gaarder, K. (1977). Biofeedback treatment of tardive dyskinesia: Two case reports. *Am. J. Psychol.*, **134**, 1149

108 Korein, J. and Brudney, J. (1976). Integrated EMG feedback in the management of spasmodic torticollis and focal dystonia: a prospective study of 80 patients. In Yahr, M. D. (ed.) *Basal Ganglia*, pp. 385–426. (New York: Raven Press)

109 Farrar, W. B. (1976). Using electromyographic biofeedback in treating orofacial dyskinesia. *J. Prosthet. Dent.*, **35**, 384

110 Nashold, B. S. (1969). The effects of central tegmental lesions on tardive dyskinesia. In Crane, G. E. and Gardner, R. (eds.) *Psychotropic Drugs and Dysfunctions of the Basal Ganglia*, pp. 111–113. (Washington, D.C.: Public Health Service Publication)

111 Calne, D. B. (1975). *Therapeutics in Neurology*, pp. 209–211. (Oxford: Blackwell Scientific Publications)

112 Simpson, G. M. and Kline, N. S. (1976). Tardive dyskinesia: Manifestations, incidence, etiology and treatment. In Yahr, M. D. (ed.) *Basal Ganglia*, pp. 427–432. (New York: Raven Press)

113 Rubovits, R. and Klawans, H. L. (1972). Implications of amphetamine-induced stereotyped behavior as a model for tardive dyskinesia. *Arch. Gen. Psychol.*, **27**, 502

114 Klawans, H. L. and Weiner, W. J. (1974). The effect of d-amphetamine on choreiform movement disorders. *Neurology*, **24**, 312

115 Klawans, H. L. and Weiner, W. J. (1976). The pharmacology of choreatic movement disorders. *Prog. Neurobiol.*, **6**, 49

116 Klawans, H. L. and Moskovitz, C. (1977). Cyclizine induced chorea. Observations on the influence of cyclizine on dopamine-related movement disorders. *J. Neurol. Sci.*, **31**, 237

117 Chase, T. N. (1972). Drug-induced extrapyramidal disorders. In Kopin, I. J. (ed.) *Neurotransmitters*. Research Publications Association for Research in Nervous and Mental Disease. Vol. L, pp. 448–471. (Baltimore: The Williams & Wilkins Company)

118 Carlsson, A. (1978). Mechanism of action of neuroleptic drugs. In Lipton, M. A., DiMascio, A. and Killam, K. F. (eds.) *Psychopharmacology: A Generation of Progress*, pp. 1057–1070. (New York: Raven Press)

119 Crane, G. E. (1973). Clinical psychopharmacology in its 20th year. *Science*, **181**, 124

120 Swett, C., Cole, J. O., Shapiro, S. and Slone, D. (1977). Extrapyramidal side-effects in chlorpromazine recipients. *Arch. Gen. Psychiatry*, **34**, 942

121 Schmidt, W. R. and Jarcho, L. W. (1966). Persistent dyskinesias following phenothiazine therapy. *Arch. Neurol.*, **14**, 369

122 Clyne, K. E. and Juhl, R. P. (1976). Tardive dyskinesia. *Am. J. Hosp. Pharmacol.*, **33**, 481

123 Gerlach, J. and Thorsen, K. (1976). The movement pattern of oral tardive dyskinesia in relation to anticholinergic and anti dopaminergic treatment. *Int. Pharmacopsychiatry*, **11**, 1

124 Sayers, A. C., Bürki, H. R., Ruch, W. and Asper, H. (1976). Anticholinergic properties of antipsychotic drugs and their relation to extrapyramidal side-effects. *Psychopharmacology*, **51**, 15

125 Gerlach, J. (1977). Relationship between tardive dyskinesia, L-dopa-induced hyperkinesia and parkinsonism. *Psychopharmacology*, **51**, 259

126 Casey, D. E. (1978). Managing tardive dyskinesia. *J. Clin. Psychol.*, 748

127 Granacher, Jr., R. P. (1978). Tardive dyskinesia. *Am. Fam. Phys.*, **17**, 163

128 Gelenberg, A. J. (1976). Computerized tomography in patients with tardive dyskinesia. *Am. J. Psychiatry*, **133**, 578

129 Roberts, M. A. and Caird, F. I. (1976). Computerized tomography and intellectual impairment in the elderly. *J. Neurol. Neurosurg. Psychiatry*, **39**, 986

130 Baldessarini, R. J. and Tarsy, D. (1978). Tardive dyskinesia. In Lipton, M. A., DiMascio, A. and Killam, K. F. (eds.) *Psychopharmacology : A Generation of Progress*, pp. 993–1004. (New York: Raven Press)

131 Kolata, G. B. (1979). Mental disorders: a new approach to treatment. *Science*, **203**, 36

8

Essential tremor

T. J. Murray

INTRODUCTION

Essential tremor has been of considerable interest for well over 100 years. Although a relatively benign disorder in most patients, it can be disturbing because it is embarrassing and may interfere with motor tasks. Many patients find it embarrassing to get haircuts, speak in public or hold a coffee-cup because of the tremulousness. In just those situations when the patient would like to be able to reduce the tremor, the tension of the moment and the increased concentration tends to worsen it. It may interfere with hand-writing and fine motor tasks, and hinder social relationships[1].

Although some authors have regarded it as a rare disease, it is now becoming evident that it is relatively common. Sevitt[2] states that there are 80 000 consultations for essential tremor, and 1.4 million for senile tremor in the United Kingdom annually.

The frequency of the disorder has become more apparent since the advent of levodopa (L-Dopa) therapy for parkinson's disease and the observation that propranolol helps essential tremor[3,4]. Many of the patients seen in Parkinson's clinics in the late 60s were patients with essential tremor referred for assessment and management. 4.5% of patients referred for therapy of Parkinson's disease are found to have essential tremor[5,6].

The increasing interest in essential tremor has led to a number of controversies. There are divergent views on its incidence, the characteristics of the tremor and whether or not it is significantly helped by propranolol therapy. There is also conflicting data as to whether essential tremor is primarily a peripheral or central defect, or both, and whether propranolol acts peripherally or centrally in this disorder. In this chapter we will attempt to review the features of this tremor and address some of these points.

EARLY DESCRIPTIONS OF THE TREMOR

M. Critchley[7] suggests that the first comment on tremor comes from Ecclesiastes (XII 3), 'The keepers of the house shall tremble', which he interprets as a tremor of the hands in the elderly. The first familial tremor was recorded by Most in 1836[8]. A case of Sanders' (1872)[9] with 'paralysis agitans' beginning at age 12 and persisting to death at age 66, was probably essential tremor. Trousseau[10] in 1885 commented on the onset of 'senile tremor' in adolescence and middle life. M. Critchley[7] refers to 45 papers on this condition prior to World War I. Dana[11] in 1887 gave the first systematic description of familial essential tremor in the English language.

The Russian neurologist, Minor[12-15], published a series of papers between 1921 and 1929 on essential tremor and the syndrome is still referred to by some authors as Minor's disease. When M. Critchley[7] wrote his extensive review of the subject in 1949 he referred to 117 papers on the subject and the number has quadrupled since then.

THE TREMOR

Essential tremor is mostly distal in the limb, rhythmical, and with a frequency rate of 6–12 Hz[16]. It may appear fine or coarse, depending on the frequency and the amplitude of the tremor.

Essential tremor involves the hands, the arms and often the head. In some patients it may affect the legs, chin, tongue, laryngeal muscles and eyes. It may begin in one hand, often intermittently with bursts of this superimposed tremor on an underlying physiological tremor. The tremors eventually become continuous and they seem to spread from one part to another. In virtually all patients the hands are involved first and most markedly, although occasional patients may have tremor only in the head, or only in the voice[17]. The diaphragm may also be involved[7].

The head tremor may be sideways *(le tremblement négatif)* or a flexion extension movement *(le tremblement positif)*[18].

Brown and Simonson found that 6 of 31 cases of organic voice tremor had no limb or head tremor and they felt this was part of the essential tremor syndrome[19]. Hachinski described three women with voice tremor only[17].

Although there are some variations, the characteristic essential tremor is absent at rest, increased by maintaining the limb in a posture or position (static, postural or attitude tremor) and during active movement (kinetic or intention tremor). It may be accentuated on approaching a goal in point to point movement (terminal tremor). The tremor is absent when at complete rest or when walking or standing with the arm passively hanging at the side.

Essential tremor may begin at any age. It has commonly been referred to as 'juvenile tremor' in the early decades, essential tremor in the middle years, and 'senile tremor' in the elderly. It is more common in advancing years, particularly over the age of 50 but may occur in children. Paulson[20] noted the tremor may disappear in children, only to reappear later as adults.

Essential tremor is probably present equally in both sexes[7] but was noted to be more common in females in other studies[21,2]. E. Critchley, on the other hand, felt it was more common in males[5]. The incidence is unknown but Hornabrook[18] noted there were 17 cases per 1000 in the 50–59 age group in New Guinea, and in Great Britain it is probably similar to the prevalence of Parkinson's disease[2].

The tremor often begins on one side but eventually becomes bilaterally symmetrical. If it is unilateral it is more often on the right side[5]. It is absent at rest and is increased by posturing or maintaining the limb in an attitude against gravity. There may be some independence of the tremor in each limb and Barlow and Schwab[22] have noted that the tremor is decreased if one limb supports the other.

The tremor is aggravated by emotional stress, excitement, physical fatigue, and extremes of temperature. M. Critchley[7] noted that cold was worse than heat. The tremor may also be aggravated by local pain in the limb, in the withdrawal period after alcohol and in some patients by tea, coffee, tobacco and hunger. It has also been described as increasing with sexual intercourse or erotic excitement in some patients[7]. Almost all patients with essential tremor find it worse in the presence of strangers and they often feel that people are staring at them. The tremor is often worse early in the morning.

The tremor is a progressive disorder, advancing slowly from one limb to another, usually over many years. The tremor may plateau for many years, and occasionally may have prolonged remissions.

There is a great deal of variation in the tremor from patient to patient. The typical postural tremor may sometimes have a mild tremor that is occasionally present at rest and inhibited by action, but it is usually absent at rest and increased by sustained postural attitude of the hand or limb. It may be accentuated at the terminal aspect of the action[23], and it is these patients that have the tremor evident in their handwriting.

In an occasional patient the frequency may be as high as 18 Hz but the mean frequency in men is 10.4 Hz and in women 9.6 Hz[24]. There is a decrease in the tremor frequency with age as with Parkinson's tremor. Those under age 40 years have an average frequency of 11.5 Hz and over age 40, 9.2 Hz. The frequency varies from 6 Hz in early life to 10 Hz in the 20–45-year age group and to 6 Hz in old age[16]. Although a number of treatments may decrease the amplitude of the tremor, none, including alcohol or propranolol, affect the frequency.

The tremor amplitude varies from one period to another, and has been noted to have a periodicity in some patients[16]. This may cause an irregular appearance in the tremor. There can be a regular cyclic variation of the tremor every 1–1.5 seconds. The difficulty or handicap due to the tremor varies with the amplitude rather than the frequency.

Based on the demonstration that the frequency pattern with age and essential tremor follows that of physiological tremor, Marshall[16] suggested the following hypothesis: physiological tremors are due to a servo-mechanism and essential tremor can be considered a failure of the dampening mechanism of the servo-control allowing for greater oscillation than usual. As the servo-mechanism begins to fail, bursts of essential tremor can be seen, and later the tremor becomes continuous[15].

Marshall[16] showed that there were two patterns of essential tremor:

(1) A smooth regular form following age changes of physiological tremor, but resembling Parkinsonian tremor with its smooth regular wave form.

(2) Small irregularities in pattern which Bertrand[21] felt were unlike tremor effects.

Perhaps essential tremor is exaggerated physiological tremor with episodic increases in amplitude superimposed on a lower amplitude tremor of this same frequency[16]. Later the wave form varies and the clinical pattern may change as time goes on.

Lee and Stein[25] felt that essential tremor was probably related to a disturbance in the olivo-cerebello-rubral system, on the basis of their methods of introducing mechanical disturbances into reflex loops and observing the resetting mechanism in essential tremor and in Parkinson patients. All patients with essential tremor showed evidence of resetting of their tremor when a mechanical input was applied to their reflex loops. The reflex mechanisms and the resetting was much more evident in essential tremor than in Parkinson's tremor.

Kreiss[26] said it was not an exaggerated physiological tremor. M. Critchley and Greenfield[27] wondered if it were a *forme fruste* or mild presentation of an underlying neurological disorder. E. Critchley[5] seems to favour this latter interpretation.

Molina-Negro and Hardy[28] assessed over 400 patients with tremor of various forms and concluded from their EMG and cinephotographic studies that there were two forms of tremor (tremor being defined as 'an involuntary, rhythmical and symmetrical movement about an axis of equilibrium'): a postural tremor and a tremor of attitude. Both of the above types of tremor are present with the limb immobile, and absent during movement. (They regard cerebellar tremor as an ataxia rather than a tremor.) They also note that head tremor disapppears, if the head is supported and the neck relaxed. It becomes worse if head movement is restrained. It was noted by Hornabrook that the women of Papua with head tremor who carried a string bag with a supporting band over their foreheads had accentuation of their tremor[18].

THE EFFECT OF ALCOHOL

Physicians and patients have long noted that alcohol even in small or moderate amounts, may dramatically reduce the tremor. In some patients the effect may be so marked that the patient begins to use alcohol as a means of therapy. The effect is shortlived, however, and repeated and frequent drinking may result. We have seen many patients with essential tremor who overindulge as a form of therapy. One ophthalmic surgeon had a small drink of vodka between each case in his office to reduce his embarrassment and concern over his tremulous hands. He understandably was anxious to avoid tremulousness in front of those to whom he might suggest he should operate on their eyes. When he responded well to propranolol therapy he stopped his drinking completely.

Rajput[29] tested the effect of one ounce of absolute alcohol in patients with essential tremor. This reduced the tremor in 62% of cases. The response is not specific, however, as 46.6% of Parkinson patients have a similar improvement. One patient with ataxia telangiectasia and one patient with a tremor from a cervical cord lesion also had reduction in tremor with alcohol. All of the patients who improved with alcohol improved with propranolol. He concluded that the reduction in tremor with alcohol was not specific to essential tremor and was not a diagnostic test of essential tremor. He suggests that it could be used as an office test to predict the effect of propranolol.

In another study[5] 13 out of 19 patients with essential tremor experienced relief with alcohol. Growdon et al.[30] studied the effect of alcohol on essential tremor to assess whether it has a central or peripheral basis. As intra-arterial isoproterenol can produce a similar tremor, a peripheral basis for such tremors is possibly due to an oscillation of peripheral servo-mechanisms. Blockade of large sensory fibres does not block the tremor, so a central mechanism is also possible. These authors gave alcohol and noted a reduction in tremor. They then put identical blood values of alcohol locally into the arm the next day and got no effect. They concluded that this indicates a central mechanism for alcohol in reducing essential tremor.

It appears that patients with essential tremor may become alcoholic from overindulgence in alcohol because it gives them shortlived relief. It is also likely that alcohol can worsen essential tremor after many years. It is uncertain whether 'alcoholic tremor' is the exaggeration of physiological tremor, a subclinical essential tremor made manifest by drink, or a slightly different form of essential tremor.

PATHOLOGY OF ESSENTIAL TREMOR

The histological basis of essential tremor is unknown and no localization of any pathology has been definitely determined[31]. Perhaps the first autopsy was by Cestan in 1899[32]. He showed no definite pathological changes. Further autopsies were done by Berganasco in 1907[33] and Maas in 1914[34], neither author showing any definite pathology. Hassler[35] did autopsies on two brothers and showed some neuronal loss but one was an alcoholic and both were over age 70. Some non-specific changes were also demonstrated by Myle and van Bogaert[36]. However, 'It cannot be claimed that our knowledge of the pathology is much advanced by these reports[7].'

ASSOCIATED DISORDERS

There has been a long controversy over whether essential tremor is a monosymptomatic disorder or a manifestation of a degenerative process that may include other degenerative features.

McDonald Critchley[7] felt that, in the majority of cases, it is a monosymptomatic condition and stated: 'In its nature as a constitutional monosymptomatic peculiarity it can scarcely be regarded as a disease'.

Ashenhurst[37] felt that it was a monosymptomatic condition in his 34 cases but Larsson and Sjogren[38] concluded, 'it cannot generally be labelled monosymptomatic'. Davis and Kunkle[39] and Jager and King[40] felt that it was a monosymptomatic condition. E. Critchley[5] felt that minimal signs of Parkinson's disease and additional neurological symptoms were commonly observed in patients with essential tremor.

Minor[12-15] mentioned, 'status macrobioticus multiparus' characterized by the triad of tremor, longevity and fecundity. This unusual association has been quoted by authors for many years but it's not the experience of many others interested in this disorder. Larsson and Sjogren[38] did not note fecundity or longevity in their careful study of families. It was also not found in our studies of essential tremor[41,42].

Katzenstein[43] added features of high intelligence, professional attainment and placid temperament. M. Critchley added they had, 'lusty virile personalities, who both work and play hard, eat heavily and drink deeply'[7]. Babinski, Louis XV and Oliver Cromwell are said to have had essential tremor[7].

Many disorders resemble essential tremor—thyrotoxicosis, anxiety, lithium tremor, alcohol tremor, diabetic tremor, choreiform movement disorders, hypoglycaemia and adrenergic stimulation. It was noted by E. Critchley[5] that leg involvement had a variety of associations such as tremor, painful limp, dyskinetic movement, ataxia, foot clubbing, and cervical muscular atrophy.

Critchley and Greenfield in 1948[27] suggested some cases of essential tremor plus other neurological signs may represent a *forme fruste* of a presenile atrophy such as olivo-ponto-cerebellar atrophy.

An association of tremor and nystagmus was noted by Nettleship in

1911[44], and van Bogaert and Savitsch in 1937[45]. Newhauser et al.[46] recently reported essential tremor in association with nystagmus and duodenal ulceration.

Rajput[47] has shown that hypertension is more frequent in essential tremor patients than the controlled population. Essential tremor females over the age of 40 years are more likely to suffer from hypertension. They conclude that sympathetic overactivity is the major contributory factor in the genesis of essential tremor and the hypertension. They noted in 66 cases that there were six patients with spasmodic torticollis, six with multiple system atrophy, three with cerebellar dysfunction, three with epileptic seizures and two with an associated resting tremor. In those patients with multiple system atrophy, cerebellar involvement was the most prominent feature. McDonald Critchley quotes Pelnar and Mussafia as noting the association of tics and tremor[7].

Shuddering attacks were noted in six infants related to essential tremor patients, and this may be a benign manifestation of the syndrome[48]. All of the patients with shuddering attacks had a family history of essential tremor. I found no cases of shuddering attacks in 26 families surveyed by questionnaire.

As noted before by Poirier[49] some patients have different types of tremor either concomitantly or in succession. Some had pill rolling when the arms were held out. Although the cases were few, using Baye's formula a patient with essential tremor had 35 times the risk of developing Parkinson's tremor than the general population who did not have essential tremor in this study.

Only eight Parkinson patients and four familial spinocerebellar degeneration cases were found in studies in Papua[18], but 175 cases of essential tremor were found. Three patients seemed to have features of Parkinson's disease and essential tremor. Some patients had stiffness as part of the general muscle tenseness associated with the essential tremor. Some had such tremor and contractions of the neck and face muscles which resembled spasmodic torticollis. Facial muscle involvement was seen in 53 out of the 135 cases and involved the jaw, muscles of speech and tongue but never the facial muscles themselves.

Charcot–Marie–Tooth disease can be associated with essential tremor and seven cases were reported with a review of the literature by Salisachs[50]. The relationship between spasmodic torticollis and essential tremor was also noted by Conch[51].

Other associations have included hyperhydrosis, cramps, dyskinetic movements, ataxia, and spasmodic torticollis[5]. Essential tremor in association with Klinefelter's syndrome has also been reported[53].

Neuhauser[46] noted the association of essential tremor, nystagmus and duodenal ulceration, and a narcolepsy-like syndrome. In 12 of the 17 affected family members there was essential tremor. They were of Swedish-Finnish ancestry. The essential tremor began about age 30 to 40 and was controlled transiently by alcohol. It resulted in alcoholism in several of the cases. Severe cases showed cerebellar signs suggesting a relationship to spinocerebellar degeneration syndromes.

In our series followed long-term[42] the most commonly noted association was mild parkinsonian features when the patients reached age 60–70, even if they have had typical essential tremor for 20–30 years before this. These patients often show mild bradykinesia, rigidity and develop a resting tremor superimposed on the other features of essential tremor.

GENETICS

The disorder occurs in both familial and sporadic forms. The familial form is usually autosomal dominant. One-third to a half of the patients have a family history of a similar tremor. In the series of E. Critchley[5] 12 of 42 cases had an autosomal dominant inheritance, four were indeterminant, and 26 were sporadic. M. Critchley[7] suggested that there may be anticipation, with the disorder occurring at a younger and younger age with succeeding generations, but this has not been our experience.

M. Critchley[7] felt there might be a dominant inheritance but with variable penetrance. An inherited predisposition, with an impaired dampening mechanism was suggested by Marshall[16]. This might explain why it can manifest with minor or subclinical precipitating factors. Sporadic cases are common but the basis of the sporadic cases is uncertain. Sex chromosome abnormalities have been noted in patients with essential tremor with supernumerary X syndromes found in 5 out of 13 cases[53].

MEASUREMENT OF ESSENTIAL TREMOR

One of the difficulties in assessing therapeutic response is the difficulty in knowing what parameters are most significant. The change in tremor amplitude by recordings is not always adequate as some patients do not feel there has been a significant response to therapy, although the physician can record a definite change. Winkler and Young[4] commented that patient satisfaction is due to relief from disability rather than relief from tremor. There was less enthusiasm in those who wished a cosmetic improvement, more from those who wanted relief from disability. We have noted that patients who were overly embarrassed tended to be dissatisfied unless there was a complete response. The significant placebo effect makes it difficult to use only subjective evaluations of therapeutic response. A combination of both objective and subjective evaluations seems most appropriate, and the parameters under discussion should be defined before analysing the results. At the present time in our own studies we use: the physician examination,

May's test and spiral tests, handwriting (see Figure 8.1) a questionnaire for subjective evaluation by the patient, a separate evaluation by family members, and objective recording of the tremor.

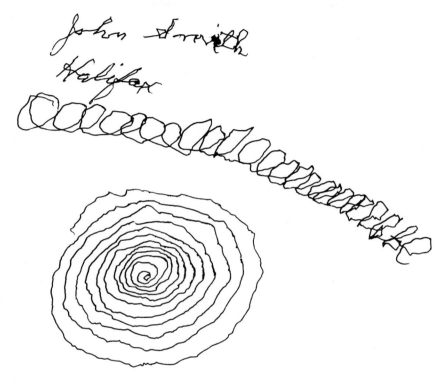

Figure 1   Handwriting and spiral tests from a patient with essential tremor for 23 years.

Although 'objective' measurements of tremor would seem most appropriate in evaluating tremor and the effect of therapy, all such measurements have drawbacks to date. An ideal tool would measure amplitude and frequency of the tremor with the person in a natural setting, unrestricted in activity or movement and carrying out normal activities affected by changes in emotion, environment and attention. As yet there is no method of objectively recording tremor that is acceptable as a measurement of the clinical reality, although attempts are being made to develop more realistic evaluation tools[54].

It seems clear that propranolol can reduce the amplitude of essential tremor. It can improve handwriting and fine manipulative tasks, it can reduce the overall tremor in some patients, and reduce the exacerbations of tremor under stress in other patients. The therapeutic response, however, must also be evaluated in the light of the subjective evaluation of the patient.

In some instances a statistically significant improvement in tremor amplitude is not a clinically significant result as far as the patient is concerned.

TREATMENT

Propranolol

In 1952 Barcroft et al.[55] noted that the administration of adrenaline increased the tremor in Parkinson's disease. They suggested that drugs that acted as adrenergic blockers might be beneficial in tremor. Studies by Herring[56], Marsden and Owen[57], Strang[58], Vas[59], and Abramsky[60] confirmed this suggestion. Marsden[61] also showed that propranolol would block the adrenalin effects on physiological tremor.

In 1971 Winkler and Young[3] reported a double blind study of propranolol in essential tremor, showing benefit in 20 out of 25 cases. The original observation was made by Winkler who noted that a patient with cardiac disease had relief from his essential tremor when his cardiac condition was treated with propranolol. Since then there have been numerous studies showing the benefit of this therapy[1,2,20,23,42,62-67] although not all patients respond, and the degree of improvement is variable and seldom complete. There have also been a number of studies which did not confirm the benefits of propranolol[68-71]. The drug has been reported as beneficial in three out of five children with essential tremor[20]. Some of the variable responses may be explained by inadequate or inappropriate evaluation techniques, too low a dose of propranolol, too short a time period of observation, or the use of an arbitrary dosage schedule which did not take into account the degree of β-blockade or serum levels. The observations have also been complicated by the fact that virtually all patients in such studies had some placebo effect. It has been noticed, however[1,41,42], that the placebo effect wears off whereas the propranolol effect persists longer.

The response to propranolol is usually a reduction in the amplitude of tremor but with no change in frequency. The hand and arm tremor respond best, the head tremor less well[41,42]. The vocal tremor may respond[17]. Some patients notice little change in the tremor overall but have less accentuation of the tremor with stress or anxiety.

The effect of propranolol, when it works, can be seen within 12–24 hours. The half-life of propranolol is only $2\frac{1}{2}$ hours, so some recommend using doses of this drug every 2–3 hours. However, the pharmacological half-life is longer and increasing the dose lengthens the response so that the dosage may only have to be administered two or three times per day[72-74].

Although it was initially suggested that the effect in essential tremor was due to blockade of peripheral β-andrenergic receptors[61] there is now evidence to suggest that it is mediated through central mechanisms. Young[76] studied essential tremor and concluded that peripheral β-adrenergic tremor-ogenic receptors are functioning normally in patients with essential tremor, that their function was not necessary for the production of essential tremor and they concluded that the effect of long-term propranolol was not mediated through the peripheral β-adrenergic blocking activity. They felt that the peripheral receptor may be responsible for the tremor of anxiety. The use of isoproterenol increased tremor in a profused arm and this was blocked by propranolol. The underlying essential tremor was not affected initially, however. Oral propranolol, which crosses the blood–brain barrier, did reduce the essential tremor over several days, as a central effect occurred. Local propranolol in the arm did not reduce the essential tremor indicating a central basis for the tremor, and indicating also that propranolol affects the tremor by a central action.

Perhaps there are different mechanisms underlying central essential tremor and peripheral mechanisms which are superimposed on the central tremor. These peripheral factors may be influenced by circulating adrenaline. Oral propranolol may then affect both the peripheral and central mechanisms. Zilm[77] also felt that the effect of propranolol on alcohol withdrawal tremor is also through central rather than peripheral mechanisms. McAllister[78], however, felt that the treatment response was correlated with the degree of β-blockade and that this observation supports Marsden's theory that peripheral receptors are involved.

Savaki et al.[79] studied the effect of propranolol on auditory evoked potentials and concluded that there was a depression of all components of the evoked auditory responses. This may be due to effects of propranolol on glucose utilization and membrane stabilization within the central nervous system.

McAllister[78] noted that the results of treating essential tremor with propranolol were inconsistent in many published series and suggested that this may have been due to the intravenous doses being too low to give effective plasma or tissue levels, and that the oral doses were not checked by plasma drug levels. They carried out a study which correlated the effects of propranolol with the intensity of β-receptor blockade and with the drug levels. Although they treated only six cases and three normals, their observations are pertinent. They noted that there was suppression of tremor in all cases, but it was directly related to the intensity of β-receptor blockade. It also varied with the drug plasma levels. The results were best when there was virtually complete β-receptor blockade and with propranolol plasma levels of 80–100 mg/ml. Tremor suppression, even when maximal, varied between 18–85% and was not related to the severity of the disease in the patient. The oral dosage necessary to keep the same plasma levels and degree of β-blockade gave similar results. Oral doses of 160 to 480 mg per day were required. Thus propranolol consistently reduces tremor, but the amount varies and depends on the sensitivity of the individual to β-blockade.

Perhaps this data explains the conflicting results in published studies in the past, as many studies used low doses of the drug, and most are in range of 80–120 mg per day.

Shand[80] noted that large doses of propranolol have a longer half-life so three or even two doses per day may be sufficient. Variations between individuals may be due to differences in receptor sensitivity or to pharmacokinetic factors. It was felt that determining drug levels in the future will be necessary to get the best therapeutic response.

McClure[81] studied the D and DL forms of propranolol and noted that both D and DL forms reduced essential tremor to the same degree. Since the peripheral beta receptor blocking action is due to the L-isomer, the finding that the D and DL forms have the same ability to reduce tremor suggests that essential tremor is not mediated by beta adrenergic receptor blockade. This may mean that the observation of McAllister that the therapeutic response was correlated with the degree of β-adrenergic blockade, may just be a factor of dosage.

Weinstock[82] found that propranolol may have a benefit in tremorine-induced tremor associated with raised plasma catecholamines, or with increased sensitivity of β-adrenoreceptors to stimulation by catecholamines.

It has also been noticed that slow intravenous profusion of 30 μg/kg of propranolol in 15–30 minutes could reduce nerve conduction speed and suppress repetitive muscular activities in subjects with chronic idiopathic tetany[83].

In the use of propranolol, the patient should be given a sufficient dose and a sufficient trial to obtain maximal benefits. Although we suggested that a 3-month trial on 120 mg/day was adequate to judge any useful response[41,42], the work of McAllister[78] suggests that the dosage should be increased before a therapeutic trial is deemed to be unsuccessful. On the basis of their data it might be reasonable to increase the dose to as high as 500 mg/day.

The best results are in patients who do not show the extrapyramidal characteristics seen in the elderly, who have had the tremor less than 15 years, and who are under the age of 55[1]. Teravainen[84] found that the best results in his series were in patients over 40 and with a tremor frequency below 10 Hz. There was no sex difference in the responses. Unfortunately, excellent and dramatic responses are seen in only a small number of patients[41,42].

When the patient does not respond to propranolol in adequate doses over a number of months, or if the response is insufficient to warrant long-term therapy, we withdraw the drug slowly over one week. This is based on the observation that cardiac patients treated with propranolol may develop angina, arrhythmias or even a myocardial infarction on sudden withdrawal of the drug. Although we now cautiously withdraw the drug once it has been instituted, we have not observed any problems on withdrawal of the drug either rapidly or slowly.

The commonest side-effects of the drug are fatigue, lethargy, Raynaud's phenomena, depression, insomnia, vivid dreaming and, rarely, rash, thrombocytopenia and alopecia. Bradycardia, particularly in the elderly may be symptomatic. Occasionally confusion and the picture of an organic brain syndrome may be seen which reverses when the drug is stopped.

Some information on the effect of propranolol on the nervous system is coming from its use and study in other conditions. Propranolol has been used extensively and is well accepted as a form of therapy in angina pectoris, cardiac arrhythmias and hypertension. It may also be of value in migraine, thyroid storm, cyanotic spells in tetralogy of Fallot, idiopathic hypertrophic subaortic stenosis, thyrotoxicosis, prophyria, anxiety, and various forms of tremor. There have been reports of the usefulness of propranolol in the tremor resulting from severe head injury[85] in two children, although my personal results in this situation in three adults were negative. Some patients with schizophrenia respond to propranolol[73].

In alcohol withdrawal states there have been some promising results with propranolol[86–88]. Drew[87] reports excellent control of the tremor in alcoholics and most of his patients said the tremor was a major reason for drinking and continuing to drink. The propranolol also reduced anxiety and improved sleep and the sense of well being. Teravainen[84], however, showed no difference in the response of alcohol withdrawal tremor to placebo or propranolol.

Kissel[89] studied 25 Parkinson patients and reported good results with propranolol in all except two who had thalamotomy. They were all treated with 60–180 mg of propranolol daily combined with levodopa. The treatment of tremor was better than with either drug used alone. The action of propranolol may be directly on the tremorogenic neurohumoral system, due to a central effect independent of its action on catecholamine metabolism[90]. Practolol, which does not cross the blood–brain barrier, has no effect on tremor. Kissel[89] concluded that this effect is due to the membrane stabilizing property of the drug rather than to its β-adrenergic blocking properties.

Tremors from increased catecholamine secretion and physiological tremor, are reduced by propranolol[61]. The use of propranolol in anxiety has led to a number of questions about its central versus peripheral effect in neurological situations. Granville-Grossman[91], Turner et al.[92] and Suzman[93] noted that the response of anxiety to propranolol resulted from the reduction in autonomic symptoms, as there is little evidence that the psychic component of anxiety is reduced. D-Propranolol does not help anxiety but has only 1/60 of the β-blocking activity of the racemic form. Since practolol, a cardioselective β-blocker, passes poorly through the blood–brain barrier, but has much the same anxiety relieving properties, there is probably a peripheral rather than central basis for the anxiety effect, but this effect may explain part of the reduction of essential tremor with propranolol, especially in stress situations[41,42].

Bonn and Turner[94] treated anxiety with the D form. β-Blockade is primarily by the L-isomer, but there is little β-blockade with the D form. These authors did a double blind study in ten cases and showed that placebo was equal to D-propranolol. Thus the D form, which does not block peripheral autonomic effects had no effect on anxiety. This study supports the central action theory as regards the effect on anxiety.

Kirk[95] has reported good results when propranolol is used to treat lithium tremor and this had been earlier observed by Floru in 1971[96]. Kellett, however[97], used both propranolol and practolol and obtained results that were poorer than placebo in this situation and concluded that the drug was not useful in the treatment of lithium tremor. It should be mentioned, however, that Kellett used only 40 mg of propranolol daily and it is questionable whether a significant result could be expected with this dosage. LaPierre[98] reported good results in five cases but his observations were uncontrolled.

Lest it be felt that the mechanism must be explained in terms of central or peripheral β-blockade only, it should be remembered that propranolol has other pharmacological effects as well. Freshman[99] noted the reversal of abnormal platelet aggregability and a change in exercise tolerance with propranolol. Blessing[100] noted that a patient of his developed myotonia while taking propranolol for ischemic heart disease which cleared when the drug was stopped. Propranolol has been shown to have membrane stabilizing effects[79,89].

Other drug therapy

Over the years a number of forms of therapy were used for essential tremor, with generally fair to poor results. The relationship of essential tremor to emotional factors led to a long period (which still continues) when tranquillizers and sedatives were used. They have limited effect on the tremor although they may have some effect on the underlying anxiety which can worsen the tremor. The two most commonly used drugs of this sort are diazepam and phenobarbital, neither of which have any significant effect in the long term. Haloperidol, useful in other movement disorders, has no value in essential tremor therapy.

Benzhexol has also been used by Sevitt[2] in essential tremor but when compared with propranolol fewer patients responded, and those that responded to both drugs did better on propranolol. All of the patients in this study responded to propranolol.

Mephenesin has been said to reduce tremor in 70–80% of patients for a 20–30-minute period and amantadine has been of some value in some patients.

Chlordiazepoxide, anticholinergic drugs, levodopa and tetrabenazine are no better than placebo[5] and levodopa may actually worsen the tremor[101].

Tryptophan and pyridoxine are of no value[102] and anticholinergic drugs are of no help[103]. Oxprenolol has had marginal, if any effect, over placebo[104].

Behaviour modification

Behaviour therapy has been used in the treatment of essential tremor[105] using Jacobson's progressive relaxation method.

Patients themselves try a number of forms of therapy initially to reduce the tremor and often learn the factors that aggravate and relieve the tremor through their own experimentation. A number of patients have tried yoga, transcendental meditation, relaxation exercises, and self-hypnosis to try and reduce the tremor. The results are variable and inconsistent and the initial enthusiasm of patients for any of these forms of therapy tends to wane with time.

Surgical

Guiot and his co-workers[106] first published the results of thalamotomy for essential tremor in 1960. Electrocoagulation in the area of the left ventro-lateral nucleus of the thalamus and also the internal capsule medial and anterior to the globus pallidus gave complete relief of the tremor. An initial lesion of the ventrolateral nucleus gave a partial response and they concluded that the capsule lesion was necessary for the complete cessation of tremor. Blacker et al.[107] suggested the lesion be made in the lower part of the ventrolateral nucleus and the subthalamus. All of their cases developed some contralateral hypotonia. There was no residual neurological deficit. A number of reports confirmed the beneficial effects of thalamotomy— Cooper[108], Laitinen[109], Obrador[110] and Bertrand[21].

Cooper[108] felt that the contralateral cerebral lesion improved essential tremor by interrupting the dentatothalamic tract from the cerebellum to the thalamus, and in this manner, modified cortical activity. He felt essential tremor was due to faulty feedback of proprioceptive information from the cerebellum to the cortex via the thalamus.

Despite some promising reports of good results with thalamotomy lesions, this procedure is seldom warranted for a tremor that is essentially benign, and which would usually require bilateral lesions. The experience with bilateral thalamotomies in Parkinson's disease should temper any enthusiasm for a surgical approach to benign essential tremor, as the complications are much higher than in unilateral lesions and the risks acceptable only in the unusual case who has severe tremor that limits normal activities. In patients with a significant disability from the tremor, however, thalamotomy can often result in a dramatic improvement.

RED NUCLEUS TREMOR

This type of tremor is doubtful as a distinct entity. The traditional description of this tremor would state that it affects limbs at rest (as in Parkinson's disease) and is classified by Marshall as a static tremor. It may have associated rigidity and bradykinesia of mild degree. There is not a satisfactory clinical pathological correlate and the tenuous association with the red nucleus is based primarily on other signs of a midbrain lesion in this situation[111].

Fahn[112] says that the midbrain or rubral tremor is really due to a lesion in the tegmentum of the midbrain resulting in a slow 3–5 Hz coarse tremor of the contralateral limbs. It may occur at rest but characteristically is worsened by action. Although it is primarily an intention or action tremor, it also has a postural component. It may be due to involvement of the cerebellofugal pathways rather than a red nucleus lesion.

PROGNOSIS

In most cases the tremor is an annoyance but not disabling. With time it tends to slowly worsen. Rajput[47] noted that in his 66 patients five retired early because of tremor, one was demoted because of it and five further patients considered early retirement because of the tremor. These 11 patients constituted 45.8% of the employable patients in their series.

Rajput concluded that the unfavourable prognostic signs were: (a) onset at a younger age, (b) family history of multiple system atrophy, (c) tremor involving the head and upper limbs, (d) coarse tremor. In his study he concluded that essential tremor is not a benign condition in many instances.

The overall prognosis in essential tremor, with the patient noting an increasing tremor which slowly interferes with fine hand tasks, has not been altered significantly by propranolol or other drugs, and surgery seems too radical an approach for most cases. An effective long-term therapy is still required in this embarrassing and annoying disorder.

References

1 Dupont, E., Hansen, H. and Dalby, M. (1973). Treatment of benign essential tremor with propranolol. *Acta Neurol. Scand.*, **49**, 75

2 Sevitt, I. (1974). A comparison of propranolol and benzhexol in essential tremor. *Practitioner*, **213**, 91

3 Winkler, G. F. and Young, R. R. (1972). The control of essential tremor by propranolol. *Trans. Am. Neurol. Assoc.*, **96**, 64

4 Winkler, G. F. and Young, R. R. (1974). Efficacy of chronic propranolol therapy in action tremors of the familial, senile or essential varieties. *N. Engl. J. Med.*, **290**, 984

5 Critchley, E. (1972). Clinical manifestations of essential tremor. *J. Neurol. Neurosurg. Psychiatry*, **35**, 365

6 Hoehn, M. M. and Yahr, M. D. (1967). Parkinsonism: onset, progression and mortality. *Neurology (Minneap.)*, **17**, 427

7 Critchley, M. (1949). Observations on essential (heredofamilial) tremor. *Brain*, **12**, 9

8 Most, R. (1836). *Encl. Méd. Praxis*, **2**, 555. Quoted by Dana. (11)

9 Sanders, W. R. (1872). *Reynold's Syst. Med.* Vol. 2nd Edn., p. 241. (London: Macmillan)

10 Trousseau, A. (1885). Tremblement sénile et paralysis agitans. *Clin. Méd. Hôtel Dieu*, Paris II: 47, 280, 7th ed. (Paris: Bailliére)

11 Dana, C. L. (1887). Hereditary tremor, a hitherto undescribed form of motor neurosis. *Am. J. Med. Sci.*, **94**, 386

12 Minor, L. (1922). Uber hereditären Tremor. *Zentralbl. Gesamte Neurol. Psychiatry*, **28**, 514

13 Minor, L. (1925). Uber das erbliche Zittern. *Zentralbl. Gesampte Neurol. Psychiatry*, **99**, 586

14 Minor, L., (1927). Zur Kasuistik des sogennanten 'essenziellen' oder hereditären Zittern, *Zentralbl. Gesampte Neurol. Psychiatry*, **110**, 204

15 Minor, L. (1929). Neve Beobachtungen über das erbliche Zittern, *Russ. K. Klin.*, **12**, 713

16 Marshall, J. (1962). Observations on essential tremor: *J. Neurol. Neursurg. Psychiatry*, **25**, 122

17 Hachinski, V. C. (1975). The nature of primary vocal tremor. *Can. J. Neurol. Sci.*, **2**, 195

18 Hornabrook, R. W. (1976). Essential tremor in Papua, New Guinea. *Brain*, **99**, 659

19 Brown, J. R. and Simonson, J. (1963). Organic voice tremor. *Neurology (Minneap.)*, **13**, 520

20 Paulson, G. W. (1976). Benign essential tremor in childhood. *Clin. Pediatr.*, **15**, 67

21 Bertrand, C., Hardy, J., Molina-Negro, P. and Martinez, S. N. (1969). Optimum physiological target for the arrest of tremor. *Third Symposium on Parkinson's Disease*, held at the Royal College of Surgeons of Edinburgh, pp. 251–259. (Livingstone: Edinburgh)

22 Barlow, J. S. and Scwab, R. S. (1971). Mutual limb stabilization in relation to tremor characteristics in parkinsonian and essential or heredofamilial tremor. *Neurology*, **21**, 78

23 Mai, J. and Pedersen, L. (1976). Clonus depression by propranolol. *Acta Neurol. Scand.*, **53**, 395

24 Marshall, J. (1968). *Handbook of Clinical Neurology*. Vol. 6. Vinken, P. J. and Bruyn, G. W. (eds.), p. 819. (New York: Wiley)

25 Lee, R. and Stein, B. Personal communication.

26 Kreiss, Ph. (1912). Über hereditären Tremor: *Dtsch. Z. Nervenheilkd*, **44**, 111

27 Critchley, M. and Greenfield, J. G. (1948). Olivo-ponto-cerebellar atrophy. *Brain*, **71**, 343

28 Molina-Negro, P. and Hardy, J. (1975). Semiology of tremors. *Can. J. Neurol. Sci.*, **2**, 23

29 Rajput, A. H., Jamison, H., Hirsh, S. and Quraishi, A. (1975). Relative efficacy of alcohol and propranolol in action tremor. *Can. J. Neurol. Sci.*, **2**, 31

30 Growdon, J. H., Shanani, B. T. and Young, R. R. (1975). The efficacy of alcohol on essential tremor. *Neurology*, **25**, 259

31 Herskovits, E. and Blackwood, W. (1969). Essential (familial hereditary) tremor: a case report. *J. Neurol. Neurosurg. and Psychiatry*, **32**, 509

32 Cestan, R. (1899). Tremblement héréditaire et atrophie musculaire tardive chez un malade porteur d'un foyer ancien de paralysie infantile: *Prog. Med. (3.s).*, **9**, 1. *Abs. Rev. Neurol.*, 7, 236

33 Bergamasco, I. (1907). Intorno ad un caso di tremore essenziale simulante in porte il quadro della sclerosi mutlipla. *Riv. Patol. Nerv. Ment.*, **12**, 4

34 Maas, O. (1914). Vorstellung von Zitterkranken. *Neurology (261)*, **33**, 328

35 Hassler, R., Mundinger, F. and Riechert, T. (1970). Pathophysiology of tremor at rest derived from the correlation of anatomical and clinical data. *Confin. Neurol.*, **32**, 79

36 Myle, G. and van Bogaert, L. (1940). Etudes anatomo-cliniques de syndromes hyper-cinétiques complexes. *Mschr. Psychiat. Neurol.*, **103**, 28

37 Ashenhurst, E. M. (1973). The nature of essential tremor. *Can. Med. Assoc. J.*, **109**, 876

38 Larsson, T. and Sjögren, T. (1960). Essential tremor in a clinical and genetic population study. *Acta Psychiat. Neurol. Scand.*, **36** (Suppl. 144)

39 Davis, C. H. and Kunkle, E. C. (1951). Benign essential (heredofamilial) tremor. *Arch. Intern. Med.*, **87**, 808

40 Jager, B. V. and King, T. (1955). Hereditary tremor. *Arch. Intern. Med.*, **95**, 788

41 Murray, T. J. (1972). Treatment of essential tremor with propranolol. *Can. Med. Assoc. J.*, **107**, 984

42 Murray, T. J. (1976). Long-term therapy of essential tremor with propranolol. *Can. Med. Assoc. J.*, **115**, 892

43 Katzenstien, E. (1948). Uber familiären Tremor. *Arch. Suisses. Neurol. Psychiat.*, **61**, 380

44 Nettleship, E. (1911). On some cases of hereditary nystagmus. *Trans. Ophthalmol. Soc. UK*, **31**, 159

45 van Bogaert, L. and De Savitsch, E. (1937). Sur une maladie congénitale et hérédo-familiale comportant un tremblement rhymique de la tête, des globes oculaires, et des membres supérieurs, *Encéphale*, **32** (1), 113

46 Neuhauser, G., Daly, R. F. and Magwell, N. C. (1976). Essential Tremor, Nystagmus and Duodenal Ulceration. A new dominantly inherited condition. *Clin. Genet.*, **9**, 81

47 Rajput, A. H., Jamieson, H. and Hirsh, S. Personal communication

48 Vanasse, M., Andermann, F. and Bédard, P. (1976). Shuddering attacks in children. An early clinical manifestation of essential tremor. *Neurology*, **26**, 1027

49 Poirier, L. P. Recent views on tremors and their treatment. In Williams, D. (ed.) *Modern Trends in Neurology*, Vol. 5. (London: Butterworths)

50 Salisachs, P. (1976). Charcot-Marie-Tooth disease associated with essential tremor: Report of 7 cases and a review of the literature. *J. Neurol. Sci.*, **28** (1), 17

51 Conch, J. R. (1976). Dystonia and tremor in spasmodic torticollis. *Adv. Neurol.*, **14**, 245

52 Baughman, F. A. Jr. (1969). Klinefelter's syndrome and essential tremor. *Lancet*, **2**, 545

53 Baughman, F. A. Jr., Higgins, J. V. and Mann, J. D. (1973). Sex chromosome anomalies and essential tremor. *Neurology*, **23**, 623

54 Siegfried, J. and Thomann, R. M. (1976/1977). A therapeutic approach and objective test in the treatment of tremor. *Appl. Neurophysiol.*, **39**, 50

55 Barcroft, H., Peterson, E. and Schwab, R. S. (1952). Action of adrenaline and nor-adrenaline on tremor in Parkinson's disease. *Neurology (Minneap.)*, **2**, 154

56 Herring, H. B. (1964). Action of pronethalol on parkinsonian tremor. *Lancet*, **2**, 892

57 Marsden, C. D. and Owen, D. A. L. (1967). Mechanisms underlying emotional variations in parkinsonian tremor. *Neurology (Minneap.)*, **17**, 711

58 Strang, R. R. (1965). Clinical trial with a β-receptor antagonist (propranolol) in parkinson-ism. *J. Neurol. Neurosurg. Psychiatry*, **28**, 404

59 Vas, C. J. (1966). Propranolol in parkinsonian tremor. *Lancet*, **1**, 182

60 Abramky, O., Carmon, A. and Lavy, S. (1971). Combined treatment of parkinsonian tremor with propranolol and levodopa. *J. Neurol. Sci.*, **14**, 491

61 Marsden, C. D. (1971). Propranolol in neurocirculatory asthenia and anxiety. *Postgrad. Med. J.*, **47** (Suppl.) 100

62 Tolosa, E. S. and Lowenson, R. B. (1975). Essential tremor: treatment with propranolol. *Neurology*, **25**, 1041

63 Barbeau, A. (1973). Traitement du tremblement essential familial par le propranolol: *Union Méd. Can.*, **102**, 899

64 Morgan, M. H., Hewer, R. L. and Cooper, R. (1973). Effect of the beta-adrenergic blocking agent propranolol on essential tremor. *J. Neurol. Neurosurg. Psychiatry*, **36**, 618

65 Gillingan, B. S. (1972). Propranolol in essential tremor. *Lancet*, **2**, 980

66 Gillingan, B. S., Veale, J. L. and Wodak, J. (1972). Propranolol in the treatment of tremor. *Med. J. Aust.*, **1**, 320

67 Pakkenberg, H. (1972). Propranolol in essential tremor. *Lancet*, **1**, 633

68 Scopa, J., Longley, B. P. and Foster, J. B. (1973). Beta-adrenergic blockers in benign essential tremor. *Curr. Ther. Res.*, **15**, 48

69 Sweet, R. D., Blumberg, J. and Lee, J. E. (1974). Propranolol treatment of essential tremor. *Neurology*, **24**, 64

70 Balla, J. I. (1973). Treatment of essential tremor with propranolol. *Lancet*, **1**, 205

71 Foster, J. B., Longley, B. P. and Stewart-Wynn, E. G. (1973). Propranolol in essential tremor. *Lancet*, **2**, 1455

72 Atsmon, A., Blum, I., Stiener, M., Latz, A. and Wijsenbeck, H. (1972). Further studies with propranolol in psychotic patients. *Psychopharmacology*, **27**, 249

73 Yorkston, N. J., Malik, M. K. and Harvard, C. W. (1975). Propranolol in the control of schizophrenic symptoms. *Br. Med. J.*, **4**, 633

74 Hasson, L., Olander, R. and Aberg, H. (1971). Twice-daily propranolol treatment for hypertension. *Lancet*, **2**, 713

75 Wilkinson, P. R., Dixon, N. and Hunter, K. R. (1974). Essential tremor. *J. Int. Res.*, **2**, 220

76 Young, R. R., Growdon, J. H. and Shahani, B. T. (1975). Beta-adrenergic mechanisms in action tremor. *N. Engl. J. Med.*, **293**, 950

77 Zilm, D. H. and Sellers, E. M. (1976). Effect of propranolol on tremor with alcohol withdrawal. *N. Engl. J. Med.*, **294**, 785

78 McAllister, R. G., Markesberry, W. R., Ware, R. W. and Howell, S. M. (1977). Suppression of essential tremor by propranolol: correlation of the effect with drug plasma levels and intensity of beta-adrenergic blockade. *Ann. Neurol.*, **1**, 160

79 Savaki, H., Kadekoro, M. and Jehle, J. (1978). α and β-adrenoreceptor blockers have opposite effects on energy metabolism of the central auditory system. *Nature*, **276**, 521

80 Shand, D. G. (1975). Drug therapy. Propranolol. *N. Engl. J. Med.*, **293**, 280

81 McClure, C. G. (1976). The effect of d-propranolol on action tremors. *Trans, Am. Neurol. Assoc.*, **101**, 269

82 Weinstock, M., Zavadil, A. P. and Rosin, A. J. (1978). The role of peripheral catecholamines in oxotremorine tremor in the rat and its antagonism by beta adrenaceptor blocking agents. *J. Pharmacol. Exp. Ther.*, **206**, 91

83 Anctil, R., Hugues, F. C. and Marche, J. (1970). Action du propranolol sur la conduction nerveuse chez l'homme. *Thérapie*, **25**, 579

84 Teravainen, H., Fogelholm, R. and Larsen, A. (1976). Effect of propranolol on essential tremor. *Neurology*, **26**, 27

85 Ellison, P. H. (1978). Propranolol for severe post-head injury action tremor. *Neurology (Minneap.)*, **28**, 197

86 Carlsson, C. and Johansson, T. (1971). The psychological effect of propranolol in the abstinence phase of chronic alcoholics. *Br. J. Psychiatry*, **119**, 605

87 Drew, L. R., Moon, J. R. and Buchanan, F. N. (1973). Inderal (propranolol) in the treatment of alcoholism. *Med. J. Aust.*, **2**, 282

88 Tyrer, P. (1972). Propranolol in alcohol addiction. *Lancet*, **2**, 707

89 Kissel, P. and Tridon, P. (1974). Levodopa-propranolol therapy in parkinsonian tremor. *Lancet*, **1**, 403

90 Dewhurst, W. G. and Marley, E. (1965). Action of sympathominetic and allied amines on the central nervous system of the chicken. *Br. J. Pharmacol.*, **25**, 705

91 Granville-Grossman, K. L. and Turner, P. (1966). The effect of propranolol on anxiety. *Lancet*, **1**, 788

92 Turner, P., Granville-Grossman, K. L. and Smart, J. V. (1965). Effect of adrenergic receptor blockade in the tachycardia of thyrotoxicosis and anxiety state. *Lancet*, **2**, 1316

93 Suzman, M. M. (1976). Propranolol in the treatment of anxiety. *Postgrad. Med. J.*, **52** (Suppl. 4) 168

94 Bonn, J. A. and Turner, P. (1971). D-Propranolol and anxiety. *Lancet*, **1**, 1355

95 Kirk, L. and Baastrup, P. C. (1973). Propranolol treatment of lithium-induced tremor. *Lancet*, **2**, 1086

96 Floru, L. (1971). Klinische Behandlungsversuche des Lithium-bedingten tremors durch einen β-Rezeptorenantagonisten (Propranolol) *Int. Pharmacopyschiatry*, **6**, 197

97 Kellett, J. M., Metcalfe, M., Bailey, J. and Coppen, A. J. (1975). Beta blockade in lithium tremor. *J. Neurol. Neurosurg. Psychiatry*, **38**, 719

98 LaPierre, Y. D. (1976). Control of lithium tremor with propranolol. *Can. Med. Assoc. J.*, **114**, 619

99 Freshman, W. H. (1974). Reversal of abnormal platelet aggregability and change in exercise tolerance in patients with Angina Pectoris following oral propranolol. *Circulation*, **50**, 887

100 Blessing, W. and Walsh, J. C. (1977). Myotonia precipitated by propranolol therapy. *Lancet*, **1**, 73

101 Barbeau, A. (1969). Levodopa therapy in Parkinson's disease: a critical review of nine years' experience. *Can. Med. Assoc. J.*, **101**, 791

102 Morris, C. E., Prange, A. J., Hall, C. D. and Weis, E. A. (1971). Inefficacy of tryptophan/pyridoxine in essential tremor. *Lancet*, **2**, 165

103 Magee, K. R. (1965). Essential tremor. Diagnosis and treatment. *Clin. Med.*, **I**, 33

104 Thompson, M. K. (1972). Effect of oxprenolol on parkinsonian tremor. *Lancet*, **2**, 814

105 Wake, A., Takahashi, Y. and Onishi, T. (1974). Treatment of essential tremor by behavior therapy. Use of Jacobson's progressive relaxation method. *Psychiatry Neurol. (Jap.)*, **76**, 509

106 Guiot, G. (1960). The principles of stereotaxy. *Marco Med.*, **39**, 1236

107 Blacker, H. M., Bertrand, C. and Martinez, N. (1968). Hyptonia accompanying the neurosurgical relief of essential tremor. *J. Nerv. Ment. Dis.*, **147**, 49

108 Cooper, I. S. (1962). Heredofamilial tremor abolition by chemothalamectomy. *Neurology (Minneap.)*, **12**, 129

109 Laitinen, L. (1965). Stereotaxic treatment of hereditary tremor. *Acta Neurol. Scand.*, **41**, 74

110 Obrador, S. A. (1957). A simplified neurosurgical technique for approaching the damaged region of the globus pallidus in Parkinson's disease. *J. Neurol. Neurosurg. Psychiatry*, **20**, 47

111 Denny-Brown, D. (1962). Degeneration of skeletal muscle. *Rev. Can. Biol.*, **21**, 507

112 Fahn, S. (1972). Differential diagnosis of tremors. *Med. Clin. N. Am.*, **56**, 1363

9

Treatment of parkinsonism

A. Williams and D. B. Calne

INTRODUCTION

The treatment of Parkinson's disease is one of the notable stories of modern neurology, its importance lying not only in the large number of patients who have benefited from drug therapy, but also in the considerable impetus it has provided in furthering the cause of neuropharmacology. Unfortunately, all present treatment is palliative and patients with Parkinson's disease must await patiently a new approach which might arrest or prevent the disease.

This review will concentrate on the practical management of patients with this disease.

HISTORICAL ASPECTS

Belladonna alkaloids, the first useful drugs for the treatment of Parkinson's disease, were introduced by Charcot[1]. In the 1950s these drugs were replaced by synthetic anticholinergic drugs which had fewer systemic side-effects.

Neurosurgical procedures for the alleviation of tremor and rigidity were introduced by Meyers in the 1940s[2] and later stereotactic procedures were adopted[3,4] with a lesion in the ventrolateral nucleus of the thalamus being the target of choice[5].

In 1955 Klein and Stanley reported that reserpine produced a syndrome of rigidity and akinesia in man[6] and later, in animals, this was related to depletion of brain dopamine and found to be reversed by administration of levodopa (L-Dopa)[7]. It was suggested that dopamine was a neurotransmitter in the central nervous system and it was found in high concentration in the basal ganglia[8,9]. Ehringer and Hornykiewicz demonstrated in

171

1960[10] that the concentration of dopamine and its major metabolite, homovanillic acid, was reduced in the basal ganglia of patients with Parkinson's disease, and soon after it was shown that experimental lesions in the substantia nigra reduced dopamine levels in the striatum[11]. Immediately, attempts were made to treat patients with low doses of intravenous or oral levodopa[12,13], but it was not until much higher oral doses were given by Cotzias, et al.[14] that the remarkable beneficial effects of this drug became clear. Later peripheral decarboxylase inhibitors were introduced[15], to avoid many of the peripheral side-effects of levodopa.

DIAGNOSIS

Correct therapy for any disease relies on accurate diagnosis. The diagnosis of Parkinson's disease rarely poses problems except in early cases where a complaint of mild tremor, weakness, clumsiness, or dysaesthesiae in a limb may need an experienced physician to pick up subtle changes in tone, handwriting, posture or degree of arm swing. Sometimes, particularly when bradykinesis is unilateral, it may be difficult to differentiate from a mild hemiparesis, especially as 'equivocal' plantar responses are common in parkinsonism. Tremors can be difficult to categorize because that of Parkinson's disease may be maximal on action and an essential, familial, or senile tremor may be prominent at rest. Close attention to the clinical features, family history and response to medication, including alcohol, is usually decisive; one should not rely on the cogwheel phenomena in the absence of true rigidity or on dubious masking of facial expression for the diagnosis of Parkinson's disease. An occasional difficulty arises when faced with the severe akinesia associated with some forms of schizophrenia, depression or myxoedema, but concomitant clinical features should enable the distinction to be made.

On rare occasions parkinsonism is associated with diseases for which alternative management is desirable. For instance, Wilson's disease can mimic parkinsonism in the young person, and rarely, parkinsonism is a feature of normal pressure hydrocephalus, a cerebral tumour, or severe hypoparathyroidism. More commonly the parkinsonism is part of another disease for which there is no adequate treatment, although in these instances a typical tremor is unusual. Examples are the Shy–Drager syndrome, progressive supranuclear palsy, familial calcification of the basal ganglia, the Westphal variant of Huntington's disease, Hallevorden–Spatz disease and striato-nigral degeneration.

It is important, when possible, to diagnose the specific cause of parkinsonism because this may affect management or explain response to therapy. In particular, one should identify postencephalitic patients and cases following administration of antipsychotic medication. Arteriosclerotic

Parkinson's disease is rare although the gait apraxia of cerebrovascular disease is sometimes diagnosed as parkinsonism.

Lastly, one should always consider accompanying medical or psychiatric illness, particularly depression, because it may exacerbate the severity of the parkinsonian deficits or affect response to medication.

TREATMENT

Therapy begins at the end of the first diagnostic interview (whether or not specific drugs are started) when the patient should have his education begun about Parkinson's disease. This accomplishes two tasks: first, it reduces anxiety and the chances of a reactive depression to the diagnosis; second, by improving a personal relationship with the patient, it encourages compliance later with drug regimens. The patient may suspect that he has a brain tumour or psychiatric disease and can be suitably reassured. Others may be worried about a hereditary basis of the disease and can also be strongly reassured. Nearly all patients appreciate a short explanation of the pathology and biochemistry of the disease and of the goals and expectations for treatment. It may be helpful to give the patient access to a suitable monograph on the subject[16] and, at some stage, to give them the addresses of local or nationwide organizations concerned with Parkinson's disease. It is helpful to have the patient's closest relative present at these discussions.

Prognosis should also be touched upon, both for life and future work. Clearly this depends upon the stage at which one sees the patient and it is difficult to be exact since the expectation for life ranges between about 4 and 35 years. Prognosis is relatively better for those patients who present with tremor alone or who respond well to medication.

Lastly, if drugs are prescribed, the nature of possible side-effects should be explained to the patient. The various drugs available for the treatment of Parkinson's disease will now be discussed.

Anticholinergics

Rationale

Choline acetyltransferase, an enzyme employed as a marker for cholinergic neurons, is present in normal concentration in the basal ganglia of patients with Parkinson's disease[17]. However, due to the loss of dopamine containing neurons, there is a functional overactivity of acetylcholine. This imbalance may be the cause of some of the symptoms of Parkinson's disease and also explains the benefit from anticholinergic drugs and the adverse effects of cholinergic agonists such as physostigmine[1]. Certain anticholinergic drugs may also help by reducing the active reuptake of dopamine from the synaptic cleft[18].

Uses[19]

The commonly used anticholinergics and their dose ranges are shown in Table 1. The antihistamines probably only achieve their beneficial action by virtue of their prominent anticholinergic properties.

Table 1   Commonly prescribed drugs for the treatment of Parkinson's disease

	Usual daily dose range
Anticholinergics	
Trihexyphenidyl	4–20 mg
Benztropine mesylate	0.5–8 mg
Biperiden	4–8 mg
Procyclidine	5–20 mg
Cycrimine	2.5–20 mg
Diphenhydramine[a]	50–200 mg
Chlorphenoxamine[a]	50–200 mg
Orphenadrine[b]	50–200 mg
Levodopa-containing preparations	
Levodopa	1–8 g
Carbidopa/levodopa (10/100 or 25/250 Sinemet[b])	40/400–200/2000 mg
Benserazide/levodopa[a] (25/100 or 50/200 Prolopa[c] or Madopar[b])	100/400–500/2000 mg
Dopamine agonists	
Bromocriptine	40–80 mg
Miscellaneous	
Amantadine	100–200 mg

a Also have strong antihistiminic properties
b Trade name
c Not FDA approved drugs for the treatment of Parkinson's disease in the USA

These drugs have a modest beneficial effect on tremor and rigidity but they have little or no effect on bradykinesia. They are also sometimes effective in alleviating the drooling of saliva experienced by many patients. Paradoxically, abrupt withdrawal of anticholinergics can, in some patients, lead to a severe increase in akinesia[20], so these drugs should be reduced gradually. This class of drugs may be the most effective in patients with postencephalitic disease and may then be given in significantly higher doses than those indicated in Table 1. Some patients find that one drug in this class is better tolerated or more efficacious than another. It was common practice to give anticholinergics at the same time as dopaminergic blocking agents when treating a psychosis, but this manoeuvre is now generally regarded as unnecessary[21].

Contraindications

These drugs should be avoided in patients who have a significant disturbance of bladder or bowel function, memory disorder, or narrow angle glaucoma. The most common side-effects are a dry mouth and blurred vision. More serious are retention of urine, severe constipation, confusion, and psychosis. Severe toxic states can be reversed by giving physostigmine.

Amantadine

Rationale

Amantadine, an antiviral agent, was discovered to be a mild antiparkinsonian agent by serendipity[22]. Its mechanism of action remains uncertain, and only at very high doses has it been found to increase synthesis, augment release and inhibit reuptake of dopamine[23,24], as well as having some anticholinergic properties[25].

Uses[26–31]

Amantadine is of the same order of potency as anticholinergic drugs but in addition has some effect on bradykinesia. It can be used in conjunction with both anticholinergics and levodopa. It is usually begun as a dose of 100 mg a day, increasing to twice a day. Improvement is seen within a week. Sometimes, the beneficial response to amantadine is lost after 2 or 3 months but may return after a period off the drug.

Contraindications

These include cardiac failure, epilepsy, confusion, and bladder dysfunction. Care should be taken in renal failure because the drug is not metabolized so it will accumulate.

Side-effects

The most common adverse reactions are confusion, psychosis, livedo reticularis, and ankle oedema. Amantadine also has some side-effects in common with the anticholinergic drugs. On rare occasions it has been reported to precipitate cardiac failure. On withdrawal, convulsions have been noted as well as a temporary increase in parkinsonism.

Levodopa

Rationale

Dopamine itself cannot be given to correct the deficiency in parkinsonism because it does not readily cross the blood–brain barrier. However, levodopa, the immediate metabolic precursor for dopamine, does enter the brain, where it is decarboxylated to dopamine. The beneficial action of flooding the striatum with dopamine is probably consequent upon the input to the striatum from the substantia nigra being tonic in nature and also upon a degree of denervation supersensitivity of the postsynaptic dopamine receptors.

Uses[32-39]

Levodopa is effective for the treatment of about 80% of patients with Parkinson's disease. It is particularly helpful in alleviating akinesia and rigidity, but is also effective for the treatment of tremor. Its use delays the onset of severe disability by about 3 or 4 years and has reduced the apparent mortality rate significantly[40,41].

Pharmacokinetics

Levodopa is rapidly absorbed from the small bowel. Plasma levels peak between 30 and 120 min after an oral dose and the plasma half-life is between 1 to 3 hours[42]. Absorption is dependent upon the rate of gastric emptying and hence may be influenced by food, intrinsic gut motility and anticholinergic drugs. Hyperacidity of gastric juice and competition for absorption by other amino acids may also interfere with absorption. About 1% of administered levodopa enters the brain unaltered, the remainder being lost through extracerebral metabolism.

Contraindications

There are no absolute contraindications. Levodopa should be avoided in any patient with a well documented psychotic episode whether drug related or not. Patients with known cardiac disease, hypotension, or closed angle glaucoma should always be given levodopa with a decarboxylase inhibitor.

Side-effects

Side-effects of levodopa can be divided into those produced outside the blood–brain barrier (which includes the medullary emetic centre) and those of more central origin. The peripheral effects can be reduced by using levodopa in conjunction with a decarboxylase inhibitor. In particular nausea, vomiting and anorexia are decreased. Cyclizine is a satisfactory additional antiemetic which can be used to counteract these symptoms and has not been shown to exacerbate parkinsonism. Cardiac dysrhythmias, such as sinus and atrial tachycardia, and premature ventricular contractions have been reported although they are rare; these dysrhythmias probably result from direct β-adrenergic receptor stimulation and can often be controlled by propranolol. Postural hypotension, a side-effect where both peripheral and central mechanisms play a part, is decreased by giving dopa decarboxylase inhibitors; many patients who show an initial hypotension improve spontaneously.

Centrally mediated side-effects include involuntary movements (dyskinesia) and psychiatric reactions. Dyskinesia develops in many patients, often within a few months of initiation of treatment and coinciding with optimal improvement. Choreoathetoid movements are usual but myoclonus and dystonia may be seen. The involuntary movements can be decreased by a reduction in the dose of levodopa; however, this also attenuates therapeutic efficacy. The dose at which dyskinesia occurs varies from patient to patient, and the movements may develop after several years of treatment without any increase in dosage. The psychiatric effects include agitation, confusion, depression, delirium, hypomania, delusions, paranoia, hallucinations, lethargy, vivid dreams, hypersexual behaviour, and overt psychosis.

Levodopa in combination with decarboxylase inhibitors

Rationale

Decarboxylase inhibitors which do not cross the blood–brain barrier block the conversion of levodopa to dopamine extracerebrally, and therefore decrease adverse reactions deriving from formation of catecholamines at the periphery. Two such inhibitors are available: carbidopa and benserazide. The advantage of using these drugs with levodopa is that most peripheral side-effects of levodopa, such as nausea and cardiovascular reactions, are reduced. Consequently, the combination allows tolerance of a more rapid build-up of initial dosage; in some cases a therapeutic intake of levodopa can be given which was previously precluded by peripheral side-effects.

Availability

Carbidopa is the only decarboxylase inhibitor approved for use in the United States. It is available as Sinemet in tablets containing 10 mg of carbidopa with 100 mg of levodopa and also as 25 mg of carbidopa to 250 mg of levodopa (10/100; 25/250). It is generally desirable to have at least 100 mg daily of inhibitor, therefore patients on low doses of Sinemet may require supplements of carbidopa (which is available as separate 25 mg tablets).

Pharmacokinetics[43]

Co-administration of levodopa and a peripheral inhibitor of dopa decarboxylase decreases levodopa requirements by around 75–80%. Therefore, when changing from levodopa to Sinemet it is easiest to stop the levodopa one evening and the next day introduce Sinemet containing 1/4 to 1/5 of the original levodopa dose.

Uses[44–50]

No side-effects appear to exist other than those of the concomitantly administered levodopa, and thus the combination is the most satisfactory method of administering levodopa.

Bromocriptine

Rationale

Bromocriptine is an ergopeptine with dopamine agonist properties[51]. The reasons for attempting to develop drugs which directly effect the dopamine receptor are threefold[52]; first, they may be more specific for the dopamine receptor; second, they may be more specific for certain subclasses of dopamine receptor and may lead to the possiblity of decreasing unwanted effects of levodopa such as dyskinesia and psychosis; third, they by-pass dopa decarboxylase, an enzyme which is necessary to the production of dopamine from levodopa, which is depleted in the brain of patients with parkinsonism. Bromocriptine does not have all of these advantages, but it may lead the way to the development of more selective agonists.

Uses[53–58]

Bromocriptine has been shown to have an antiparkinsonian effect comparable to that of levodopa. It is not usually used as a first-line drug. Nevertheless, there are a number of patients who show better control of their Parkinson's disease when the two drugs are used in combination. In particular, some patients with the on–off phenomenon or those experiencing end of dose akinesia are often helped by the addition of bromocriptine. Also, some patients who develop dyskinesia on low doses of levodopa can occasionally get a beneficial response from bromocriptine without the precipitation of such severe involuntary movements. Patients who have persistent nausea on levodopa or Sinemet may occasionally be helped by bromocriptine.

Dosage

After a test dose of 1 mg, intake is built up to a dose of around 15 mg four times daily, over 4 weeks. Occasional patients may get increased benefit from doses up to 100 mg a day.

Pharmacokinetics

Peak plasma levels after oral dosage are reached at 2–3 h. The plasma half-life of bromocriptine is longer (4–6 h) than that of levodopa.

Contraindications

A previous history of psychosis, and severe coronary or peripheral vascular disease are contraindications.

Side-effects

The most important initial side-effect is hypotension, which can be profound. Usually, it occurs at low doses and tachyphylaxis rapidly develops. Nausea and constipation occur but are rarely troublesome. The most serious late side-effects are psychiatric and are similar to those described for levodopa, although frank psychosis may be somewhat more common and severe. Dyskinesia is less common than in patients receiving levodopa, though it does occur with bromocriptine. An unusual adverse reaction is the development of hot, warm, oedematous feet (erythromelalgia) which is associated with a mononuclear infiltrating vasculopathy in the skin. Other side-effects include nasal stuffiness, blurred vision, digital vasospasm, and impairment of liver function tests which are usually transient.

Other drugs

A number of other drugs used for Parkinson's disease have limited value.

Deprenyl

Deprenyl is an inhibitor of monoamine oxidase B which is an important enzyme for the catabolism of dopamine. Levodopa can be safely combined with this inhibitor without development of dangerous hypertensive reactions. Although more enthusiastic claims have been made[59], it seems that this drug's main advantage is prolonging the action of levodopa and it may thus be of some help to patients with end of dose akinesia or the immobility that is sometimes particularly troublesome during the night or early morning[60].

Propranolol

Some patients with Parkinson's disease have a prominent action tremor and this can occasionally be improved by a β-adrenergic blocking agent such as propranolol[61].

Baclofen

Baclofen is a GABA analogue used for the treatment of spasticity. It has been claimed that this drug helps dystonia of the foot, which is sometimes a problem in Parkinson's disease. However, hallucinations can be precipitated by withdrawal[62].

Amphetamine

Amphetamine is an old treatment for Parkinson's disease and in some patients it may have a mildly beneficial action. It has been claimed to be particularly helpful for the treatment of the oculogyric crises encountered in postencephalitic parkinsonism.

SURGICAL MANAGEMENT

The surgical procedure of choice for Parkinson's disease is ventro-lateral thalamotomy, with the patient conscious in order to evaluate the effects of temporary lesions before placing the final lesion[63]. Very few patients with Parkinson's disease are considered for this procedure now that potent drugs are available. The only candidate is the patient with severe unilateral tremor who has had a full trial of all available medications without success. In such cases, if the tremor is seriously disabling, the risk of an operation is justified. Bilateral operations are not warranted because the risk of complications, particularly severe speech disturbance, is unacceptably high.

DRUGS WHICH ARE CONTRAINDICATED IN PARKINSON'S DISEASE

A number of drugs may upset patients with Parkinson's disease. Agents which deplete the brain of catecholamines, such as reserpine or tetrabenazine, or drugs which block the dopamine receptors, such as the butyrophenones and the phenothiazines, are contraindicated. Monoamineoxidase inhibitors (other than a selective MAO B inhibitor) should not be given to patients who are also taking levodopa because they may precipate hypertension. Some physicians feel that benzodiazepines and barbiturates are contraindicated in Parkinson's disease; however, only a small minority of patients deteriorate on these drugs and they can safely be used in most cases. Pyridoxine should be avoided when patients are taking levodopa without a decarboxylase inhibitor[64] because it decreases the efficacy of levodopa; pyridoxine-free multivitamin preparations are available. Papaverine[65] and methyl-dopa[66] may also exacerbate parkinsonism.

SUPPORTIVE MEASURES

In addition to support from the physician, a number of other paramedical personnel should participate in the management of patients with Parkinson's disease. It is important to have a social worker involved with the patient to give personal support, advice about financial affairs and help with placement in a nursing facility or arrangement for outside help in the home. Problems may arise at work and decisions may have to be made about retirement. Occupational therapists may be helpful by giving simple aids to assist in performing the tasks of daily living and also in adapting the home to the needs of the patient. At some stages help and advice from nurse practitioners in the clinic or visiting nurses at home may be necessary. Physical therapy may be important, especially when there are periods of forced immobility. It should be directed to keeping the joints supple, particularly at the shoulder, and to giving the patients help and practice with their gait. It is also useful for the physiotherapist to teach a number of planned exercises for the patients to perform at home.

MANAGEMENT

The individual drugs that can be used for Parkinson's disease have been discussed and now some guidelines for the management of individual patients will be given.

The newly diagnosed patient

Although levodopa is clearly the most effective treatment for Parkinson's disease, long-term side-effects and pharmacological concerns about the effect of chronic administration suggest that it is probably wise not to begin levodopa treatment as soon as the diagnosis is made[67,68]. Therefore, in patients who have mild complaints and for whom the disease is having no serious impact on their occupation or social life, it is best to withhold medication. Patients who demand therapy or who have significant symptoms should start with an anticholinergic and, if necessary, amantadine can later be added.

Some patients, because of their personality or because of a demanding occupation, require a consideration of levodopa treatment despite relatively mild disease. In these cases it is reasonable to start off with Sinemet in doses of 10/100, three or four times a day, and observe if there is any improvement, where necessary increasing to 25/250 four times daily. When there is significant benefit, treatment should be continued at the lowest dose that will keep the patient's symptoms controlled. If improvement is inadequate, which is particularly common in patients who only have tremor as their major manifestation, it is prudent to stop the drug and keep it in reserve for a later date.

Sooner or later the patient will unequivocally need levodopa and then it is reasonable to start Sinemet 10/100 three or four times a day building up to whatever dose is necessary. There is no need to stop an anticholinergic or amantadine at this stage. While definitive evidence is lacking, it seems likely that long-term side-effects of levodopa are reduced if the patient is on the lowest possible dose and although it was common practice to tolerate considerable involuntary movement, it now seems desirable to keep dyskinesia minimal, even at the expense of a significant parkinsonian deficit during much of the day.

Treatment of special forms of parkinsonism

Postencephalitic forms of parkinsonism respond poorly to levodopa because of psychiatric complications and involuntary movements[69]. Their best treatment is usually high doses of anticholinergics, though sometimes small additional doses of levodopa can be helpful. Drug-induced parkinsonism generally occurs early in the course of treatment with neuroleptics, is relatively mild, and often clears spontaneously, even when the causal drug is continued[21]. Occasionally it is severe or persistent and should be treated by either discontinuation or a major reduction in the dose of the neuroleptic. An anticholinergic in this situation may be helpful, but levodopa or bromocriptine are not.

PROBLEMS

A number of common problems in the management of patients will now be considered.

No response to therapy

A review of the diagnosis should be made as the patient may have one of the forms of striatonigral degeneration, progressive supranuclear palsy of the Shy–Drager syndrome. If facilities are available, it is worth checking plasma levels of levodopa or bromocriptine to make sure that there is not a pharmacokinetic explanation for the lack of response, although this is exceedingly rare.

Excessive dyskinesia

This difficult problem can only be controlled by a reduction of the dose of levodopa, but since this may cause unacceptable immobility, the patient often prefers to be dyskinetic. In a few patients with severe dyskinesia a better functional response can be attained with less dyskinesia by using bromocriptine. An alternative approach is to combine the levodopa with a dopamine receptor blocking drug; in the past this has always been unsuccessful because of a concomitant increase in the parkinsonian deficit. However, recent reports with a new drug, tiapride, indicated possible success in reducing dyskinesia, though the dose of levodopa may have to be increased to offset a slight increase in parkinsonism[70]. One form of dyskinesia which requires a somewhat different approach is the dystonia that some patients with Parkinson's disease develop in the early mornings, usually in one foot; this may respond to bromocriptine, with a reduction in the dose of levodopa.

Wearing-off phenomena

Some patients who are receiving levodopa, particularly after several years, develop akinesia, or dyskinesia, several hours after their last dose of levodopa and before their next dose is due[71,72]. The reasons for this are unclear and do not have a simple relationship with a low plasma concentration of levodopa. This problem can sometimes be helped by giving smaller dosages, closer together, without necessarily changing the daily intake. An alternative management is to add bromocriptine, with a corresponding reduction in the dose of levodopa.

On–off phenomenon

This problem all too frequently develops in patients who have been on levodopa for several years; in addition, it occasionally develops within a few weeks of starting the drug. Classically, the 'on–off' phenomenon is a sudden switch between either good control or dyskinesia, to severe akinesia[32,72,73]. This change has devastating physical and emotional consequences for the patient and there is no satisfactory form of treatment. Some are improved by the addition of bromocriptine, or reintroduction of amantidine, but many are not and adjustment of the timing of levodopa dosage only occasionally helps. This syndrome and possibly some of the late non-responders to levodopa may be helped by a period off, or on a reduced dose of levodopa. Such management is so far unproven; theoretically it may help to re-establish the sensitivity of the dopamine receptors which can be rendered subsensitive by chronic treatment with levodopa[68].

Psychosis

Psychosis in the parkinsonian patient is usually drug induced, though occasional instances of the coexistence of Parkinson's disease and schizophrenia may be seen. Management of either problem is extremely difficult since it may be impossible to discontinue levodopa without endangering the patient's life. Whenever possible, antiparkinsonian medication should be stopped because any of the drugs used may be responsible; the last introduced agent may not be the culprit. When a drug is responsible, psychosis usually responds quickly provided the drug is stopped as soon as symptoms become obvious. The only exception is the prolonged psychosis sometimes seen after bromocriptine therapy, which can last up to 6 weeks. Antipsychotic medication should be avoided, especially if the Parkinson's disease is severe, because it may precipitate bulbar dysfunction and lead to aspiration. Nevertheless, it may sometimes be necessary to use antipsychotics, which should be given cautiously and only in slowly increasing dosages. Thioridazine is probably the best drug as it has considerable anticholinergic properties. Other antipsychotic medications, which spare the striatal dopamine receptor and preferentially affect mesolimbic receptors, may be available in the foreseeable future. Similar considerations apply to patients who become confused; however, dementia may be due to the Parkinson's disease and on occasion improves with levodopa treatment.

Depression

Depression is a common feature of parkinsonism and may be either reactive or part of the disease process; it is rarely due to medication. Many mild depressions respond to psychotherapy by the neurologist, patient's family, and other professional or patient help groups. In some patients drug treatment with tricyclics, such as amitriptyline or imipramine, is helpful. Tricyclics should be built up to conventional doses but if the patient does not respond within 6–8 weeks the advice of a psychiatrist should be sought. In rare instances electroconvulsive therapy may be justified and may be effective in both helping the depression and the parkinsonism[74].

Sleep disturbances may respond to chloral hydrate or diphenhydramine, but it is best to try to avoid hypnotics. Flurazepam or a barbiturate may be tried.

Autonomic disturbances

Many patients with Parkinson's disease have problems due to malfunction of their autonomic nervous system. A mild neurogenic bladder is common and may be exacerbated by anticholinergics. Full investigation is indicated to exclude a contributing obstructive lesion, which is particularly common in men of this age group and may require surgical treatment; if absent, the addition of urecholine may be helpful. Impotence is also common in Parkinson's disease and occasionally patients develop hypersexuality on treatment. Severe postural hypotension is unusual in the untreated patient and should lead to a suspicion of the Shy–Drager syndrome, but hypotension is common in the early stages of treatment with levodopa. It may rarely be necessary to use tight stockings and very exceptionally fluorocortisone may be helpful.

Constipation is very common in Parkinson's disease and occasionally causes impaction or precipitates volvulus. Anticholinergics and bromocriptine may exacerbate the sluggish bowel. Patients should be encouraged to have a high residue diet, if necessary supplementing with bran. Artificial bulk agents can help, such as metamucil, dioctyl sodium sulphosuccinate or methylcellulose. Alternatively, laxatives may be given, such as bisacodyl, orally or as an enema.

Concomitant medical problems

Most medical and surgical problems that occur in patients with Parkinson's disease should be treated promptly in the conventional manner. Surgical treatment for a badly osteoarthritic hip can have a remarkably beneficial effect on a 'parkinsonian' gait and removal of a subdural haemotoma or treatment of a urinary infection may help a patient's confusion.

Surgical procedures should not be undertaken lightly as there is an increased risk deriving from postoperative immobility. Respiratory problems are usually due to poor chest expansion, aspiration, and occasionally vocal cord paralysis. Full clinical assessment and breathing exercises should be undertaken preoperatively. It is conventional to stop levodopa 12 hours before general anaesthesia although in severe parkinsonism this may not be appropriate, in which case the patient should be given extra decarboxylase inhibitor to reduce any risk of cardiac dysrhythmia. Anti-parkinsonian medication should be given immediately postoperatively via a nasogastric tube, or when this is impossible by intravenous infusion of levodopa (rectal levodopa is poorly absorbed). Chest and limb physical therapy should be started and the patient mobilized as soon as possible. Many patients develop temporary retention of urine or postoperative confusion.

Terminal patients

Sooner or later all patients will become severely disabled and unresponsive to therapy. Nursing home or hospital care will then become necessary and should be expedited rather than prolonging an unreasonable burden on the patient's family. Availability of the physician will provide a welcome anchor for the patient and his relatives. Communication with many patients is difficult at this stage, often because of dysarthria rather than dementia.

CONCLUSION

Treatment of the symptoms of Parkinson's disease delays the onset of severe disability by several years and there is hope for refinement of therapy in the future. Unfortunately there is no treatment which arrests or prevents the disease, so many patients will eventually become severely disabled and die. In this situation the physician must consider every aspect of the patient's needs, and while drug therapy is of paramount importance, he should not ignore the numerous additional approaches available for alleviating physical, mental, social and domestic problems.

Note: Recently a preparation combining carbidopa 25 mg with levodopa 100 mg (Sinemet 25/100) has become available in several countries.

Acknowledgement

We are very grateful to Ms Ann Miller and Ms Betsy Bliss for typing this manuscript, and collating the references.

References

1 Duvoisin, R. C. (1967). Cholinergic-anticholinergic antagonism in parkinsonism. *Arch. Neurol.*, **17**, 124

2 Meyers, R. (1940). Surgical procedure for postencephalitic tremor, with notes on the physiology of premotor fibres. *Arch. Neurol. Psychiatry*, **44**, 455

3 Spiegel, E. A. and Wycis, H. T. (1954). Ansotomy in paralysis agitans. *Arch. Neurol. Psychiatry*, **71**, 598

4 Cooper, I. S. (1955). Chemopallidectomy, an investigative technique in geriatric parkinsonians. *Science*, **121**, 217

5 Hassler, R. R. (1956). Dis extrapyramidalen Rindensysteme und die zentrale Regelung der Motorik. *Dtsch. Z. Nervenheilk.*, **175**, 283

6 Kline, N. S. and Stanley, A. M. (1955). Use of reserpine in a neuropsychiatric hospital. *Ann. N.Y. Acad. Sci.*, **61**, 85

7 Carlsson, A., Linqvist, M. and Magnusson, T. (1957). 3,4,-Dihydroxy-phenylalanine and 5-hydroxytryptophan as reserpine antagonists. *Nature (London)*, **180**, 1200

8 Carlsson, A., Lindqvist, M., Magnusson, T. and Waldeck, B. (1958). On the presence of 3-hydroxytyramine in brain. *Science*, **127**, 471

9 Carlsson, A. (1959). The occurrence, distribution and physiological role of catecholamines in the nervous system. *Pharmacol. Rev.*, **11**, 490

10 Ehringer, H. and Hornykiewicz, O. (1960). Verteilung von Noradrenalin und Dopamin (3-Hydroxytyramin) in gehirn des Menschen und ihr terhalten Beierkranhungen des extrapyramidalen System. *Klin. Wochenschr.*, **38**, 1236

11 Anden, N. E., Roos, B. E. and Werdinius, B. (1964). Effects of chlorpromazine, haloperidol and reserpine on the levels of phenolic acids in rabbit corpus striatum. *Life Sci.*, **3**, 149

12 Birkmayer, W. and Hornykiewicz, O. (1961). Der L-dioxy-phenylalanin (Levodopa)-Effekt bei der Parkinson-akinese. *Wien. Klin. Wochenschr.*, **73**, 787

13 Barbeau, A., Sourkes, T. L. and Murphy, G. (1962). Les catecholamines dans la maladie de Parkinson. In de Ajuriaguerra, J. (ed.) *Monamines et Systeme Nerveux Central*, pp. 247–262. (Paris: Masson)

14 Cotzias, G. C., van Woert, M. H. and Schiffer, L. M. (1967). Aromatic amino acids and modification of parkinsonism. *N. Engl. J. Med.*, **276**, 374

15 Birkmayer, W. and Mentasti, M. (1967). Weitere experimentelle Untersuchungen uber den Catecholaminstoff-wechsel bei extrapyramidalen Erkrankungen. *Arch. Psychiatr. Nervenkr.*, **210**, 29

16 Duvoisin, R. C. (1978). *Parkinson's Disease: A Guide for Patient and Family*, p. 196. (New York: Raven Press)

17 McGeer, P. L. and McGeer, E. G. (1971). Cholinergic enzyme systems in Parkinson's disease. *Arch. Neurol.*, **25**, 265

18 Coyle, J. T. and Snyder, S. H. (1969). Antiparkinsonian drugs: inhibition of dopamine uptake in the corpus striatum as a possible mechanism of action. *Science*, **166**, 899

19 Yahr, M. D. and Duvoisin, R. C. (1968). Medical therapy of parkinsonism. *Mod. Treat.*, **5**, 283

20 Granger, M. E. (1961). Exacerbations in parkinsonism. *Neurology*, **11**, 538

21 Sovner, R. and DiMascio, A. (1978). Extrapyramidal syndromes and other neurological side-effects of psychotropic drugs. In Lipton, M. A., DiMascio, A. and Killam, K. F. (eds.) *Psychopharmacology; A Generation of Progress*, pp. 1021–1032. (New York: Raven Press)

22 Schwab, R. S., England, A. C. Jr., Poskanzer, D. C. and Young, R. R. (1969). Amantadine in the treatment of Parkinson's disease. *J. Am. Med. Assoc.*, **208**, 1168

23 Stromberg, U. and Svensson, T. H. (1971). Further studies on the mode of action of amantadine. *Acta Pharmacol.*, **30**, 161

24 Von Voigtlander, P. F. and Moore, K. E. (1971). Dopamine: release from the brain *in vivo* by amantadine. *Science*, **174**, 408

25 Nastuk, W. L., Su, P. C. and Doubilet, P. (1976). Anticholinergic and membrane activities of amantadine in neuromuscular transmission. *Nature (London)*, **264**, 76

26 Schwab, R. S., Poskanzer, D. C., England, A. C. Jr. and Young, R. R. (1972). Amantadine in Parkinson's disease. Review of more than two years experience. *J. Am. Med. Assoc.*, **222**, 792

27 Parkes, J. D., Zilkha, K. J., Calver, D. M. and Knill-Jones, R. P. (1970). Controlled trial of amantadine hydrochloride in Parkinson's disease. *Lancet*, **1**, 259

28 Godwin-Austen, R. B., Frears, C. C., Bergmann, S., Parkes, J. D. and Knill-Jones, R. P. (1970). Combined treatment of Parkinsonism with levodopa and amantadine. *Lancet*, **2**, 383

29 Zeldowicz, L. R. and Huberman, J. (1973). Long-term therapy of Parkinson's disease with amantadine, alone and combined with levodopa. *Can. Med. Assoc. J.*, **109**, 588

30 Fahn, S. and Isgreen, W. P. (1975). Long-term evaluation of amantadine and levodopa combination in parkinsonism by double-blind crossover analysis. *Neurology*, **25**, 695

31 Timberlake, W. H. and Vance, M. A. (1978). Four-year treatment of patients with parkinsonism using amantadine alone or with levodopa. *Ann. Neurol.*, **3**, 116

32 Cotzias, G. C., Papavasiliou, P. S. and Gellene, R. (1969). Modification of parkinsonism — chronic treatment with levodopa. *N. Engl. J. Med.*, **280**, 337

33 Yahr, M. D., Duvoisin, R. C., Shear, M. J., Barrett, R. E. and Hoehn, M. M. (1969). Treatment of parkinsonism with levodopa. *Arch. Neurol.*, **21**, 343

34 Klawans, H. L. Jr. and Garvin, J. S. (1969). Treatment of parkinsonism with levodopa. *Dis. Nerv. Syst.*, **30**, 737

35 Mawdsley, C. (1970). Treatment of parkinsonism with levodopa. *Br. Med. J.*, **1**, 331

36 Sweet, R. D. and McDowell, F. H. (1975). Five years treatment of Parkinson's disease with levodopa: therapeutic results and survival of 100 patients. *Ann. Intern. Med.*, **83**, 456

37 Yahr, M. D. (1975). Levodopa: drugs five years later. *Ann. Intern. Med.*, **83**, 677

38 Marsden, C. D. and Parkes, J. D. (1977). Success and problems of long-term levodopa therapy in Parkinson's disease. *Lancet*, **1**, 345

39 Fahn, S. and Duffy, P. (1978). Parkinson's disease. In Goldensohn, E. S. and Appel, S. H. (eds.) *Scientific Approaches to Clinical Neurology*, pp. 1119–1158. (Philadelphia: Lea & Febiger)

40 Joseph, C., Chassan, J. B. and Koch, M. L. (1978). Levodopa in Parkinson's disease: a long-term appraisal of mortality. *Ann. Neurol.*, **3**, 116

41 Diamond, S. G., Markham, C. H. and Treciokas, L. J. (1976). Long-term experience with levodopa: efficacy, progression and mortality. In Birkmayer, W. and Hornykiewicz, O. (eds.) *Advances in Parkinsonism*, pp. 444–445. (Basel: Editiones Roche)

42 Calne, D. B., Karoum, R., Ruthven, C. R. J. and Sandler, M. (1969). The metabolism of orally administered levodopa in parkinsonism. *J. Pharmacol.*, **37**, 57

43 Tissot, R., Bartholini, G. and Pletscher, A. (1969). Drug-induced changes of extracerebral dopa metabolism in man. *Arch. Neurol.*, **20**, 187

44 Calne, D. B., Reid, J. L., Vakil, S. D., Rao, S., Petrie, A., Pallis, C. A., Gawler, J., Thomas, P. K. and Hilson, A. (1971). Idiopathic parkinsonism treated with an extracerebral decarboxylase inhibitor in combination with levodopa. *Br. Med. J.*, **3**, 729

45 Papavasiliou, P. S., Cotzias, G. C., Duby, S. E., Steck, A. J., Fehling, C. and Bell, M. (1972). Levodopa in parkinsonism: potentiation of central effects with a peripheral inhibitor. *N. Engl. J. Med.*, **286**, 8

46 Yahr, M. D. (1973). *Treatment of Parkinsonism—The Role of Dopa Decarboxylase Inhibitors. Advances in Neurology*. Vol. 2, p. 303. (New York: Raven Press)

47 Barbeau, A. and Roy, M. (1976). Six-year results of treatment with levodopa plus benzerazide in Parkinson's disease. *Neurology*, **26**, 399

48 Marsden, C. D., Parkes, J. P. and Rees, J. E. (1973). A year's comparison of treatment of patients with Parkinson's disease with levodopa combined with carbidopa versus treatment with levodopa alone. *Lancet*, **2**, 1459

49 Mars, H. (1973). Modification of levodopa effect by systemic decarboxylase inhibition. *Arch. Neurol.*, **28**, 91

50 Markham, C. H., Diamond, S. G. and Treciokas, L. J. (1974). Carbidopa in Parkinson's disease and in nausea and vomiting of levodopa. *Arch. Neurol.*, **31**, 128

51 Corrodi, H., Fuxe, K., Hokfelt, T., Lidbrink, P. and Ungerstedt, U. (1973). Effect of ergot drugs on central catecholamine neurons: evidence for a stimulation of central dopamine neurons. *J. Pharm. Pharmacol.*, **25**, 409

52 Calne, D. B. (1978). Dopaminergic agonists in the treatment of parkinsonism. In Klawans, H. L. (ed.) *Clinical Neuropharmacology*. Vol. 3, pp. 153–166. (New York: Raven Press)

53 Teychenne, P. F., Calne, D. B., Leigh, P. N., Greenacre, J. K., Reid, J. L., Petrie, A. and Bamji, A. N. (1975). Idiopathic parkinsonism treated with bromocriptine. *Lancet*, **2**, 473

54 Lees, A. J., Shaw, K. M. and Stern, G. M. (1975). Bromocriptine in parkinsonism. *Lancet*, **2**, 709

55 Kartzinel, R., Perlow, M., Teychenne, P., Gielen, A. C., Gillespie, M. M., Sadowsky, D. A. and Calne, D. B. (1976). Bromocriptine and levodopa (with or without carbidopa) in parkinsonism. *Lancet*, **2**, 272

56 Lieberman, A., Kupersmith, M., Estey, E. and Goldstein, M. (1976). Treatment of Parkinson's disease with bromocriptine. *N. Engl. J. Med.*, **295**, 1400

57 Kartzinel, R. and Calne, D. B. (1976). Studies with bromocriptine: Part 1. 'On-off' phenomena. *Neurology*, **26**, 508

58 Parkes, J. D., Debono, A. G., Marsden, C. D. and Asselman, P. (1976). Clinical pharmacology of bromocriptine in parkinsonism. In Bayliss, R. I. S., Turner, P. and Maclay, W. P. (eds.) *Pharmacological and Clinical Aspects of Bromocriptine (Parlodel)— Proceedings of a Symposium held at The Royal College of Physicians, London, 14 May, 1976*, pp. 27–33. (Tunbridge Wells: MCS Consultants)

59 Birkmayer, M., Riederer, P., Ambrozil, L. and Youdim, M. B. H. (1977). Implications of combined treatment with MOPAR and L-Deprenyl in Parkinson's disease. *Lancet*, **1**, 440

60 Lees, A. J., Shaw, K. M., Kohout, L. J., Stern, G. M., Elseworth, J. D., Sandler, M. and Youdim, M. B. H. (1977). Deprenyl in Parkinson's disease. *Lancet*, **2**, 791

61 Owen, D. A. L. and Marsden, C. D. (1965). Effect of β-blockade in parkinsonian tremor. *Lancet*, **2**, 1259

62 Lees, A. J., Shaw, K. M. and Stern, G. M. (1978). Baclofen in Parkinson's disease. *J. Neurol. Neurosurg. Psychiatry*, **41**, 707

63 Cooper, I. S. (1965). Surgical treatment of parkinsonism. *Ann. Rev. Med.*, **16**, 309

64 Duvoisin, R. C., Yahr, M. D. and Coté, L. J. (1969). Pyridoxine reversal of levodopa effects in parkinsonism. *Trans. Am. Neurol. Assoc.*, **94**, 81

65 Duvoisin, R. C. (1975). Antagonism of levodopa by papaverine. *J. Am. Med. Assoc.*, **231**, 845

66 Duvoisin, R. C. (1975). Alpha-methyldopa and parkinsonism: induction or exacerbation. *Neurology*, **25**, 376

67 Yahr, M. D. (1976). Evaluation of long-term therapy in Parkinson's disease: mortality and therapeutic efficacy. In Birkmayer, W. and Hornykiewicz, O. (eds.) *Advances in Parkinsonism*, pp. 435–443. (Basel: Editiones Roche)

68 Lee, T., Seeman, P., Rajput, A., Farley, I. J. and Hornykiewicz, O. (1978). Receptor basis for dopaminergic supersensitivity in Parkinson's disease. *Nature (London)*, **273**, 59

69 Calne, D. B., Stern, G. M., Lawrence, D. R., Sharkey, J. and Armitage, P. (1969). Levodopa in post-encephalitic parkinsonism. *Lancet*, **1**, 744

70 Price, P., Parkes, J. D. and Marsden, C. D. (1978). Tiapride in Parkinson's disease. *Lancet*, **2**, 1106

71 Muenter, M. D., Sharpless, N. S., Tyce, G. M. and Darley, F. L. (1976). Patterns of Dystonia ('1-D-1' and 'D-1-D') in response to levodopa therapy for Parkinson's disease. In Birkmayer, W. and Hornykiewicz, O. (eds.) *Advances in Parkinsonism*, pp. 350–360. (Basel: F. Hoffman-LaRoche Company Ltd.)

72 Barbeau, A. (1976). Pathophysiology of the oscillations in performance after long-term therapy with levodopa. In Birkmayer, W. and Hornykiewicz, O. (eds.) *Advances in Parkinsonism*, pp. 424–434. (Basel: Editiones Roche)

73 Marsden, C. D. and Parkes, J. D. (1976). 'On-off' effects in patients with Parkinson's disease on chronic levodopa therapy. *Lancet*, **1**, 292

74 Asnis, G. (1977). Parkinson's disease, depression and ECT: a review and case study. *Am J. Psychiatry*, **134**, 191

10

Stereotactic and peripheral surgery for the control of movement disorders

C. Bertrand

INTRODUCTION

In the wave of enthusiasm which followed the initial results of stereotactic surgery in the early 1950s, it became widely used and, in some centres, large lesions were performed without precise anatomic and physiological controls. Gradually, the indications and limitations of stereotactic surgery and other procedures such as peripheral denervation have been better understood. The need for a careful preoperative assessment, for painstaking physiological controls including both recording and stimulation, for a precise target and accurate tailored lesions, has become well recognized; the few adjoining zones which must be avoided have been circumscribed so that more constant results and rare complications can be expected. Long-term follow-ups have helped to establish the persistence of postoperative improvement for specific symptoms adding further to the predictability of surgery.

This chapter will deal particularly with the experience of our group (C. Bertrand, S. N. Martinez, Pedro Molina-Negro and J. Hardy), especially since stereotactic surgery was introduced in our department in 1954[1-3]. Stereotactic procedures were performed for involuntary movements besides other forms of surgery such as rhizotomies, ramicectomies, neurectomies, myotomies and initially a few corticectomies. Most stereotactic lesions have been centred in ventral thalamus or immediately underneath in zona incerta, in globus-pallidus internus and the ansa lenticularis, or in the field of Forel[4]. Stereotactic surgery of the cerebellar nuclei will not be discussed since, up to now, it seems that the hypotonia obtained from surgery of the basal ganglia is sufficient and that there are less side-effects; nor have we placed any lesion within the pulvinar. It must be underlined that we have no personal experience in stereotactic surgery of these two regions. We have not used implanted stimulating electrodes for chronic problems of this kind.

SURGICAL PHYSIOPATHOLOGY

Stereotactic surgery

The history of surgery of movement disorders and the general physiological basis for the various targets used have been reviewed recently by Molina[5]. Because of my former training in the surgery of epilepsy, we used stimulation from the very beginning during stereotactic surgery mostly to identify surrounding structures, particularly primary motor, sensory and visual pathways. It soon became evident that there existed a restricted target zone for tremor immediately underneath the ventro-lateral thalamus. Mere introduction of the electrode through that point would abolish tremor but this did not occur in surrounding areas[6].

Microelectrode recording was introduced in human stereotactic surgery by Albe-Fessard et al.[7] and added to our method by Hardy. It has been established that with a system of proportional measurements or, better still, computerized averaging techniques, the relationship of structures to the intercommissural line is relatively constant, small deviations being detected by stimulation and recording. For instance, with decimal segments of the AC PC line as a yardstick, the point where tremor is arrested, is situated immediately underneath the 8/10th to the 9/10th segments of the AC PC line, five segments lateral to the midline, in the zona incerta, as demonstrated by Velasco et al.[8] in an analysis of cases from our department (20–22 mm behind AC, 12.5 mm lateral to the AC PC midline and within 2.5 mm underneath the horizontal plane through the AC PC line for an AC PC line of 25 mm). Although less dependable, penetration of another point in posterior VOI suppresses the increment of electromyographic discharges in the involved muscles which accompanies lateral gaze in cases of dystonia[9,10]. This small zone is situated in the 6/10th segment of the AC PC line, 1/10th segment above it and 4/10th segments lateral to the midline (15 mm behind AC, 10 mm lateral to the midline and 2.5 mm above the horizontal plane through the AC PC line when that line measures 25 mm).

The classical motor cortico-spinal fibres have been well identified by other workers[11,12] and by our group[13-16] in the third quarter of the posterior limb of the internal capsule. They lie at a safe distance postero-lateral and underneath the thalamic targets. They are easily detectable by increasing stimulation and they have never been involved by our circumscribed lesions.

Likewise, the sensory nuclei and the underlying lemnisci are easily identified both by stimulation and recording, especially using evoked potentials. There is no problem in avoiding them[15,17].

The subthalamic nucleus with its high voltage rhythmic activity at a frequency of 12–14 Hz with the sparse high voltage cell discharges, is readily identified following the diminution of activity recorded once the electrode leaves the thalamus[4]. In only one instance in a child was this activity obtained above the AC PC line. With these precautions, there has been no instance of choreic or ballistic movements following surgery.

While motor and sensory pathways are situated well away from the usual targets, the cortico-bulbar fibres lie close to the thalamus in a coronal plane which passes through the midpoint of the AC PC line, where the thalamus is much more narrow. Lesion of these and adjoining fibres may cause dysarthria and slowness of contra-lateral movements. They are in the same coronal plane as VOI, the posterior portion of which is the target for dystonias. Partial manifestations of this syndrome were found in 5% of cases where dystonia was the indication for surgery; in most instances, the lesions were bilateral[9, 10, 18, 19].

Peripheral surgery

Anterior rhizotomy of C1, C2, and C3 bilaterally and a portion of C4, at least unilaterally, has helped many patients with torticollis, especially when combined with denervation of one of the sterno-cleido-mastoid muscles[20, 21]. However, it leaves an ungainly neck and the roots of the phrenic nerve at C4 limit the downward extension of the rhizotomy so that fairly strong contractions of the posterior nuchal muscles may still be present. A few months ago we operated on a patient suffering from athetosis with torticollis on whom we had performed a thalamotomy in 1961 and an anterior rhizotomy of C1, C2, C3 on the right and C1, C2, C3 and the upper portion of C4 on the left in 1966. As often happens after rhizotomy, she still had contractions of the left splenius and complexus group of muscles which have been relieved by ramicectomy of the posterior rami of C2, C3, C4, C5 and C6. During this last procedure, these rami could still be stimulated probably from anastomoses with the lower rami or the distal portion of the roots. Ramicectomy of C1 and the posterior rami of the other cervical roots has the great advantage of being a lesser procedure, directly oriented to the involved muscles; it can be extended as far down as C7 according to the results of blocking before operation and of stimulation during the procedure[10, 12]. Total abolition of responses must be obtained with these precautions, only peripheral derivation is required usually for torticollis.

PREOPERATIVE INVESTIGATION

While the assessment varies somewhat for the different types of movement disorders, certain requisites should be mentioned. Surgery is usually considered when the disorder handicaps or at least seriously inconveniences the patient and when it is not amenable to medical therapy over the long term, for instance marked tremor of attitude (essential or familial tremor) of the dominant hand in a young person. In the personal history, it may be important to find out from the relatives whether there has been temporary episodes of loss of memory or of mental confusion following the use of drugs or in situations of stress, especially in cases of Parkinson's disease[4]. This is frequently not mentioned spontaneously and it is a contraindication to surgery. In view of the close relationship between late dystonias and familial tremor the family history must be well detailed in these cases[22,23].

In the course of physical examination, palpation of the muscles during abnormal movements is of great help in determining the group of muscles predominantly involved, although evidently not as precise as electromyography.

Movies or video tapes are the best records: they allow repeated study and arrest of movements; they are a great help in the assessment of the progression of the disease or of the results of treatment; and they may be sufficient initially to decide whether a patient should come up for consideration for surgery.

Electromyography is particularly useful in establishing the characteristics of tremors or dystonic movements and in determining which muscles are mainly involved, whether the movement disorder, for instance torticollis, is restricted enough to be amenable solely to peripheral denervation or whether a stereotactic procedure contralateral to the direction of the movements or even a combined approach is required.

It is often repeated together with local infiltration to verify that involved muscles, such as the sterno-cleido-mastoid on one side or the posterior nuchal group of muscles on the other, have been blocked effectively in order to judge what improvement can be expected from permanent denervation. When the trapezius is involved, as in some forms of laterocollis, temporary blocking is most helpful in determining how much limitation of abduction and elevation of the arm may result from denervation since this varies considerably in different individuals. When blocking the spinal nerve, there may be transitory diminution of the volume of the voice and difficulty in swallowing if the infiltration is too deep and involves the recurrent laryngeal nerve. To block CI and the posterior rami of C2, C3 and C4, the patient lies on the opposite side, the needle is first placed against the occipital bone and then laterally on the posterior surface of the articular facettes. One should aspirate frequently to avoid injecting in the large venous plexuses. In our first group of cases there were two instances of a drop in blood pressure, faintness, nausea and nystagmus presumably from diffusion into the brain stem circulation. This was rapidly corrected by intravenous corticoids. For this reason, an intravenous solution of 5% glucose is installed beforehand[10,19]. Sometimes, stimulation is used, mostly to determine the optimum site for nerve blocking. Pre- and postoperative myotactic reflex studies are

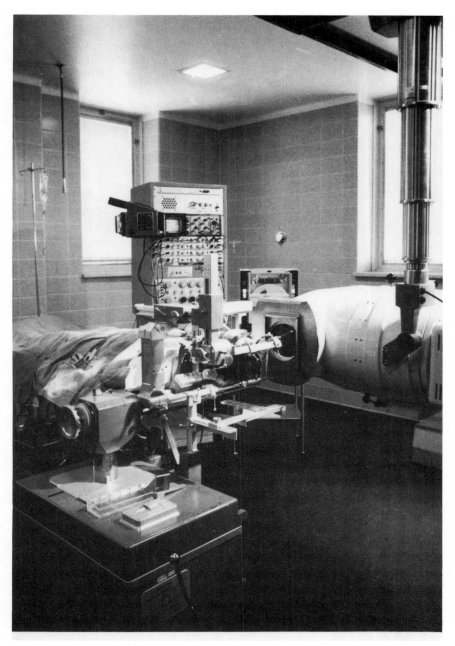

Figure 1 Photography of stereotactic operating room during a procedure showing the teleguided stereotactic apparatus, the electromyographic stimulating and recording unit, video tape, TV and X-ray facilities

valuable in the prognosis of the long-term effects. When there is good postoperative contralateral hypotonia there exists a definite hypoexcitability of the γ-motor neurons. When the lesion involves cortico-bulbar and adjoining cortico-spinal fibres hyperexcitability of the α-motor neurons is evident.

SURGICAL TECHNIQUES

Stereotactic surgery

At the time our technique was introduced 25 years ago[1-3], that of Spiegel and Wycis[24], of Leksell[25] and of Riechert[26] were already in use. Our purpose was to shorten the duration of stereotactic procedures without any sacrifice to accuracy by simplifying orientation and fixation of the apparatus and by using a central beam for direct accurate measurements. These same basic principles remain in our present instrumentation. The use of a central beam or alternately of tele-radiology have gained almost universal acceptance. Our technique has been described elsewhere[2,4] and will not be repeated in detail, especially since there exists at present quite a few apparatuses which combine accuracy together with rapid enough fixation for the entire pro-cedure to be done under local anaethesia while the patient is fully conscious. This is essential for physiological preoperative studies and immediate control of the results obtained (Figure 1).

Other inherent elements in our method should be mentioned: we like to use a parasagittal approach to the basal ganglia so that modifying one of the measurements, such as depth, does not alter the other parameters. Under these circumstances, a trephine is used to penetrate the skull and dura so that venous lakes may be seen if present. The burr-hole is centred anterior to the coronal suture where these lakes are infrequent. Filling of the ventricles must be sufficient to visualize both the anterior and the posterior com-missures since the commissures and the AC PC line are still the common references for measurements. Television is most useful to know when the proper amount of filling has been obtained. The patient is asked to create positive pressure by tightening of the abdominal muscles so that air is aspirated within the third ventricle and the aqueduct when the pressure is released. Air should not be forced all the way to the fourth ventricle and the sub-arachnoid spaces where it may cause headache, nausea or even vomit-ing.

After the target has been identified on our proportional scale using decimal portions of the AC PC line as units, fine electrode recording not only identifies the borders of penetration and exit from the globus pallidus or the thalamus, as the case may be, but also provides safety in avoiding certain structures such as the sub-thalamic nucleus or the sensory pathways in nucleus ventralis posterior. When a pallidal lesion is required the upper and lower limit of the pallidum are also verified with the microelectrode. As it is penetrated, the low-voltage activity of the internal capsule is replaced by moderate spikes with a tendency to rhythmic discharges.

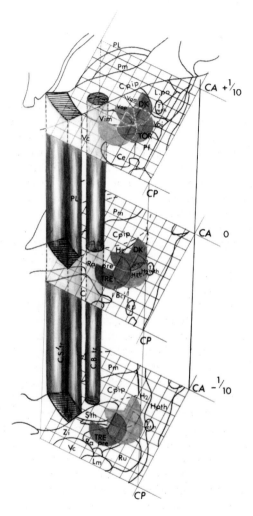

Figure 2 Schematic drawing which demonstrates the relationship of the cortico-bulbar tract (C.B. tr) and of the cortico-spinal tract (C.S. tr) to the thalamic nuclei and to target areas for torticollis and dystonias (TOR), for dyskinesias (DK) and for tremor (TRE). The more deeply shaded areas indicate the level where the lesion is most extensive in each instance. The intermediate horizontal section is at the level of the AC PC line, the top one at 1/10th of the length of the AC PC line above it (2.5 mm for an AC PC line of 25 mm) and the bottom one at 1/10th of the length of the AC PC line below the intermediate section. The proximity of the cortico-bulbar fibres to the anterior target is evident

Recording is followed by stimulation with a triple-lead monopolar electrode to identify sensory, motor and specially cortico-bulbar pathways which may lie lateral to the proposed lesion, especially in cases of dystonia with posterior VOI as a target.

A leucotome is still used because it allows the operator to sculpture the lesion according to the findings of recording and stimulation as well as the anatomic placement; more specifically, the lateral quadrants can be spared when the lesion might encroach upon the internal capsule (Figure 2). This is not possible with instruments producing a concentric lesion. Temporary suppression of a function may also be obtained by merely opening the wire in a given direction without oscillation. With these precautions, postoperative complications are exceptional. Proximity of the cortico-bulbar fibres is practically the only possible source of problem in stereotactic surgery of the thalamus. Many years have elapsed since a postoperative hemorrhage or infection has occurred.

Peripheral surgery

As already mentioned, the treatment of dystonic movements, particularly spasmodic torticollis, may require only peripheral denervation of appropriate muscles or this may have to be combined with a unilateral stereotactic procedure[10].

Denervation of the sterno-cleido-mastoid muscle is done with light anaesthesia and stimulation. One must be aware not only of the possibility of smaller branches well above the main trunk to the sterno-mastoid, but also of recurrent branches from the division of the nerve going to the trapezius which occasionally course back to the lower portion of the sterno-cleido-mastoid muscle: this may explain the occasional reappearance of contractions in the muscle after all branches have apparently been sectioned.

With the patient lying on his side, with his head flexed, C1 and the posterior rami of the other cervical roots are approached through an inverted hockey stick incision starting mesial to the mastoid, curving laterally and extending downwards vertically, just posterior to the transverse processes of the cervical vertebrae. Above the upper border of the horizontal portion of the trapezius, one must be wary of a branch to that muscle which comes to lie underneath the skin, in the lower portion of the incision. It is easily identified by stimulation. The most difficult part of the operation is the identification of C1 which is very small and is first detected by stimulation. It is avulsed as it emerges over the posterior arch of the atlas, under the horizontal segment of the vertebral artery. The posterior rami, including those of the greater occipital nerve are also localized by stimulation as they curve around the articular facettes. The posterior ramus of C2 usually divides immediately in two large branches and it must be avulsed close to its origin where it is near the vertebral artery. The posterior rami are avulsed as far down as is necessary to obtain denervation of all the involved muscles, even down to C7 in severe cases. They are quite variable in size, distribution and anastomoses. No laminectomy is required. There is little limitation of movements and little change in the appearance of the neck since the anterior group of muscles are not involved, with the exception of the contra-lateral sterno-cleido-mastoid. In more severe cases, the trapezius and even the levator scapulae may have to be denervated or the scaleni sectioned.

Tenotomy or myotomy are done much less frequently but they are also useful procedures in certain cases, for instance partial section of the pectoralis major to facilitate movements of the arm away from the chest. Recently, we have had occasion to perform an anterior multi-level fusion of the lower cervical and upper dorsal spine in a patient with a severe dystonia who had a good result from bilateral thalamotomies and pallidotomies but who still had a tendency to antero-flexion of the lower neck musculature, in spite of partial section of prevertebral musculature. Such radical solutions are rarely indicated but it is essential to choose whatever treatment will enhance the functional capacity of the patient.

With the improvement of medical therapy, section of the obturator nerves in patients with scissor gait is required much less frequently but it remains useful when necessary. Myelotomy or anterior lombo-sacral rhizotomy are both effective for spastic paraplegia in flexion, although I have a preference for the latter procedure, which is more definitive.

SPECIFIC INDICATIONS AND RESULTS

Tremor of attitude (essential tremor, familial tremor)

Tremor of attitude is usually first noticed during adolescence and progresses very slowly. At present it is the most frequent indication for stereotactic surgery[4,27]. Since it is not accompanied by any other deficit, surgery is only considered when tremor is detrimental to everyday activities. The target used is the same as that for parkinsonian tremor, that is between the 8/10th and the 9/10th segments of the AC PC line, five segments lateral to the midline and within one segment below the AC PC line, (for a 25 mm AC PC line, 20–22 mm behind AC, 12 to 14 mm lateral to the midline and 2 mm below the AC PC line). The results are most satisfactory and one may expect marked relief of tremor in 90% of cases with total relief in a high percentage of these. Occasionally, the patient initially experiences a slight diminution in dexterity or an increase in fatiguability of the lower limb but the initial hypotonia is rapidly compensated for. Many of these patients have returned to or taken jobs requiring high agility: chemists, mechanics, plumbers. Except in rare cases, the lesion is done only unilaterally. If tremor is equal on both sides, the major hand is the one for which a contra-lateral thalamotomy is performed. Otherwise, it is done contra-lateral to the more severely involved side. When there is tremor of the head, electromyography combined with nerve blocking is most useful to determine the relief to be expected. A good result will be obtained only when there is clear predominance of the tremor on one side.

Intention tremor of multiple sclerosis

Although the large amplitude tremulous movements sometimes encountered in multiple sclerosis are associated with hypotonia and cerebellar signs, they respond very well to a contra-lateral thalamic lesion. It does make these patients' lives much less unpleasant; they become able to use their limbs purposefully on one side and they are not constantly agitated. It is most important to warn them that the other symptoms of multiple sclerosis will not be improved. Some of these patients are quite insistent that surgery should be performed on the other side, but this should be resisted unless the remaining tremor on the other side is such that the patient's situation is untenable.

Hemiballismus

Hemiballismus following a cerebro-vascular accident usually responds to medical therapy. Only a few patients with hemiballismus were operated on in our clinic; in one case, the movements were particularly violent as it was part of a rapidly progressive encephalitis. Although the large amplitude movements were relieved in these patients, a few still exhibited some choreic movements after surgery.

Choreathetosis

Few cases of choreathetosis should be considered for surgery since they usually present marked motor and cortico-bulbar manifestations with dysarthria and slowness of movements. In fact, it seems that the mixture of choreic and dystonic movements which is so difficult to reproduce experimentally, results from a lesion of cortico-bulbar and adjoining cortico-spinal fibres together with a portion of the adjoining sub-thalamic nucleus. Surgery can be beneficial for patients in which choreiform movements predominate. Again it should be done only unilaterally. When writhing movements are very strong and painful, a unilateral lesion combined with peripheral denervation is very helpful, especially when the neck is severely involved. In the preoperative assessment, one must evaluate carefully the amount of underlying weakness of voluntary movements. Thus one may give a more realistic prognosis of the results of surgery which usually produces only moderate improvement in these cases.

Spasticity

No appreciable benefit can be expected from stereotactic lesions in cases of spasticity, as confirmed in a recent review by Siegfried[28]. Some improvement has been reported following cerebellar and cord stimulation for both athetosis and athetosis with spasticity, but further data are needed. Partial section of sensory rootlets, advocated by Gros et al.[29], seems to be helpful in cases in which useful voluntary movements are present, for instance in Little's disease.

Parkinson's disease

It is well known that surgery does not improve akinesia. In 1973, in a chapter on Parkinson's disease we wrote:

> Patients for whom surgery is definitely indicated are those with tremor and rigidity with slow progression predominating on one side, who are seriously inconvenienced in their daily life or sufficiently annoyed by certain manifestations such as tremor. These patients are usually under 65 years of age, mentally alert and have few central signs: there is good convergence of the eyes, good equilibrium, no speech difficulty expect possibly a tendency towards festination or tachyphemia. These patients are motivated towards rehabilitation although their handicap is only moderate. They are anxious to improve their ability to function in daily life and are moderately well controlled by standard drugs[4].

This statement has to be qualified further since most cases now respond well to medical therapy. Surgery is performed if tremor becomes very annoying or incapacitating, or in the infrequent situation when rigidity fails to respond to medical treatment, especially if there are painful cramps in the leg most severely involved.

As mentioned previously, transitory mental confusion or a tendency to propulsion or retropulsion are contraindications. The hypotonia which follows surgery might increase imbalance in relation to the other more rigid unoperated side, if the patient already has trouble with equilibrium. The fact remains that besides suppressing all or most of the tremor, surgery improves rapidly alternating movements of the hand enabling the patient to use his hand more efficiently, probably by removing the barrier created by antagonistic muscles. With proper selection a good result can be expected in over 80% of cases. It remains a precious adjunct to medical therapy.

Dystonias

In the discussion of surgical therapy of dystonias, one must first establish a clear distinction between dystonia musculorum deformans of childhood and the dystonias of adults. The childhood variety is usually more evenly bilateral, more peripheral with clasp-knife rigidity. Because of this and the age of the patient, surgery is only considered when all forms of conservative therapy fail. It can give appreciable relief on the most affected side; occasionally, when bilateral lesions are required the result is dramatic.

In the past few years, we have been dealing mostly with the late forms of dystonias. As substantiated by numerous reports, including ours[10,22,23], there is a strong relationship between familial tremor and dystonias. This is not surprising since, in the macaque, the lesion behind the substantia nigra near the fibres of the third nerve used to produce tremor, dovetails with the one for torticollis. Furthermore, of the three post-traumatic cases of Benedict's syndrome including a large dilated pupil which required a thalamotomy in our department, two had contralateral large amplitude tremor and one had torticollis. The most frequent manifestation of late dystonias, spasmodic torticollis, is usually self limiting. In the more severe forms, reciprocal innervation is more disorganized. There may be marked deformation of the spine all the way down to the lumbar region and gradual involvement of the peripheral musculature. We have encountered only four cases of the more rare and severe myoclonic type, all of which obtained marked relief from surgery.

It is somewhat ironic after all the discussions of the past decade concerning the relative merits of stereotactic surgery and of rhizotomy that our present approach to this problem involves a combination of stereotactic surgery and/or peripheral denervation. If nerve blocks combined with electromyography demonstrate that only certain groups of muscles are involved, for instance the sterno-cleido-mastoid on one side together with the posterior nuchal group of muscles on the other side, peripheral denervation may suffice. This happens more frequently as well-defined cases of torticollis are referred for surgery: two of the 19 cases reported last year had only peripheral denervation, whereas seven out of 27 cases have now been so treated.

When the dystonia is more diffuse, unilateral thalamotomy is necessary and sometimes also pallidotomy. In the late dystonias, there is nearly always unilateral involvement or at least marked preponderence of discharges on one side. It is paramount to perform the stereotactic procedure contralateral to the involved paravertebral musculature. If there still remains an appreciable amount of abnormal movements, in the more severe forms, peripheral denervation may be done a few days later. Bilateral lesions are rarely required. If this is the case one should wait a few months before doing the contralateral procedure. Our results have been reported recently in some detail[10,19]. Briefly, of the last 27 cases, seven have been subjected only to peripheral denervation—three with an excellent result and four with marked improvement, (i.e. there still remains an occasional contraction of the involved muscles but not enough to consider stereotactic surgery). Twenty have undergone unilateral thalamotomy and/or pallidotomy with or without peripheral denervation (almost equally), two of the latter have shown no appreciable change, nine had an excellent result and nine are markedly improved—one of these has some cortico-bulbar manifestations although he is able to practice active sports such as tennis and skating. If the patient has been warned that the relief may not be complete, he is most grateful for the definite improvement in posture and relief from severe muscle contractions such that many of these patients can return to an active life.

COMMENTS

The numerous open procedures on the brain and spinal cord used in the 1930s for control of involuntary movements, are now mostly of historical interest, while surgery of branches of the peripheral nerves to denervate specific muscles of the limbs are still performed. These central procedures have been useful in demonstrating that surgery could modify abnormal movements, and specially in increasing our knowledge of human physiology. Aspiration of the head of the caudate nucleus together with the underlying anterior limb of the internal capsule was last used in our department in 1950 in a severe case of choreathatosis with jacksonian seizures. The abnormal movements were only slightly improved and partial denervation of the biceps and deltoid were required later on. However, the patient's seizures were abolished. This was the origin of our interest in stereotactic lesions of cortico-spinal fibres in epilepsia partialis continua[30, 31] and of bilateral lesions of the field of Forel for intractable epilepsy; the latter produced very inconstant results[32].

From these lesions of the field of Forel, from the numerous lesions of the globus pallidus, of the ansa lenticularis and of the adjoining anterior portion of the posterior limb of the internal capsule, it has been definitely established that there are no motor fibres in the anterior third of the posterior limb of the internal capsule. As a more anterior target, posterior VOI, was chosen to interrupt the vestibulo-interstitio-thalamo-cortical pathway described by Hassler and Hess for dystonias[33]—cortico-bulbar complications became more frequent. The thalamus becomes much narrower at that level and these fibres lie close to it in the internal capsule. In a review of 625 consecutive thalamotomies, complications occurred in 2% of cases, nearly all of which had bilateral lesions[18]. However, when taking into account only cases of severe dystonia with bilateral lesions, the percentage was almost 10%. In 1968 Selby[34], reviewing his own cases as well as those of Krayenbuhl and Gillingham reported that, 'most surgeons comment that this dreaded complication may occur in some 25–33% of cases'. Recently Copper[35], using bilateral spherical lesions, mentioned 18%. This complication may have been the major deterrent to the use of stereotactic surgery for dystonias. Performing only unilateral stereotactic lesions in most cases, with above threshold stimulation to detect the proximity of cortico-bulbar fibres, also avoiding the lateral quadrants while making a carefully planned lesion with a leucotome, it has been constantly below 5%. When this complication has occurred in the past few years it has been partial, that is without dysarthria, consisting mostly of slowness of movements of the upper limb and very little tendency to pronation of the limbs. In the two cases reported by Zoll[36], VPL was also involved with sensory as well as motor signs. From our experience we certainly do not believe that a lesion of VPL contributes to this syndrome. Nor do we agree with Hassler and Diekman[37] that, with the size of lesions necessary to obtain a permanent result, they can be centred differently for different types of dyskinesias.

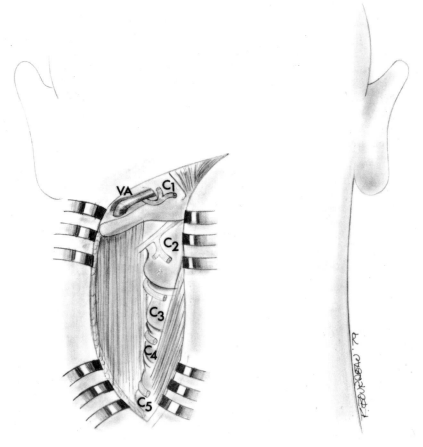

Figure 3 Schematic drawing made from a peroperative photograph of the approach to C1 and the posterior rami of C2 to C6

However, we are convinced that the fibres ascending to VOI can be reached at a lower and more posterior point. A marked hypotonia is also obtained with the safer and more posterior subthalamic target, used in Parkinson's disease so that this complication should also occur in only 2% in unilateral lesions for dystonias, but more frequently in bilateral lesions where compensatory mechanisms are less effective.

All thalamic lesions from VOI to VIM produce some degree of hypotonia in the contralateral limbs. While this is useful in increasing the rapidity of movements of the hand, it seems temporarily to diminish muscle awareness or muscle sense. Occasionally, patients operated on for 'tremor of attitude', in which muscle tone is normal before operation, require a short period of adaptation. In Parkinson's disease, it is beneficial to the gait of the patient only if rigidity is excessive; otherwise postoperatively, there may be a transitory period of imbalance[4].

Pallidal lesions, which are safely away from the cortico-bulbar fibres also produce a definite hypotonia. On the other hand, there may be a period of drowsiness or indifference, especially when performed in the major hemisphere in older patients with Parkinson's disease. From our early series of cases, it appears that the results on tremor and rigidity maintain well over the years. At present, thalamic lesions are used much more frequently[4]. In younger patients with severe dystonias, a pallidal lesion is added to the thalamic lesion whenever necessary to enhance muscle relaxation and there has been no evidence of long-term detrimental effects on mental processes[9,10,19].

From the results obtained from lesions made at different locations, together with those from stimulation and recording techniques, it is possible to draw a map of the basal ganglia and adjoining structures at the level of the AC PC line and immediately above and below that line, to distinguish the areas in which a lesion can be safely centred from those which must be avoided. The cortico-bulbar fibres and probably some cortico-spinal fibres immediately adjoining them are the only ones which should cause concern to the surgeon during stereotactic surgery when using physiological safeguards together with proportional or computer-averaged measurements[18] (Figure 3).

As a corollary, it has been shown that, within the posterior limb of the internal capsule, there are at least two different groups of fibres which have to do with voluntary movements:

(1) The cortico-bulbar and immediately adjoining cortico-spinal fibres situated in the coronal plane passing through the midpoint of the intercommissural line.

(2) The others, much more postero-lateral, in the third quarter of the posterior limb of the internal capsule, make up the classical motor cortico-spinal tract[13]. A third group has been identified at the level of the cortex which gives rise to flaccid paralysis when injured[13]. It is now well

recogniized that the symptoms which follow a haemorrhage in the internal capsule result from massive involvement of various groups of cortico-spinal fibres.

SUMMARY AND CONCLUSION

With careful selection of cases, and the use of computerized or proportional measurements together with stimulation, recording and well-oriented lesions, stereotactic surgery is quite safe and can bring appreciable relief to patients suffering from involuntary movements. Under these conditions, complications do not exceed 2%. They are greater with bilateral lesions which should be used only in problem cases such as severe dystonias. Stereotactic surgery is particularly useful for tremor of attitude, for intention tremor of multiple sclerosis and for the severe tremor or rigidity of Parkinson's disease which is not responsive to medical therapy.

Stereotactic surgery alone or (if necessary) combined with ramicectomy and peripheral denervation, is most useful in late dystonias, especially in cases of spasmodic torticollis. For the latter, when the condition is well localized as determined by electromyography and nerve blocks, ramicectomy and peripheral denervation is usually sufficient. In all elective procedures for the relief of involuntary movements, the aim must evidently be to obtain the maximum improvement compatible with a high degree of safety.

References

1 Bertrand, C. (1955). Une nouvelle modification technique pour la chirurgie des mouvements involontaires. *Union Med. Can.*, **84**, 150

2 Bertrand, C. and Martinez, N. (1959). An apparatus and technique for surgery of dyskinesias. *Neurochirurgia (Stuttg.)*, **2**, 35

3 Bertrand, C. (1958). A pneumotaxic technique for producing localized cerebral lesions. *J. Neurosurg.*, **15**, 251

4 Bertrand, C., Martinez, S. N., Hardy, J., Molina-Negro, P. and Velasco, F. (1973). Stereotactic surgery for parkinsonism: Miroelectrode recording, stimulation, and oriented sections with a leucotome. *Progress, Neurological Surgery*. Vol. 5, pp. 79–112 (Basel: Karger)

5 Molina-Negro, P. (1979). Neurology of brain functional disorders. In Rasmussen, T. and Marino, R. Jr., (eds.) *Functional Neurosurgery*, pp. 25–44 (New York: Raven Press)

6 Bertrand, C., Hardy, J., Molina-Negro, P. and Martinez, N. (1969). Optimum physiological target for the arrest of tremor. *3rd Symp. Parkinson's disease*, pp. 251–259 (Edinburgh: Livingstone)

7 Albe-Fessard, D., Arfel, G., Guiot, G., Hardy, J., Vourc'h, G., Herzog, E. and Aleonard, P. (1961). Identification et délimitation précise de certaines structures sous-corticales de l'homme par l'électrophysiologie. *C. R. Acad. Sci.*, **253**, 2412

8 Velasco, F. C., Molina-Negro, P., Bertrand, C. and Hardy, J. (1972). Further definition of the subthalamic target for arrest of tremor. *J. Neurosurg.*, **36**, 184

9 Bertrand, C. (1976). The treatment of spasmodic torticollis with particular reference to thalamotomy. In Morley (ed.) *Current Controversies in Neurosurgery*, pp. 455–459. (Philadelphia, Saunders)

10 Bertrand, C., Molina-Negro, P. and Martinez, S. N. (1978). Combined stereotactic and peripheral surgical approach for spasmodic torticollis. In Gildenberg, P. L. (ed.) *Appl. Neurophysiol.*, **41**, 122

11 Brion, S. and Guiot, G. (1964); Topographie des faisceaux de projection du cortex dans la capsule interne et dans le pédoncule cérébral. Etude des dégénérescences secondaires dans la sclérose latérale amyotrophique at la maladie de Pick. *Rev. Neurol. (Paris)*, **110**, 123

12 Smith, M. C. (1960). Nerve fibre degeneration in the brain in amyotrophic lateral sclerosis. *J. Neurol. Neurosurg. Psychiatry*, **23**, 269

13 Bertrand, C., Martinez, S. N., Robert, F., Bouvier, G. and Mathieu, J. P. (1972). L'origine des fibres corticospinales motrices: A propos d'un cas de quadriplégie flasque par lésion corticale bilatérale. *Rev. Can. Biol.*, **31**, 263

14 Bertrand, C. (1966). Functional localization with monopolar stimulation. 2nd Symp. Parkinson's disease, part II. *J. Neurosurg.*, **14**, 403

15 Bertrand, C., Martinez, N. and Hardy, J. (1964). Localisation des fonctions lors de la chirurgie stéréotaxique par une voie d'abord frontale parasagittale. *Neuro-chirurgie, (Paris)*, **10**, 389

16 Martinez, N., Bertrand, C. and Botana-Lopez, C. (1967). Motor fiber distribution within the cerebral peduncle. *Confin. Neurol.*, **29**, 117

17 Bertrand, C., Martinez, N. and Hardy, J. (1963). Electro-physiological studies of the human thalamus and adjoining structures. *J. Neurol. Neurosurg. Psychiatry*, **26**, 1552

18 Bertrand, C., Molina-Negro, P. and Martinez, S. N. (1979). Stereotactic targets for dystonias and dyskinesias: their relationship to cortico-bulbar fibers and other adjoining structures. In Poirier, L. J., Sourkes, T. L. and Bédard, P. J. (eds.) *Advances in Neurology*, pp. 395–399, (New York: Raven Press)

19 Bertrand, C. (1978). Torticollis revisited. First William Cone Memorial Lecture. *III Foundation Lectures, Montreal Neurological Institute, Montreal.* (In press)

20 Hamby, W. and Schiffer, S. (1969). Spasmodic torticollis: Results after cervical rhizotomy in 50 cases. *J. Neurosurg.*, **31**, 323

21 McKenzie, K. G. (1955). The surgical treatment of spasmodic torticollis. *Clin. Neurosurg.*, **2**, 37

22 Couch, J. R. (1976). Dystonia and tremor in spasmodic torticollis. In Eldridge and Fahn (eds.) *Advances in Neurology. XIV Dystonia.* (New York: Raven Press)

23 Marsden, C. D. (1976). Dystonia. The spectrum of the disease. In Yahr (ed.) *The Basal Ganglia.* Vol. 55, p. 351. (New York: Raven Press)

24 Spiegel, E. A. and Wycis, H. T. (1952). Stereoencephalotomy. Part I. *Methods and stereotaxic atlas of the human brain.* Vol. 2. (New York: Grüne and Stratton)

25 Leksell, L. (1949). A stereotaxic apparatus for intracranial neurosurgery. *Acta Chir. Scand.*, **99**, 229

26 Riechert, T. and Mundinger, F. (1955). Beschreibung und Andwendung eines Zielgerates für stereotaktische Hirnoperationen. II model. *Acta Neurochir. Supp. III*, pp. 308–337

27 Bertrand, C., Hardy, J., Molina-Negro, P. and Martinez, S. N. (1969). Tremor of attitude. In spiegel, E. A. (ed.) *Confin. Neurol.*, **31**, 37. (Basel/New York: Karger)

28 Siegfried, J. (1979). Neurosurgical treatment of spasticity. In Rasmussen, T. and Marino, R. (eds.) *Functional Neurosurgery*, pp. 123–128. (New York: Raven Press)

29 Gros, C., Ouaknine, G., Vlahovitch, B. and Frerebeau, Ph. (1967). La radicotomie sélective postérieure dans le traitement neuro-chirurgical de l'hypertonie pyramidale. *Neurochirurgie, (Paris).* Vol. 13, pp. 505–518

30 Bertrand, C., Martinez, S. N. and Hardy, J. (1964). Stereotactic procedures in the treatment of certain specific forms of epilepsy. *Lobulo Temporal (Symposium Internacional)*, (Mexico), pp. 114–120

31 Martinez, N., Bertrand, C. and Hardy, J. (1964). Traitement de l'épilepsie partielle continue par section stéréotaxique capsulaire. *Neuro-chirurgie, Paris*, **10**, 551

32 Jelsma, R. K., Bertrand, C. M., Martinez, S. N. and Molina-Negro, P. (1973). Stereotaxic treatment of frontal-lobe and centrencephalic epilepsy. *J. Neurosurg.*, **39**, 42

33 Hassler, R. and Hess, W. R. (1954). Experimentell und anatomische befunde über die Drehbewegungen und ihre nervösen Apparate. *Arch. Psychiatr. Nervenkr.*, **192**, 488

34 Selby, G. (1968). Parkinson's disease. In Vinken and Bruyn (eds.) *Handbook of Clinical Neurology. Diseases of the Basal Ganglia.* Vol. 6 (Amsterdam: North Holland)

35 Cooper, I. S. (1976). Dystonia. Surgical approach to treatment and physiologic implications. See discussion 486. In Yahr (ed.) *The Basal Ganglia.* (New York: Raven Press)

36 Zoll, J. G. (1978). Inversion or pronation of the foot following thalamotomy for Parkinson's disease. In Gildenberg, P. L. (ed.) *Appl. Neurophysiol.*, **41**, 232

37 Hassler, R. and Dieckmann, G. (1970). Stereotactic treatment of different kinds of spasmodic torticollis. *Confin. Neurol.*, **32**, 135

11

Treatment of Wilson's disease

A. Barbeau

INTRODUCTION

Of all disorders of movement known to us, the first one where a rational treatment became available is one of the rarest. Hepatolenticular degeneration, better known as Wilson's disease, was first recognized and characterized both clinically and pathologically by S. A. Kinnier Wilson in 1912[1]. It has been studied in detail, particularly since it became evident that many of the defects were due to copper accumulation in cells, a situation proven to be reversible. Many excellent reviews on the management of this disorder have been published[2-7,62] and for this reason we will keep our own *mise-au-point* short.

CLINICAL PRESENTATIONS

Wilson's disease, like most inborn errors of metabolism, is inherited as an autosomal recessive trait, which means that for the disease to become manifest clinically the abnormal gene must be inherited from both parents. It therefore implies a familial incidence, a high consanguinity rate, and the absence of the disease in the parents and in other heterozygotes[8]. The calculated gene frequency is 0.001 and the carrier rate 0.002.

The clinical manifestations of Wilson's disease usually arise during childhood or adolescence, and in almost all cases before the age of 40. The usual presentation is neurological, but many cases come to initial attention through hepatic or haematological symptoms. In young people, as described by Wilson himself[1], the disease is usually acute and progressive. Symptoms of tremor, rigidity, dysarthria, akinesia, fixed facial grimaces and dysphagia appear relatively early in random fashion. In general, severe spastic rigidity clearly predominates over tremor. Gradually the patients become helpless in bed, their facial expressions vacuous and fixed[2]. The course is different, and much slower, in patients whose disease started later in life (Westphal's pseudosclerosis). Flexion–extension tremor of the wrist and 'yes' tremor of the head which can become quite violent, are the principal symptoms, with rigidity a latter and distant second. Occasionally choreiform or athetoid movements and dystonic postures can be seen, confusing the picture and the diagnosis. Finally there exists a characteristic and pathognomonic feature of the disease which was not noted by Wilson—a brown or greyish-green ring present in the Descemet membrane of the cornea which is best seen by slit-lamp examination (Kayser–Fleisher ring). The ring is found in over 90% of cases with the naked eye. Its absence does not exclude the diagnosis of hepatolenticular degeneration, but makes it highly improbable.

Although the neurological form of the disease, described above, is the most common presentation, it is not the only one. Many patients are referred initially to psychiatrists because of social adjustment problems, bizarre behaviour, anxiety–neurosis, mania, depression, psychosis, hysteria, schizo-affective disorders or even schizophrenia[4]. The associations of these psychiatric disorders with the neurological symptoms of tremor, dystonia or rigidity, particularly in young people, should always lead to efforts at eliminating the diagnosis of Wilson's disease.

In childhood, the most common mode of presentation and the most frequently misdiagnosed, is hepatic disease. It may take different forms such as chronic or recurrent hepatitis, juvenile cirrhosis, post necrotic cirrhosis or fulminant hepatitis[4] leading to hepatic failure, signs of portal hypertension, ascites, splenomegaly or bleeding oesophageal varices. As recommended by Cartwright[4], it is mandatory to exclude Wilson's disease in all patients with 'familial cirrhosis'. On the other hand, in some cases the initial episode may be an acute haemolytic anaemia, occasionally of an intermittent nature. Finally some rare patients[9] may have symptoms related to bone disease, with impaired proximal renal tubular reabsorption, aminoaciduria and phosphaturia. This phenomenon contributes to the low serum uric acid frequently seen in Wilson's disease and useful in diagnosis.

PATHOLOGY

The characteristic lesions in Wilson's disease involve the liver and the lenticular nuclei. The hepatic lesions are of variable intensity, from minimal steatosis to portal and periportal fibrosis and finally to a macronodular cirrhosis; evidence of previous hepatitis is often found on histological examination. Rubeanic acid staining permits visualization of copper granules, but is not a very reliable technique. Electron microscopic studies usually reveal important anomalies of mitochondria.

In the brain, the lesions are particularly evident in the lenticular nuclei even at macroscopy. In most cases the cerebral cortex and the dentate nuclei are also severely damaged. Histologically, tissue necrosis alternates with areas of neuronal rarefaction, degenerating neurons and proliferation of large astrocytes (Alzheimer glia). When patients are kept alive for long periods in a bed-ridden state, the destruction of the brain may be extreme[10].

The biochemical pathology of Wilson's disease is imperfectly known. As will be seen later, the brain and hepatic contents of copper are markedly increased[11,12]. It is of interest that tyrosine hydroxylase and dopa-decarbarboxylase are normal while dopamine-β-hydroxylase, a copper enzyme, is markedly inhibited[13].

BIOCHEMISTRY

The first indication of a biochemical disturbance in trace metals were found in the old German literature[14]. In 1945 Glazebrook[11], in Edinburgh, investigated a single case of Wilson's disease and found increased contents of copper in liver and brain. This has been amply confirmed, mainly through the studies of Cumings in England[12] and extended to a number of other tissues, including the kidney and the cornea. Shortly afterwards Mandelbrote and collaborators[15] demonstrated an increased urinary excretion of copper in these patients. Serum copper levels, on the other hand, are usually decreased but can be normal or slightly increased in rare cases[16,17]. The metabolism of copper has been clarified through the use of radioactive ^{64}Cu. When first absorbed from the intestine (possibly through binding with a specific cuproprotein) copper is loosely bound to serum albumin and is thus carried through the portal system to the liver where it is deposited[18]. In Wilson's disease this fraction of serum copper is increased, indicating enhanced absorption[19]. In 1948, Holmberg and Laurell[20] identified the main copper-containing protein. It is an α_2 globulin now called ceruloplasmin. The copper content of ceruloplasmin accounts for about 95 % of the serum copper. Each protein molecule of 151 000 molecular weight contains eight atoms of copper, four of which are tightly bound, four more loosely attached. In normal subjects, within a few hours, the radioactivity is associated with the newly synthesized ceruloplasmin and thus circulates through the body. In patients with Wilson's disease the situation is different; they appear to be unable to properly synthesize ceruloplasmin[21]. This deficiency is highly specific[22]. Consequently no uptake of copper into the protein occurs and most of the copper remains bound to serum albumin in a very loose bond. The copper can thus be easily dissociated from the protein moiety and is abnormally deposited in tissues wherever there are substances in the tissues which have a greater affinity for copper than serum albumin[2]. In tissues, surplus copper acts as an irritant and interferes with essential enzymes, thus causing chromatolysis and cell death. Copper deposition, in the liver contributes to the cirrhosis, in the cornea to the formation of the Kayser–Fleisher rings and in the kidney to tubular damage. The latter lesion partially explains the increased aminoaciduria in this disease, first described by Uzman and Denny-Brown[23], which also contributes to the cirrhosis. Finally the increased urinary urate excretion also produced by the tubular lesion is responsible for the low serum uric acid[24].

Despite the above-mentioned findings, the basic biochemical defect of Wilson's disease is still unclear. Abnormalities of the structure and metabolism of ceruloplasmin have been suggested, but not yet proven. A metalloprotein with abnormally high copper affinity in the liver has also been advanced[32]. Sternlieb et al[63]. have proposed that the primary defect is in the absence of one of the liver proteins involved in the excretion of copper via the bile. This defect could be lysosomal[63].

BIOCHEMICAL DIAGNOSIS

As previously mentioned, tissue copper is increased in Wilson's disease. This can be measured by direct determination of liver copper after biopsy. Normal values are below 250 μg/g dry weight. Any measurement above this is pathological. Values up to 1500 μg/g have been obtained. Copper urinary excretion in normal subjects is from 0–30 μg/24 hours. Any value above 50 μg/24 h should be considered pathological, but not necessarily diagnostic since slight increases can be seen in non-wilsonian cirrhosis. Patients with clinically evident hepatolenticular degeneration usually excrete more than 180 μg/day and much more, of course, under treatment. Finally serum copper is usually decreased in Wilson's disease but this is rarely specific or diagnostic.

The best measurement is the evaluation of serum ceruloplasmin. This can be done with spectrophotometric methods or the determination of the rate of oxidation of paraphenylenediamine[20], but is now more accurately estimated through immunological methods[27]. Normal values are from 20 to 50 mg/100 ml of serum. 95% of patients with Wilson's disease have values below 10 mg/100 ml. Only the very rare case has low normal values of ceruloplasmin[28].

The problem arises with the recognition of asymptomatic cases and of heterozygotes. Very few radiological methods are useful, but recently Nelson and collaborators[29] have claimed that computerized tomography (CT scan) revealed involvement of the basal ganglia. In a familial case still asymptomatic but later definitely involved, we found normal ceruloplasmin values with slightly increased urinary copper (70 mg/day)[30] and almost normal radioactive ^{64}Cu patterns; thus, it seems that measurement of ceruloplasmin is not necessarily sufficient. Other authors[31] have found abnormal histological findings, but little cirrhosis, in seven asymptomatic patients.

Only two of these patients had Kayser–Fleisher rings and two had normal ceruloplasmin levels. Five of the six studied had cupriuria ($> 200\ \mu g/24\ h$; range 68–592). Hepatic copper concentration was elevated in all four patients in whom it was studied and ranged from 411 to 1195 $\mu g/gm$ dry weight[32]. In some cases urinary excretion of radioactive copper can be a useful test in heterozygotes or presymtomatic cases[33].

Recently a diagnostic marker has been claimed from a study of fibroblasts. Chan and co-workers[34] found that Wilson's disease fibroblasts have an elevated intracellular copper concentration as compared to cultured control cells. A decreased ratio of copper to protein was observed in cytoplasmic protein (or proteins) having a molecular weight greater or equal to 30 000 in Wilson's disease cells. If these studies are confirmed, the early diagnosis of the disorder can be hoped for.

THERAPEUTIC APPROACHES

The biochemical changes in Wilson's disease reported above permit a rational approach to the disease. Such a rational therapy, according to Bearn[3], has two principal aims:

(1) to eliminate from the body the excessive copper that is already present,
(2) to prevent its reaccumulation.

However, a more direct method would have been to replace serum ceruloplasmin. Unfortunately such attempts proved to be unsuccessful[35,36,37]. Modification of serum ceruloplasmin levels through the use of oestrogens also failed in practice[3].

The *first* direct approach consists of a restriction in the absorption of copper[38]. This can be accomplished by reducing the dietary intake and by binding intestinal copper so that it will be excreted directly into the faeces. A certain number of foods can be proscribed because of their high copper content: liver, chocolate, cocoa, nuts, mushrooms, molasses, dried peas, broccoli and shellfish of any kind. Except for these foods, however, we do not find it advisable to impose any strict dietary control, which would be unacceptable to most patients. The other component of the intake restriction can be achieved with various methods of binding intestinal copper to prevent its absorption. The first of these tried was a carboxylic cation exchange resin (CARBO–RESIN). Unfortunately this treatment is considered unpalatable by most patients and causes frequent nausea. We have found it useful only during the initial therapeutic trial in hospital. Potassium sulphide is easier to tolerate[39]. It precipitates dietary copper in the gut as the insoluble sulphide, with resultant faecal excretion. Capsules of 20 mg once or twice a day (after main meals) are sufficient.

The *second* (and most successful) approach is to attempt increasing the urinary excretion of copper—normally below 50 µg/24 h—which in Wilson's disease can range from 180 to 500 µg/24 h, even without treatment. In 1948 Mandelbrote and co-workers, showed that the intramuscular injection of the anti-nerve gas compound British-Anti-Lewisite (BAL—2,3,dimercapto-propanol) resulted in increased urinary excretion of copper[15]. Cumings[12] suggested that BAL could be useful in Wilson's disease. Initial results, particularly in tremor cases of long standing, were satisfactory[40] but long-term use is made difficult by the necessity to administer the drug intra-muscularly, the inherent risks of local infection and pain, and especially, the difficulty in maintaining a negative copper balance[41]. Improvement is seldom if ever observed in the group of patients characterized by severe progressive lenticular degeneration with accompanying widespread destructive lesions in the brain. The second group, who suffer from the pseudo-sclerotic variety of the disease, appear to respond more favourably[3]. Similar results have been claimed after the use of other chelating agents such as versene (calcium disodium ethylenediaminetetra-acetate), but this approach is not practical for long-term use because it requires intravenous adminis-tration[42].

The introduction of penicillamine (β,β-dimethylcysteine), a powerful chelating agent, has revolutionized the treatment of Wilson's disease. Walshe[43] was the first to demonstrate this copper chelating effect which far exceeded that of BAL. Values of 4 to 8 mg of copper excreted by 24 hours are frequently observed during the initial phases! It has been calculated[38] that 1 g of penicillamine (molecular weight, 149) is responsible for the excretion of approximately 2 mg of copper in the urine. This can be followed through periodic measurements of urinary copper which usually indicate a gradually decreasing excretion, or by examination of liver content of copper through biopsy. The ultimate goal of treatment is to obtain a negative copper balance (which experience has shown, may take from 2 to 12 months of treatment) and to maintain it throughout the remainder of the patient's life. It is thus necessary to warn the patient and his family that he will require treatment continuously and that no drug vacations are foreseeable. My own approach is to use D–penicillamine (Cuprimine), in progressively increasing doses. 250 mg is given the first few days and then increased, by 250 mg/day increments, until a maximum of 2 g/day is reached. This initial treatment should preferably be carried out in hospital where all the necessary labora-tory control studies can be carried out (serum, liver and urine copper determinations, CT scans, ceruloplasmin, slit-lamp examination, etc.). Close monitoring is required to avoid, or treat immediately, some of the early complications: generalized reaction with fever, rash and adenopathy[3], thrombocytopenia and leukopenia[44], severe haemolytic anaemia[45] or even aplastic anaemia[46]. Usually these rare complications occur during the first month of treatment and can be reversed by the temporary cessation of penicillamine. After 1 month the dosage is usually decreased to 1 gram of penicillamine per day and this level maintained for years thereafter. Urinary copper excretion will increase considerably at first (to 5–7 mg/day) but will eventually settle to 2 mg/day, or below, during the maintenance phase. To avoid depletion of vitamin B_6 through chelation and consequent epileptic episodes, we normally add pyridoxine 25 mg once or twice a day. Finally, as stated above, the management of our patients includes the use of potassium sulphide (20 mg twice daily) and the avoidance of high-copper foods (see above). A very important part of the therapeutic regime is the regular visit, first monthly and thereafter every 2–3 months. This visit includes a full neurological assessment, liver function profile, serum, celuloplasmin and uric acid determination, and evaluation of urinary copper excretion (24 h period). It should be mentioned that ceruloplasmin values tend to further decrease at first but eventually settle at levels barely above the control findings, despite good clinical results. We do not find serum copper determination valuable or of prognostic significance.

Recently Hoogenraad et al[61] proposed to use oral zinc sulphate (200 mg orally three times daily) as a chelating agent. Preliminary results over 14 years in one patient seemed to be favourable. It appears that zinc sulphate may prevent storage of copper and may contribute to the mobilization and excretion of deposits of copper. In some patients, particularly of the acute type, the addition of levodopa to penicillamine, may be of some use[72].

With the penicillamine regime, the majority of patients, particularly those with the slower pseudosclerotic form, do very well (see below). Only a few problems should be mentioned as they may be observed on long-term therapy. It appears that despite D-penicillamine, successful pregnancy and delivery of patients can be accomplished[47, 48]. Skin changes have been noted in a number of patients, ranging from pemphigus-like mucocutaneous lesions[51] to cutis hyperelastica[49, 50]. Penicillamine also possesses the ability to cause autoimmune disorders, possibly through induced IgA deficiency[52]. Reported cases (with penicillamine in Wilson's disease, rheumatoid arthritis, cystinuria and heavy-metal intoxications) include immunecomplex nephropathy[53], haemolytic anaemia[54], Goodpasture syndrome[55], thyroiditis[56], a lupus erythematosus syndrome[49, 57], myasthenia gravis[58, 59] and polymyositis[60].

LONG-TERM RESULTS OF PENICILLAMINE THERAPY

The long-term results[71] with this treatment are very significant and encouraging, particularly if the diagnosis of Wilson's disease is made early[64–70]. Adequate treatment of asymptomatic patients completely prevents the development of clinical disease[65] and therefore should be started as soon as the diagnosis is made. Particularly important is the systematic screening of all family members (siblings and cousins) when a definite case is identified.

This screening battery should include, at the minimum, determination of serum ceruloplasmin, uric acid and urinary copper excretion, with a complete neurological examination and slit-lamp examination of the cornea.

The results of treatment in patients with overt disease are also impressive: in most cases symptoms and neurological signs regress and the prospects of survival are good, whereas formerly virtually all patients died. In our own series of 38 patients seen over the last 20 years, 22 are surviving virtually free of neurological symptoms after periods of 2 to 10 years of continuous treatment. Six have now died and the remaining 10 patients still indicate significant if not complete improvement of neurological symptoms. Similar results were reported by Strickland *et al.*[66] who examined the prognosis in 142 patients with Wilson's disease, including 88 who had been treated with penicillamine for up to 16 years. Of 36 symptomatic patients who had not been treated, all but one were dead, while 31 of the 35 symptomatic patients being treated with penicillamine remained alive, including 22 who had had penicillamine for 2 years or more; only six of these had residual symptoms. Thus if the disease is diagnosed and treated at an early stage, there is a good chance of complete and permanent control[64,69]. In the early phase of treatment it is not unusual to find an exacerbation of neurological symptoms and signs, particularly tremor, but eventually, sometimes after many months, there is gradual improvement in these manifestations.

Unfortunately the results are not so good in patients diagnosed later, in patients who present with the juvenile neurological (dystonic or akinetic) form and for patients whose disease is mainly hepatic, with cirrhosis, portal hypertension and renal tubular damage[66,67,70]. Little change can be seen in the cirrhosis even when liver copper content decreases. Protein supplementation may be important to prevent progression of the cirrhosis. The Kayser–Fleisher rings will usually decrease markedly after many months of treatment and may not be seen anymore[69] with the naked eye. However slit-lamp examination of the cornea is still positive in most cases.

CONCLUSIONS

Hepatolenticular degeneration (Wilson's disease) is a rare autosomal recessive disease with movement disorders and tissue copper accumulation which is now treatable, with a chance for complete and permanent control if the diagnosis is made early. This result occurs even though the cause and pathophysiology of the copper tissue accumulation is still incompletely understood. The principles of management include reduction of the intake and absorption of copper (elimination of high-copper foods; potassium sulphide) and methods to induce a greater urinary excretion of copper (D-penicillamine and possibly zinc sulphate).

References

1 Wilson, S. A. K. (1912). Progressive lenticular degeneration: a familial nervous disease associated with cirrhosis of the liver. *Brain*, **34**, 295

2 Bearn, A. G. (1956). Wilson's disease—hepatolenticular degeneration. *Postgrad. Med. J.*, **32**, 477

3 Bearn, A. G. (1957). Wilson's disease—an inborn error of metabolism with multiple manifestations. *Am. J. Med.*, **22**, 747

4 Cartwright, G. E. (1978). Diagnosis of treatable Wilson's disease (current concepts). *N. Engl. J. Med.*, **298**, 1347

5 Sass-Kortsak, A. (1975). Wilson's disease—a treatable liver disease in children. *Pediatr. Clin. N. Am.*, **22**, 963

6 Cumings, J. N. (1959). *Heavy Metals and the Brain*. (Oxford: Blackwell Scientific Publications)

7 Dastur, D. K. and Manghani, D. K. (1977). Wilson's disease: inherited cuprogenic disorder of liver, brain, kidney. In Goldensohn, E. S. and Appel, S. H. (eds.) *Scientific Approaches to Clinical Neurology*, pp. 1033–1051. (Philadelphia: Lea and Fabinger)

8 Bean, A. G. (1953). Genetic and biochemical aspects of Wilson's disease. *Am. J. Med.*, **15**, 442

9 Walshe, J. M. (1962). Wilson's disease: the presenting symptoms. *Arch. Dis. Child.*, **37**, 253

10 Schulman, S. and Barbeau, A. (1963). Wilson's disease: a case with almost total loss of cerebral white matter. *J. Neuropath. Exp. Neurol.*, **22**, 105

11 Glazebrook, A. J. (1945). Wilson's disease. *Edinburgh Med. J.*, **52**, 83

12 Cumings. J. N. (1948). The copper and iron content of brain and liver in the normal and in hepatolenticular degeneration. *Brain*, **71**, 410

13 Nagatsu, T., Kato, T., Nagatsu, I., Kondo, Y., Inagaki, S., Iizuka, R. and Narabayashi, H. (1979). Catecholamine—related enzymes in the brain of patients with parkinsonism and Wilson's disease. *Arch. Neurol.*, **24**, 283

14 Rumpel, A. (1913). Uber das Wesen und die Bedeutung der Leberveränderungen und der Pigmentierungen bei den damit verbundenen Fällen von Pseudosklerose, zugleich ein Beitrag zur Lehre von der Pseudosclerose (Westphall-Strümpell) *Dtsch. Z. Nervenheilk.*, **49**, 54

15 Mandelbrote, B. M., Stanier, M. W., Thompson, R. H. S. and Thurston, N. M. (1948). Studies on copper metabolism in demyelinating diseases of the central nervous system. *Brain*, **71**, 212

16 Bearn, A. G. and Kunkel, H. G. (1954). Abnormality of copper metabolism in Wilson's disease and their relationship to the aminoaciduria. *J. Clin. Invest.*, **33**, 400

17 Bickel, H., Neale, F. C. and Hall, G. (1957). A clinical and biochemical study of hepatolenticular degeneration (Wilson's disease). *Q. J. Med.* (N.S.), **26**, 527

18 Bearn, A. G. and Kunkel, H. G. (1955). Metabolic studies in Wilson's disease using ^{64}Cu. *J. Lab. Clin. Med.*, **45**, 623

19 Matthews, W. B. (1954). The absorption and excretion of radio-copper in hepato-lenticular degeneration (Wilson's disease). *J. Neurol. Neurosurg. Psychiatry*, **17**, 242

20 Holmberg, C. G. and Laurell, C. B. (1948). Investigations in serum copper. II. Isolation of the copper-containing protein, and a description of some of its properties. *Acta Chem. Scand.*, **2**, 550

21 Scheinberg, I. H. and Gitlin, D. (1952). Deficiency of ceruloplasmin in patients with hepato-lenticular degeneration (Wilson's disease). *Science*, **116**, 484

22 Scheinberg, I. H., Harris, R. S., Morell, A. G. and Dubin, D. (1958). Some aspects of the relation of ceruloplasmin to Wilson's disease. *Neurology*, **8**, 44

23 Uzman, L. and Denny-Brown, D. (1948). Amino-aciduria in hepato-lenticular degeneration (Wilson's disease). *Am. J. Med. Sci.*, **215**, 599

24 Mahoney, J. P., Sandberg, A. A., Gubler, C. J., Cartwright, G. E. and Wintrobe, M. M.

(1955). Uric acid metabolism in hepato-lenticular degeneration. *Proc. Soc. Exp. Biol. Med.*, **88**, 427

25 Goldstein, N. P., Randall, R. V., Gross, J. B. and McGuckin, W. F. (1965). Copper balance studies in Wilson's disease—observations on the effects of penicillamine, carbacrylamine resins, and potassium sulfide. *Arch. Neurol.*, **12**, 456

26 Tu, J. B., Blackwell, Q. and Watten, B. H. (1965). Copper balance studies during the treatment of patients with Wilson's disease. *Metabolism*, **14**, 653

27 Schorr, J. B., Morell, A. G. and Scheinberg, I. H. (1958). Studies of serum ceruloplasmin during early infancy. *J. Dis. Child.*, **96**, 541

28 Warnock, C. G. and Neill, D. W. (1958). The diagnosis and treatment of Wilson's disease. *Brain*, **81**, 258

29 Nelson, R. F., Guzman, D. A., Grahovac, Z. and Howse, D. C. N. (1979). Computerized cranial tomography in Wilson's disease. *Neurology*, **29**, 866

30 Barbeau, A., Reilly, R. W. and Kirsner, J. B. (1960). Acquisitions récentes sur la maladie de Wilson. *Union Méd. Can.*, **89**, 422

31 Werlin, S. L., Grand, R. J., Perman, J. A. and Watkins, J. B. (1978). Diagnostic dilemmas of Wilson's disease: diagnosis and treatment. *Pediatrics*, **62**, 47

32 Shapiro, J. R., Morell, A. G. and Scheinberg, I. H. (1961). Wilson's disease. *J. Clin. Invest.*, **40**, 1081

33 Gibbs, K., Hanka, R. and Walshe, J. M. (1978). The urinary excretion of radiocopper in pre-symptomatic and symptomatic Wilson's disease, heterozygotes and controls: its significance in diagnosis and management. *Q. J. Med.* (NS), **47**, 349

34 Chan, W. Y., Cushing, W., Coffman, M. A. and Rennert, O. M. (1980). Genetic expression of Wilson's disease in cell culture: a diagnostic marker. *Science*, **208**, 299

35 Sternlieb, I., Morell, A. G. and Scheinberg, I. H. (1958). The effect of intravenously administered ceruloplasmin on copper absorption in a patient with Wilson's disease. *J. Clin. Invest.*, **37**, 934

36 O'Reilly, S. (1967). Problems in Wilson's disease. *Neurology*, **17**, 137

37 Bickel, H., Schultze, H. E., Grüter, W. and Göllner, I. (1956). Versuche zur coeruloplasmin substitution bei der hepatocerebralen degeneration (Wilsonshe krankheit). *Klin. Wochenschr.*, **34**, 961

38 Scheinberg, I. H. and Sternlieb, I. (1960). The long-term management of hepato-lenticular degeneration (Wilson's disease). *Am. J. Med.*, **24**, 316

39 Ferris, G. S. and Berry, S. (1957). Hepatolenticular degeneration. *Arch. Intern. Med.*, **99**, 656

40 Denny-Brown, D. and Porter, H. (1951). The effect of BAL (2,3-dimercaptopropanol) in hepatolenticular degeneration (Wilson's disease). *N. Engl. J. Med.*, **245**, 917

41 Bearn, A. G. (1956). The place of BAL in the therapy of Wilson's disease. *Am. J. Med.*, **21**, 134

42 Zimdahl, W. T., Hyman, I. and Stafford, W. F. (1954). The effect of drugs upon the copper metabolism in hepatolenticular degeneration and in normal subjects. *J. Lab. Clin. Med.*, **43**, 774

43 Walshe, J. M. (1956). Penicillamine, a new oral therapy for Wilson's disease. *Am. J. Med.*, **21**, 487

44 Walshe, J. M. (1959). Current views on the pathogenesis and treatment of Wilson's disease. *Arch. Intern. Med.*, **103**, 155

45 Deiss, A., Lee, G. R. and Cartwright, G. E. (1970). Hemolytic anaemia in Wilson's disease. *Ann. Intern. Med.*, **73**, 413

46 Gollan, J. L., Hussein, S., Hoffbrand, A. V. and Sherlock, S. (1976). Red cell aplasia following prolonged D-penicillamine therapy. *J. Clin. Pathol.*, **29**, 135

47 Scheinberg, I. H. and Sternlieb, I. (1975). Pregnancy in penicillamine treated patients with Wilson's disease. *N. Engl. J. Med.*, **293**, 1300

48 Fukuda, D., Ishii, A., Matsue, Y., Funaki, K., Hoshiai, H. and Maeda, S. (1977). Pregnancy and delivery in penicillamine treated patients with Wilson's disease. *Tohoku J. Exp. Med.*, **123**, 279

49 Charlebois, G., Cadotte, M. and Barbeau, A. (1972). Cutis hyperelastica following prolonged administration of penicillamine in a patient with Wilson's disease. *Union Med. Can.*, **101**, 893

50 Greer, K. E., Askew, F. C. and Richardson, D. R. (1976). Skin lesions induced by penicillamine. Occurrence in a patient with hepatolenticular degeneration (Wilson's disease). *Arch. Dermatol.*, **112**, 1267

51 Hay, K. D., Muller, H. K. and Reade, P. C. (1978). D-penicillamine-induced mucocutaneous lesions with features of pemphigus. *Oral Surg.*, **45**, 385

52 Proesmans, W., Jaeken, J. and Eeckels, R. (1976). D -penicillamine-induced IgA deficiency in Wilson's disease. *Lancet*, **2**, 804

53 Jaffe, I. A., Treser, G., Suzuki, Y. and Ehrenreich, T. (1968). Nephropathy induced by D-penicillamine. *Ann. Intern. Med.*, **82**, 673

54 Harrison, E. E. and Hickman, J. W. (1975). Haemolytic anaemia and thrombocytopenia associated with penicillamine ingestion. *South. Med. J.*, **68**, 113

55 Sternlieb, I., Bennett, B. and Scheinberg, I. H. (1975). D-penicillamine-induced Goodpasture's syndrome in Wilson's disease. *Ann. Intern. Med.*, **82**, 673

56 Delrieu, F., Menkes, C. J., Sainte-Croix, A., Delbarre, F., Babinet, P. and Chesneau, A. M. (1975). Myasthénie et thyroidite auto-immune au cours d'une polyarthrite rhumatoide traitée par la D -pénicillamine. *Nouv. Presse Med.*, **4**, 2890

57 Harpey, J. P., Caille, B., Moulias, R. and Goust, J. M. (1971). Lupus-like syndrome induced by penicillamine in Wilson's disease. *Lancet*, **1**, 292

58 Bucknall, R. C., Dixon, A. S. J., Glick, E. N., Woodland, J. and Zutshi, D. W. (1975). Myasthenia gravis associated with penicillamine treatment for rheumatoid arthritis. *Br. Med. J.*, **1**, 600

59 Masters, C. L., Dawkins, R. L., Zilko, P. J., Simpson, J. A. and Leedman, R. J. (1977). Penicillamine-associated myasthenia gravis, antiacetylcholine receptor and antistriational antibodies. *Am. J. Med.*, **63**, 689

60 Bouteiller, G., Durroux, R., Vancina, R. S. and Arlet, J. (1979). La polymyosite: une complication rare du traitement par la D-pénicillamine. *Rev. Med. Toulouse*, **15**, 85

61 Hoogenraad, T. U., Kowvoet, R. and de Ruyter Korver, E. G. W. M. (1978). Oral zinc sulfate as long-term treatment in Wilson's disease (hepatolenticular degeneration). *Eur. Neurol.*, **18**, 205

62 Sass-Kortsak, A. and Bearn, A. G. (1978). Hereditary disorders of copper metabolism; In *The Metabolic Basis of Inherited Disease*, pp. 1098–1126. (New York: McGraw-Hill)

63 Sternlieb, I., Van den Hamer, C. J. A., Morell, A. G., Albert, S., Gregoriadis, G. and Scheinberg, I. H. (1973). Lysosomal defect of hepatic copper excretion in Wilson's disease. *Gastroenterology*, **64**, 99

64 Deiss, A., Lynch, R. E., Lee, G. R. and Cartwright, G. E. (1971). Long-term therapy of Wilson's disease. *Ann. Intern. Med.*, **75**, 57

65 Sternlieb, I. and Scheinberg, I. H. (1968) Management of hepatolenticular degeneration (Wilson's disease). *N. Engl. J. Med.*, **278**, 352

66 Strickland, G. T., Frommer, D. and Leu, M. L. (1973). Wilson's disease in the United Kingdom and Taiwan. I. General characteristics of 142 cases and prognosis. II. A genetic analysis of 88 cases. *Q. J. Med.*, **42**, 619

67 Cartwright, G. E. and Lee, G. I. R. (1974). The pathogenesis and evolution of Wilson's disease. *Epatologia*, **20**, 51

68 Strickland, G. T. and Leu, M. L. (1975). Wilson's disease: clinical and laboratory manifestations in 40 patients. *Medicine*, **54**, 113

69 Goldstein, N. P. and Gross, J. B. (1977). Treatment of Wilson's disease. *Clin. Neuro-pharmacol.*, **2**, 99

70 Sternlieb, I. (1972). Evolution of the hepatic lesion in Wilson's disease (hepato-lenticular degeneration) *Prog. Liver Dis.*, **4**, 511

71 Anonymous (1978). Don't forget Wilson's disease. *Br. Med. J.*, **2**, 1384

72 Barbeau, A. and Friesen, H. (1970). Treatment of Wilson's disease with levodopa after failure with penicillamine. *Lancet*, **1**, 1180

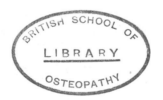

Index

abnormal involuntary movements   135
acetylcholine
  dietary precursors   38
  dopamine balance   32
  overactivity in parkinsonism   173
adrenocorticotropic hormone   72, 73
adverse reactions   122
  amantadine   175
  anticholinergics   174, 175
  bromocriptine   179
  carbamazepine   123
  carbidopa   53
  clonazepam   66
  clozapine   115
  L-dopa   25, 53, 116, 176, 177, 182
  haloperidol   112, 113, 123
  L-5-hydroxytryptophan   71, 72
  lithium   139
  α-methylparatyrosine   115, 116
  penfluridal   114
  penicillamine   214, 215
  pimozide   113
  propranolol   124, 163
  surgery   203–6
  tetrabenazine   115
akinesia and dyskinesia   24
alcohol
  benign tremor relief   138, 139
  and essential tremor relief   155
  withdrawal   163
Alzheimer glia   211
amantadine   139
  in athetosis   51
  in dystonia   94
  in parkinsonism   175
γ-aminobutyric acid (GABA)   137, 138
  and benzodiazepines   67
  blockers   67
  brain levels and dipropylacetate   69, 70

deficiency   27
  in Huntington's disease   32
  in myoclonus   67, 68
amitriptyline   112, 184
  in Tourette syndrome   120
amphetamine   29, 180
  -induced chorea   38, 39
angiotensin   26
apomorphine   31
  effect on athetoid cerebral palsy   52, 53
  in torsion dystonia   87
  in torticollis   93
  in Tourette syndrome   116, 117
arecholine   137
ataxia telangiectasia and alcohol   155
athetose double   16, 19
athetosis   14–18
  basal ganglion lesions   43
  biofeedback   54
  description   43, 81
  dopamine effects   56
  dyskinesia assessment   46, 47
  encephalitic   49
  measurement methods   44–7
  pharmacology of   43–56
  pharmacotherapy   45, 48–54
  placebo effects   45
  spasticity   47
  speech assessment   45, 46
  surgery   54, 55
  tension   47
atropine   24

baclofen   49, 50, 73, 138, 179, 180
  and Tourette syndrome   123
ballismus   18, 19
barbiturates   122
basal ganglion, familial calcification   172